Lipoedema

Gilles Laur

Lipoedema

Voices of Resilience

Springer

Gilles Laur
Medicine
Laurel Clinical
Parkwood, QLD, Australia

ISBN 978-981-96-8938-5 ISBN 978-981-96-8939-2 (eBook)
https://doi.org/10.1007/978-981-96-8939-2

This Springer imprint is published by the registered company Springer Nature Singapore Pte Ltd.
The registered company address is: 152 Beach Road, #21-01/04 Gateway East, Singapore 189721, Singapore

Prologue

There is a domain of illnesses that defy straightforward categorization, and it may be found inside the sacred halls of medicine, where science and compassion meet. Among these, lipedema is one that stands out as both a mystery and a call to action at the same time. An invitation to explore the complexities that constitute this condition is extended to readers via this book, which is an excursion into the depths of this complicated disorder.

As people who work in the healthcare industry, we are privileged to be witnesses to the travels of innumerable individuals, each of whom has their own personal narratives woven into the fabric of their life. Even when confronted with a disease as difficult as lipedema, we see that these tales include a significant amount of courage and tenacity.

While walking through the hallways of clinics, we come across patients whose voices reverberate with a single refrain: "Please assist me in comprehending." Help me find my way along this journey. They are the ones who carry the burden of lipedema, with both physical and figurative meanings. Physical agony, mental sorrow, and a culture that may not always appreciate the depth of their challenges are all things that they must come up against.

Nevertheless, there is an unconquerable energy contained inside their narratives. A soul that is persistent, that seeks solutions, and that yearns for a higher quality of life is what we are talking about here. It is a spirit that cries out for instruction, sympathy, and expertise from those who are knowledgeable.

This book is a response to the call that was made. Lipedema is not only a clinical entity; rather, it is a lived experience, and this is a testimonial to the devotion and curiosity of healthcare personnel who are motivated to comprehend lipedema. In doing so, it is a recognition of the fact that the practice of medicine is a combination of art and science.

Within these pages, we will start on a trip that will not only take us through the physiological complexity of lipedema, but will also take us through the lives of individuals who are now coping with its weight. It is a journey that will challenge preconceived notions, that will call for a strategy that incorporates several disciplines, and that will eventually result in care that is more compassionate and more efficiently delivered.

As we stand on the brink of comprehension, let us not forget that we are not the only ones who are making this journey. Partners in this endeavor include not just our colleagues and researchers but also the patients themselves. We are going to work together to solve the mysteries of lipedema. By working together, we will pave the way for a more accurate diagnosis, more tailored therapy, and eventually, a more promising future for individuals who are impacted with this condition.

Let us begin on this journey with open minds and unwavering hearts, aware that each step we take takes us closer to a world where lipedema is greeted with understanding, compassion, and professional treatment. Let us embrace this adventure with open minds and unwavering hearts. Our commitment is to do so. This demonstrates our commitment. Our dedication to the people who entrust us with their health and well-being is reflected in this promise.

Preface

Within the ever-evolving field of medical research, where the breadth and depth of knowledge continue to develop with each passing day, there are still disorders that have evaded the spotlight of full understanding. Lipedema is one of these conditions. This book arises as a lighthouse for those who are attempting to highlight the shadows created by this condition that is sometimes disregarded. It is with great expectation and a pioneering attitude that this book emerges as possible. This publication stands as the first of its type, precisely prepared to serve as an introduction guide for medical practitioners, allied health workers, and patients who find themselves at the threshold of knowledge about lipedema.

The purpose of this book is to provide a basic knowledge of lipedema by outlining its features, diagnosis, and treatment techniques. It is mainly directed toward those who have little to no prior experience with the ailment. Instead of catering to experts or experienced physicians who are well-versed in the issue, our goal is to bridge the gap for those who are on the front lines of patient care and may come across lipedema without being aware of it. In order to play a crucial role in the early detection and intervention of this illness, it is for the general practitioner, the nurse, the physical therapist, and other professionals working in the allied health sectors.

Throughout the history of medicine, lipedema has been a mysterious condition that is often misinterpreted or incorrectly diagnosed. While simultaneously cultivating a sympathetic knowledge of the patient experience, the purpose of this effort is to debunk misconceptions, provide clinical presentations that are more clear, and provide therapeutic techniques that are supported by data. We hope that by publishing this book, we will be able to offer medical professionals with the resources they need to recognize lipedema at an earlier stage in their practice, therefore improving the results for patients and establishing a new era of awareness and advocacy for people who are afflicted with this ailment.

As you read these pages, you will start on a voyage of discovery along which you will investigate the clinical signs of lipedema, as well as the historical backdrop and therapeutic paths that are accessible for treatments. By reading this book, you will be given the opportunity to broaden your clinical expertise, adopt a holistic perspective on patient treatment, and make a contribution to the expanding body of information about a disease that requires attention. We believe that by doing so, we will be able to motivate a crowd of knowledgeable practitioners who are prepared to make a substantial difference in the lives of those who are coping with lipedema.

Regarding the knowledge and treatment of lipedema, we would like to welcome you to a new frontier. Let this book serve as your guide as we investigate the complexity and difficulties associated with this illness together, with the ultimate objective of enhancing the quality of treatment provided to patients and the results achieved in the area of medicine.

Parkwood, QLD, Australia Gilles Laur

Acknowledgments

As I reflect on the journey that has led to the writing of this book, I am deeply grateful to a group of extraordinary individuals whose influence and support have been essential. First, I must express my profound gratitude to my teachers in the field of medicine. Their unwavering dedication and insightful guidance have not only shaped my professional path but have also enriched my understanding and passion for medicine. Their commitment to excellence and nurturing of my curiosity have left an indelible mark on my career and personal growth.

I am especially thankful to those who introduced me to the fascinating world of phlebology and lipedema. Exploring these specialized areas has profoundly expanded my horizons, allowing me to make meaningful contributions to our understanding and treatment of these conditions. The mentors and colleagues who guided me through these complex fields have provided me with invaluable knowledge and inspiration, for which I am eternally grateful.

Above all, my deepest appreciation goes to my family—my wife and my sons—who are my foundation and my joy. Their love, patience, and encouragement sustain me. My wife, in her infinite wisdom and compassion, has been a constant source of support and motivation. Together with our sons, she has created a loving and nurturing home that rejuvenates my spirit and fuels my endeavors. Their presence in my life brings me immeasurable joy and fulfillment, grounding and inspiring me in ways they may never fully realize.

To all of you who have touched my life through your support, wisdom, and love, thank you from the bottom of my heart. This book is not only a testament to my professional journey but also a tribute to each of you, who have made this journey possible and worthwhile.

Contents

Basic Considerations

History

Lipedema is a prevalent yet sometimes misunderstood and misdiagnosed illness that impacts millions of individuals globally. Lipedema is a persistent medical problem that mostly affects women and is characterized by the abnormal buildup of fat tissue in the lower limbs. It differs from typical obesity because it involves the even distribution of fat, sensitivity to touch, and swelling that does not leave an indentation when pressed. Lipedema often exhibits a progressive nature and exacerbates during periods of hormonal fluctuations such as adolescence, pregnancy, or menopause. The adipose tissue related to lipedema is usually unresponsive to dietary changes and physical activity, leading to dissatisfaction among those afflicted by this condition.

Lipedema may have profound emotional and psychological effects, such as feelings of self-consciousness and dissatisfaction.

The oldest documented accounts of lipedema may be traced back to the seventeenth century, when a German physician named Johann Georg Falke provided the first description of a disorder he referred to as "lipomatosis dolorosa." Falke's clientele consisted mostly of female individuals who had pain and suffering due to an excess accumulation of adipose tissue, also known as fat, in their legs. During the eighteenth and nineteenth centuries, other doctors recorded instances of a medical condition referred to as "adiposis dolorosa," "lipomatosis of the legs," or "lipohyperplasia dolorosa." Nevertheless, there remained a limited comprehension of the fundamental reasons or effective remedies for the illness.

The first documented instances of lipedema may be traced back to the late nineteenth century, when medical professionals and researchers initially characterized the ailment. Lipedema, or lipedema, is a persistent medical disorder marked by the abnormal buildup of adipose tissue in certain regions of the body, often the lower limbs, hips, and, sometimes, the arms. This leads to swelling and sensitivity in those areas.

The occurrence of lipedema throughout human history is highlighted by references in historical paintings and sculptures, spanning many millennia. An example of this is Queen Ati of the land of Punt (Fig. 1), who lived in the 15th century

G. Laur, *Lipoedema*, https://doi.org/10.1007/978-981-96-8939-2_1

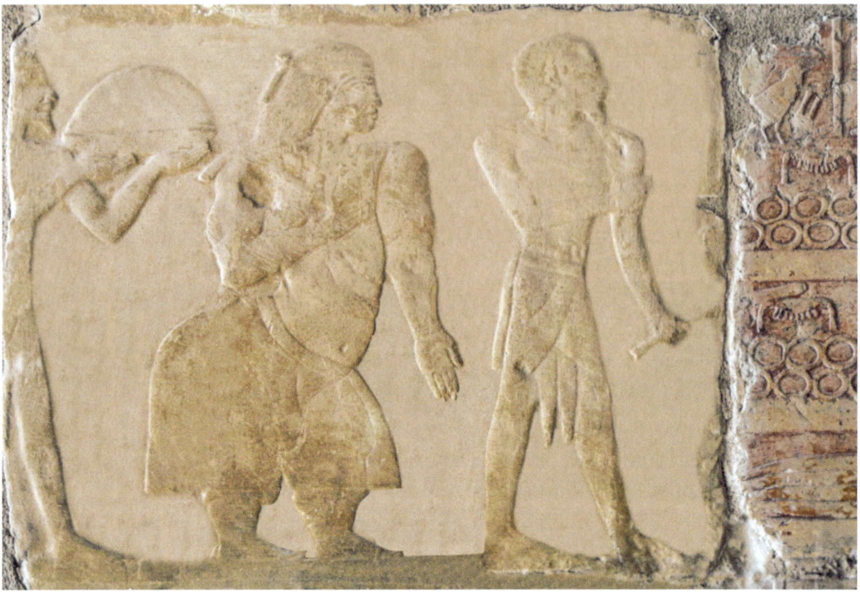

Fig. 1 Relief from Dayr al Bahari temple showing Queen Ati of Punt with her husband Perahu as they welcome the delegation by sea of Queen Hatshepsut. Fifteenth c. B.C. Luxor, Egypt

BC. The scene shows modifications in the lower legs that resemble the unique characteristics of lipedema. The portrayal of the Great Queen with these characteristics implies an early recognition of this state, maybe mirroring its depiction in religious or cultural objects.

Moreover, the ancient Egyptian relief depicting Ati, the Queen of Punt, which dates back more than 3500 years ago, provides a convincing argument. Ati, shown in the temple of Pharaoh Hatshepsut (approximately 1479 to 1458 BC), has morphological traits that contemporary observers have compared to prominent lipedema. This portrayal provides historical evidence of the state and illuminates the aesthetic ideals and cultural perspectives on physical forms in ancient Egypt.

However, the understanding of Ati's portrayal has been influenced by several prejudices, such as the "European Hottentot Complex." This notion entails doing a comparative examination of the disparaging portrayals of Ssehura, who is also referred to as the "Hottentot Venus." The aim is to demonstrate a pattern within European academics where non-European physical appearances are seen with contempt or as abnormal conditions.

By examining these ancient depictions through the lens of Afronography, which prioritizes African aesthetic principles and cultural concepts, a more profound and sophisticated comprehension is attained. This method specifically examines the ancient Egyptian representation of Ati of Punt in relation to the concept of "tiknis," a Jamaican phrase that honors certain body forms. This research illustrates the transfer of African aesthetic norms throughout generations and many cultures, providing a more thorough understanding of the historical and cultural aspects of lipedema.

The name “lipedema” was first used by Dr. Allen and Dr. Hines of the Mayo Clinic in 1940, although the ailment had been previously recognized and described. Below are many significant milestones in the acknowledgement and comprehension of lipedema:

With the accumulation and recording of further instances, specific diagnostic criteria for lipedema began to develop. Physicians diagnosed the illness by examining the clinical symptoms and excluding other possible reasons for limb swelling, such as lymphedema or venous insufficiency. The diagnostic criteria for lipedema have undergone changes throughout time, transitioning from observational descriptions to more precise clinical standards.

Early accounts of lipedema were formed by clinical observations of symmetrical swelling in the lower limbs, mostly impacting women. Historically, doctors observed that there was an identifiable pattern of excessive fat accumulation in the legs and sometimes the arms, which was often accompanied by sensitivity or discomfort.

Advancements in research and medical imaging tools, including ultrasound and magnetic resonance imaging (MRI), have contributed to a more comprehensive knowledge of the structural alterations related to lipedema. Furthermore, heightened awareness and promotion endeavors have resulted in enhanced identification and assessment of the illness.

Over the course of history, lipedema has often been confused with obesity or linked to lifestyle issues, resulting in incorrect diagnosis or insufficient recognition of the condition. As our understanding of the problem has improved, we have come to recognize its unique characteristics and the need of specialized treatment, which may include conservative treatments, compression garments, and, in some situations, surgical procedures.

Lipedema, a persistent swelling of the limbs, has been acknowledged as a distinct illness apart from other medical disorders. Historically, early categorization systems relied on clinical observations and the intensity of symptoms, which were then grouped into stages or grades. With the progression of medical knowledge and advancements in diagnostic techniques, categorization systems have become more precise. These systems now include staging systems, subtypes or variations, and the integration of imaging results. The current process of naming and categorizing involves a blend of clinical assessment, imaging examinations, and staging methods to determine the extent of the condition and provide treatment choices.

Physicians Maurice Klippel and Paul Trenaunay identified the lymphatic involvement in lipedema throughout the early twentieth century. During the 1930s, the German physician Karl Lohrmann introduced the term “lymphedema adiposum” to explain how the lymphatic system is involved in the development of this illness. Lipedema remained undiagnosed and poorly understood until the 1990s, when Dr. Etelka Földi devised a comprehensive set of diagnostic criteria for lipedema. These criteria include a thorough physical examination, ultrasound imaging, and lymphoscintigraphy.

Recently, there has been an increasing recognition of lipedema among doctors, who are becoming more aware of its significant influence on patients' quality of life. This text discusses the development of terminology related to lipedema, the influence of hormones on lipedema, and the historical management of lipedema. Discussions have taken place on the advancement of research on lipedema, with influential individuals adding to the present comprehension of the issue.

The comprehension and treatment of lipedema have been greatly impacted by patient activism. Misinterpretation of lipedema as obesity has resulted from prevailing social views, which, in turn, have led to judgment and stigma. Incorrect interpretation of the symptoms of lipedema might cause a delay or hinder the provision of appropriate therapy and assistance for affected persons. The lack of knowledge and education among the general population and healthcare professionals leads to the under-recognition of lipedema. The psychological well-being of patients with lipedema, in addition to the cultural constraints associated with body image, may have a substantial effect on their overall health. Inadequate awareness of the ailment may lead to insufficient resources, delayed diagnosis, or a dearth of specialized treatment alternatives, which may have a negative influence on patients' quality of life.

The involvement of patient advocates, support organizations, and awareness campaigns has played a crucial role in changing cultural prejudices and enhancing the acknowledgement of lipedema. These projects seek to diminish stigma and provide support for those impacted by raising awareness, pushing for improved knowledge among healthcare professionals, and fostering understanding in society. To tackle the public perspective of lipedema, it is necessary to make a focused and coordinated effort to raise awareness, encourage education, and cultivate empathy. Advocacy projects, support groups, and campaigns that raise awareness about the true nature of lipedema are essential in combating misunderstandings, diminishing social stigma, and fighting for improved acknowledgement and assistance for those afflicted.

Lipedema support networks have developed in response to the specific requirements of those who are affected by this ailment. These networks provide vital resources, foster community, and advocate for their members, creating a platform for sharing information, receiving emotional support, and engaging in joint endeavors. They have progressed via initiatives led by patients, campaigns advocating for their cause, dissemination of knowledge and information, empowerment and validation, provision of resources, cooperation with healthcare experts, and engagement in fundraising efforts.

The pursuit of comprehension and consciousness about lipedema is a continuous expedition propelled by many stakeholders, such as patients, healthcare professionals, researchers, and advocacy organizations. The main components of this ongoing endeavor encompass advocating for patients and empowering them, providing medical education and training, conducting research and making scientific advancements, raising awareness through campaigns and engaging the public, establishing collaborative networks and support groups, advocating for policies and integrating them into the healthcare system, and delivering empathetic and compassionate care.

Patients have a major role in promoting awareness and fighting for improved recognition and treatment. The purpose of advocacy initiatives is to eliminate misunderstandings, diminish social disapproval, and promote prompt identification and action. Collaborative networks that include patients, healthcare professionals, researchers, and advocacy organizations promote multidisciplinary cooperation, guaranteeing fair access to specialized care, insurance coverage for treatments, and the incorporation of lipedema into health policies and standards.

The ongoing pursuit of comprehending and acknowledging lipedema entails cooperative and multifaceted endeavors focused on enhancing the identification, diagnosis, therapy, and assistance for persons impacted by the ailment. The objective is to establish a more knowledgeable, helpful, and all-encompassing atmosphere that empowers individuals with lipedema via joint efforts and advocacy.

Lipedema is a medical illness with a lengthy and intricate history, spanning from its first descriptions to contemporary methods of diagnosis and treatment. Although there are still many unknowns concerning lipedema, recent years have seen substantial advancements, providing reasons for optimism for future growth. We aspire that this book has imparted a deeper comprehension of lipedema and the obstacles confronted by those living with it.

Suggested Reading

Child AH, Gordon KD, Sharpe P, Brice G, Ostergaard P, Jeffery S, Mortimer PS. Lipedema: an inherited condition. Am J Med Genet A. 2010 Apr;152A(4):970–6.

Kruppa P, Georgiou I, Biermann N, Prantl L, Klein-Weigel P, Ghods M. Lipedema-Pathogenesis, Diagnosis, and Treatment Options. Dtsch Arztebl Int. 2020 Jun 01;117(22–23):396–403.

Paolacci S, Precone V, Acquaviva F, Chiurazzi P, Fulcheri E, Pinelli M, Buffelli F, Michelini S, Herbst KL, Unfer V, Bertelli M., GeneOb Project. Genetics of lipedema: new perspectives on genetic research and molecular diagnoses. Eur Rev. Med Pharmacol Sci. 2019 Jul;23(13):5581–5594.

Herbst KL. Subcutaneous Adipose Tissue Diseases: Dercum Disease, Lipedema, Familial Multiple Lipomatosis, and Madelung Disease. In: Feingold KR, Anawalt B, Blackman MR, Boyce A, Chrousos G, Corpas E, de Herder WW, Dhatariya K, Dungan K, Hofland J, Kalra S, Kaltsas G, Kapoor N, Koch C, Kopp P, Korbonits M, Kovacs CS, Kuohung W, Laferrère B, Levy M, McGee EA, McLachlan R, New M, Purnell J, Sahay R, Shah AS, Singer F, Sperling MA, Stratakis CA, Trence DL, Wilson DP, editors. Endotext [Internet]. MDText.com, Inc.; South Dartmouth (MA): Dec 14, 2019.

Martin JP. La reine de Pount souffroit-elle de Cutis Laxa? [Did the Queen of Pount suffer from cutis laxa?]. Vesalius. 2010 Dec;16(2):83–7. French. PMID: 21560608.

Dadras M, Mallinger PJ, Corterier CC, Theodosiadi S, Ghods M. Liposuction in the Treatment of Lipedema: A Longitudinal Study. Arch Plast Surg. 2017 Jul;44(4):324–331.

Torre YS, Wadeea R, Rosas V, Herbst KL. Lipedema: friend and foe. Horm Mol Biol Clin Investig. 2018 Mar 09;33(1).

Halk AB, Damstra RJ. First Dutch guidelines on lipedema using the international classification of functioning, disability and health. Phlebology. 2017 Apr;32(3):152–159.

Schneider R. Low-frequency vibrotherapy considerably improves the effectiveness of manual lymphatic drainage (MLD) in patients with lipedema: A two-armed, randomized, controlled pragmatic trial. Physiother Theory Pract. 2020 Jan;36(1):63.

Epidemiology

Lipedema is a condition that affects the distribution of fat in the body, leading to an abnormal accumulation of fat in the lower extremities, hips, and buttocks. The exact prevalence of lipedema is unknown, but estimates suggest that it affects between 11% and 17% of women worldwide. Diagnosis is largely clinical and based on criteria established in 1951. However, due to the lack of awareness and underdiagnosis of the condition, these figures may be an underestimate.

Lipedema is more common in women, with estimates suggesting that it affects between 85% and 98% of all cases. It often appears during puberty, pregnancy, or menopause, suggesting a hormonal influence. Lipedema can also affect men, but it is less common, with estimates suggesting that it affects less than 1% of all cases.

The prevalence of lipedema varies across different populations and regions, with some studies suggesting higher rates in Europe and North America. The estimated prevalence in Europe varies between 0.06% and 39%. The condition is often misdiagnosed as obesity or lymphedema, leading to underreporting and a lack of accurate prevalence data. The study used an automated methodology to select a sample of the total population, using SurveyMonkey® software. The questionnaire demonstrated appropriate reliability and similarity to the general population. There was a minor difference in educational level between the study population and the census projection, possibly due to the selection of respondents with Internet access. The questionnaire took 18% slower than the original, and the dropout rate was low. The most widely accepted lipedema prevalence reported in the literature is 11% of the female population. The study achieved a diagnostic probability of 77.8% for the tool used, with specificity of 0.88 and sensitivity of 0.46.

The prevalence in the female Brazilian population was 12.3%, with an estimated prevalence of 8.8 million women aged 18 to 69 years old. The study by Dudek et al. investigated the prevalence and characteristics of lipedema in the Brazilian population using a questionnaire. The results showed that 67.5% of the women with lipedema had a BMI greater than 25 kg/cm^2, making diagnosis more difficult due to the complexity of differentiation from common obesity. The study also identified hypothyroidism in 31.6% of the Polish women, while another study with a Dutch

G. Laur, *Lipoedema*, https://doi.org/10.1007/978-981-96-8939-2_2

population reported 11.7%. The self-reported lymphedema rate was 30.6% in the Dutch sample, but only mentioned by 3.2% of the Brazilian women. The study found that putting weight on in the arms and legs easily was mentioned by 99% of the Polish sample, feelings of heavy legs by 96.9%, frequent ecchymosis by 90.8%, and difficulty losing weight from arms and legs by 86.8%. Brazilian women with lipedema had self-reported depression in 38.7% and anxiety in 61.3%, both with positive correlations. Anemia was also mentioned by 41.9% of these volunteers and was positively correlated with the disease. The study highlights the need for standardizing assessment criteria and developing instruments capable of assessing the clinical impact of lipedema and supporting definitive diagnosis. Estimates suggest that lipedema affects between 11% and 17% of women worldwide, but these figures may be an underestimate. Lipedema fat is most common in the lower limbs but can occur in any subcutaneous adipose tissue throughout the body. The disease is classified into five different types, depending on fat location, and three stages according to disease progression determined through a clinical examination. Stage 1 refers to a normal skin surface but enlarged hypodermal subcutaneous adipose tissue; stage 2 includes indentations of the skin and underlying larger mounds of subcutaneous adipose tissue; and stage 3 involves large extrusions of tissue that cause gross deformations.

Pain is the leading symptom of lipedema. A survey was conducted to gather information on sociodemographic factors, health-related matters, symptom severity, and comorbidities. The authors developed these questions based on published scholarly lipedema literature, in collaboration with a primary public healthcare physician and two members from a lipedema association group. The survey included questions on lipedema type and stage, symptom severity, and comorbidities. Participants reported any comorbidities by filling in pre-specified health problems and diseases and could also respond using free text. The severity of symptoms was assessed using a 47-question survey. Participants were asked how much they experienced certain lipedema-related symptoms over the past month, using a scale from 1 to 4—where 1 meant they did not have the symptom at all and 4 meant they were severely affected by it.

To understand participants' overall health and wellbeing, the study used two tools: the RAND-36 and the Sense of Coherence scale-13 (SOC-13). The RAND-36 is a questionnaire with 36 questions about different areas of health, like pain, energy, physical and emotional functioning, and social life. It is commonly used for people with lipedema. The SOC-13 looks at how people view life and their ability to cope with stress. It includes 13 questions that measure how well people understand, manage, and find meaning in their experiences. Each answer is scored from 1 to 7, and a higher total score means a stronger sense of control and resilience. The researchers got official permission to use both of these tools in Swedish.

The researchers used computer programs (IBM SPSS and Stata) to analyze the data. They collected basic background information about each participant, including their lipedema stage and other health conditions. They then used a method called factor analysis to find patterns in the 47-symptom survey and removed questions that did not fit well, ending up with 41 strong items.

For the RAND-36, they calculated average scores for each health area using a standard method. They also tested how reliable the questions were, with results showing good consistency (Cronbach's alpha between 0.80 and 0.92 for RAND-36 and 0.71 and 0.77 for SOC-13).

To compare different groups, the researchers used tests that are good for analyzing scores that do not follow a normal pattern, like the Mann-Whitney and Kruskal-Wallis tests. They also used the chi-squared test to see if symptom severity was related to the stage of lipedema. Finally, to compare the health scores of women in this study with those of women in the general Swedish population, they used a standard t-test. Any result with a p-value less than 0.05 was considered statistically significant. Overall, the study aimed to explore how common other health conditions are among women with lipedema, depending on how advanced their condition is.

The most common comorbidities were being overweight and obesity, with the majority of participants reporting these conditions. Nearly one-fifth of women had hypothyroidism, which was more common in more progressive stages. Hypertension was also prevalent among 25.3% of women with stage 3 lipedema, with the highest prevalence (31.6%) observed among women in this stage. Over 17% of women had fibromyalgia, and 13.5% reported depression. Moderate and severe lipedema symptoms were reported across all stages, but most often in stage 3. Moderate or severe symptoms in terms of leg heaviness, swelling, stiffness, and feeling exhausted at light physical exertion were significantly more common among women with stage 3 lipedema than those with stage 1 (Fig. 1). Easily bruising was reported among 97.5% of participants. Pain was reported in 98.7% of participants. Health-related

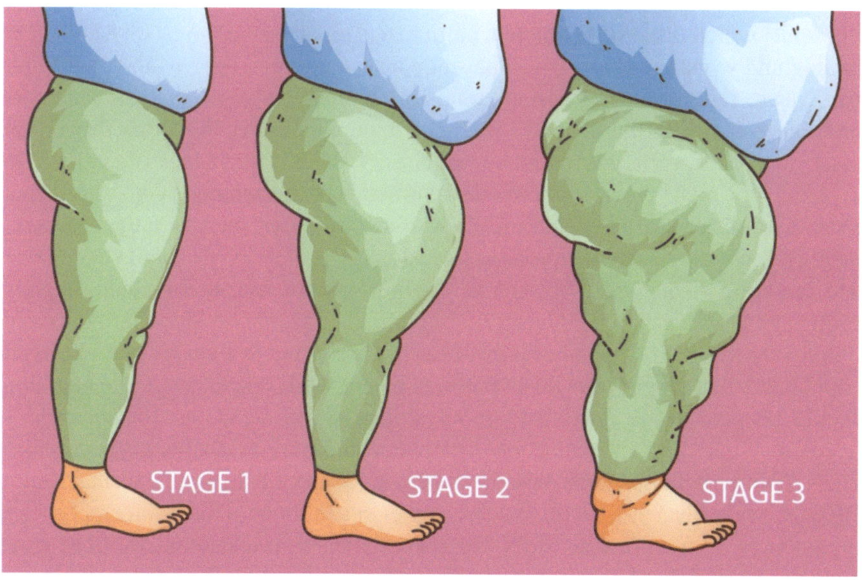

Fig. 1 Evolution of the lower limb in patients with lipedema

quality of life (HRQOL) scores across various subscales among participants were found to be the lowest in physical role functioning (mean 38.2/SD 40.5), reflecting difficulties with work or other daily activities due to physical health. Conversely, the highest scored health scale was emotional well-being, with a mean of 64.9 (SD 19.7). Women with stage 3 lipedema reported significantly lower scores in physical health compared to those with stages 1 and 2, including in terms of physical functioning, work-related activities, more severe and limiting pain, and worse general health. Worse physical health was also found among women at age 70 or older in the scales of physical functioning and physical role functioning compared to those in all younger age groups. Women who had experienced lipedema onset as adults reported poorer mental health than those with lipedema onset in their adolescence, with significantly lower scores in social functioning, emotional role functioning, emotional wellbeing, and overall lower scores in health changes over the past year. No significant differences in HRQOL were found between women with a confirmed or unconfirmed lipedema diagnosis. Compared to an age-matched general Swedish female population, women with lipedema scored significantly lower in all HRQOL scales—except for emotional role functioning on the age group 30–39, wherein our study sample reported higher scores. Overall, in most age groups, women with lipedema scored approximately 25–35 points lower in both their physical and mental health. This study focuses on the health, HRQOL, and sense of coherence (SOC) in a Swedish female lipedema population. The main findings indicate that lipedema is associated with several health problems and a lower overall HRQOL, and women with lipedema often wait decades before being correctly diagnosed by the healthcare system. Comorbidities among the participants were common, such as being overweight and having obesity.

The highest prevalence of obesity was found among women with stage 3 lipedema, which is the stage wherein participants reported the lowest physical functioning and worst levels of pain. The study also found that approximately 20% of participants reported having hypothyroidism, a higher prevalence than the estimated prevalence of 7% in the general Swedish female population. Although there is an association between hypothyroidism and obesity, there is still a lack of evidence to explain the high prevalence of the former among women with lipedema. Hypothyroidism, like lipedema, may cause health issues such as fatigue, weight gain, feeling cold, and sleep problems. Healthcare professionals should encourage and support patients with lipedema in striving for a lifestyle that includes healthy eating and physical activity. Over 17% of participants in this study reported having fibromyalgia, which is a higher prevalence than reported in females in the general populations that range from 2.4 to 6.8%. A recent work claims that more attention should be paid to the fact that fibromyalgia and lipedema (especially stage 1 lipedema) share several clinical characteristics and may be challenging to distinguish. Women with lipedema onset in adolescence scored better in the mental health HRQOL scales than those with lipedema onset in adulthood. This result emphasizes the findings from a previous study wherein women with lipedema described their bodies as painful, burdensome, unreliable, and unpredictable. The burden of comorbidities in patients with lipedema needs to be considered as a critical compounding factor to HRQOL. Therefore, healthcare professionals must be aware of and manage the complexity of lipedema and any comorbidities and their negative impact on patients' health status and quality of life. Moderate and severe lipedema symptoms and poor physical health were reported in all stages. Women with stage 3 lipedema stage primarily reported on complaints of heaviness, swelling, feeling cold, easy bruising, and hypermobility in joints. These symptoms tend to increase as lipedema progresses into higher stages and are assumed to be associated with changes in loose connective tissue such as dysfunctional blood vessels, a loss of elasticity in lipedema tissue, and an excess of interstitial fluid. Pain was reported as moderate or severe and therefore more likely to affect health and daily life. When supporting women with lipedema in managing their pain and improving their HRQOL, a careful assessment of the exact nature of their pain and the application of a holistic approach in healthcare are necessary. Furthermore, a crucial area in future research would be the evaluation of various treatment plans for lipedema pain.

Lipedema has been associated with several other health conditions, such as lymphedema, varicose veins, and joint problems. Lymphedema is a common comorbidity, affecting up to 90% of people with lipedema, as the abnormal accumulation of fat can compress the lymphatic vessels and cause swelling. Varicose veins are also common, affecting up to 70% of people with lipedema, as the added weight of the excess fat can put pressure on the veins. Joint problems, particularly in the knees and ankles, are also common, as the added weight can lead to wear and tear on the joints.

The cost of treating lipedema, a persistent and sometimes misdiagnosed illness, is high for both patients and healthcare systems. The abnormal buildup of fat that characterizes the illness, which often affects the lower limbs, causes discomfort, decreased movement, and a variety of comorbidities. Treatment for lipedema is typically delayed or wrong because it is commonly misdiagnosed or ignored. Patients have longer suffering as a consequence, and the expense of addressing the illness rises. People who have lipedema often need a variety of medical treatments, such as expert consultations, diagnostic testing, medicines, and surgical operations. Costs like this may add up over time, particularly for those with more severe conditions. The care of lipedema often entails a mix of less invasive procedures (such as liposuction, lymphatic-sparing methods, compression garments, and physical therapy).

The financial strain is increased by the fact that these therapies may be pricey and may call for several sessions. Severe lipedema may seriously impair mobility and functioning, which can reduce output at the workplace. Due to the illness, people may skip workdays, have difficulty doing duties effectively, or even lose their jobs. Additional expenses may be incurred by family members or carers who provide support and help with everyday tasks to those who have lipedema.

Lipedema may have significant psychological and social repercussions, such as anxiety, sadness, problems with body image, and a worse quality of life. These psychosocial variables may have further effects on a person's capacity for employment and raise the price of providing mental health assistance in healthcare.

Despite the significant impact of lipedema on individuals and the healthcare system, the condition remains poorly understood and underdiagnosed. There is a need for more comprehensive and standardized epidemiological studies to accurately assess the prevalence and impact of lipedema. Patient advocacy and awareness campaigns are also essential in improving diagnosis rates and reducing the economic burden of the condition. The development of new treatments and interventions, such as surgical options and lymphatic drainage techniques, also has the potential to significantly improve the quality of life of people living with lipedema.

Suggested Reading

Allen EV, Hines EA, Hines EA. Lipedema of the legs: a syndrome characterized by fat legs and orthostatic edema. Proc Staff Meet Mayo Clin. 1940;15:184–7.

Wold L, Hines EA Jr., Allen EV. Lipedema of the legs: a syndrome characterized by fat legs and edema. Ann Intern Med. 1951;34(5):1243–50. https://doi.org/10.7326/0003-4819-34-5-1243. PMid:14830102.

Whonamedit? Allen-Hines syndrome. 2021 [citado 2021 out 28]. https://www.whonamedit.com/synd.cfm/2015.html.

Kruppa P, Georgiou I, Biermann N, Prantl L, Klein-Weigel P, Ghods M. Lipedema-Pathogenesis, Diagnosis, and Treatment Options. Dtsch Arztebl Int. 2020;117(22–23):396–403. PMid:32762835.

Amato ACM. Is lipedema a unique entity? EC Clin Med Cases Reports. 2020;2:1–7.

Dudek JE, Białaszek W, Gabriel M. Quality of life, its factors, and sociodemographic characteristics of Polish women with lipedema. BMC Womens Health. 2021;21(1):27. https://doi.org/10.1186/s12905-021-01174-y. PMid:33446179.

Fife CE, Maus EA, Carter MJ. Lipedema: a frequently misdiagnosed and misunderstood fatty deposition syndrome. Adv Skin Wound Care. 2010;23(2):81–92. https://doi.org/10.1097/01.ASW.0000363503.92360.91. PMid:20087075.

Beninson J, Edelglass JW. Lipedema: the non-lymphatic masquerader. Angiology. 1984;35(8):506–10. https://doi.org/10.1177/000331978403500806. Mid:6476475.

Amato ACM, Amato FCM, Benitti DA, Santos RV. Translation, cultural adaptation, and validation of a lipedema symptoms questionnaire. J Vasc Bras. 2020;19:e20200049. https://doi.org/10.1590/1677-5449.200049. PMid:34178078.

Amato ACM, Saucedo DZ, Santos KS, Benitti DA. Ultrasound criteria for lipedema diagnosis. Phlebol J Venous Dis. 2021;36(8):026835552110023. PMid:33853452.

Cellina M, Gibelli D, Soresina M, et al. Non-contrast MR Lymphography of lipedema of the lower extremities. Magn Reson Imaging. 2020;71:115–24. https://doi.org/10.1016/j.mri.2020.06.010. PMid:32561380.

Monnin-Delhom ED, Gallix BP, Achard C, Bruel JM, Janbon C. High resolution unenhanced computed tomography in patients with swollen legs. Lymphology. 2002;35(3):121–8. PMid:12363222.

Amato ACM, Amato FCM, Benitti DA, Amato LGL. Criação de questionário e modelo de rastreamento de lipedema. J Vasc Bras. 2020;19:e20200114. https://doi.org/10.1590/1677-5449.200114.

Mandrekar JN. Receiver operating characteristic curve in diagnostic test assessment. J Thorac Oncol. 2010;5(9):1315–6. https://doi.org/10.1097/JTO.0b013e3181ec173d. PMid:20736804.

Choy M, Switzer P, De Martel C, Parsonnet J. Estimating disease prevalence using census data. Epidemiol Infect. 2008;136(9):1253–60. https://doi.org/10.1017/S0950268807009752. PMid:18047747.

Herpertz U. Krankheitsspektrum des lipodems an einer lymphologischen fachklinik – erscheinungsformen, mischbilder und behandlungsmoglichkeiten. Vasomed. 1997;9:301–7.

Amato ACM, Markus DV, dos Santos RV. Lipedema associado a obesidade, linfedema e insuficiência venosa: relato de um caso. Diagnóstico e Trat. 2020;25:4–8.

Schwahn-Schreiber C, Marshall M. Prävalenz des Lipödems bei berufstätigen Frauen in Deutschland. Phlebologie. 2011;40(03):127–34. https://doi.org/10.1055/s-0037-1621766.

Instituto Brasileiro de Geografia e Estatística – IBGE. Projeção da população brasileira. 2021 [citado 2021 out 28]. https://www.ibge.gov.br/apps/populacao/projecao/index.html ().

Heen MSJ, Lieberman JD, Miethe TD. A comparison of different online sampling approaches for generating national samples. Cent Crime Justice Policy. 2014;1:1–8.

Instituto Brasileiro de Geografia e Estatística – IBGE. SIDRA. Tabela 5919: população, por níveis de instrução. 2021 [citado 2021 out 28]. https://sidra.ibge.gov.br/tabela/5919

Nunnaly J, Bernstein I. No psychometric theory. 3rd ed. New York: McGraw-Hill; 1994.

Asmussen PD, Földi M, Strößenreuther R, et al. Földi's textbook of lymphology for physicians and lymphedema therapists. München: Elsevier Urban & Fischer; 2012.

Forner-Cordero I, Szolnoky G, Forner-Cordero A, Kemény L. Lipedema: an overview of its clinical manifestations, diagnosis and treatment of the disproportional fatty deposition syndrome – systematic review. Clin Obes. 2012;2(3–4):86–95. https://doi.org/10.1111/j.1758-8111.2012.00045.x. PMid:25586162.

Schmeller W, Hueppe M, Meier-Vollrath I. Tumescent liposuction in lipoedema yields good long-term results. Br J Dermatol. 2012;166(1):161–8. https://doi.org/10.1111/j.1365-2133.2011.10566.x. PMid:21824127.

Harwood CA, Bull RH, Evans J, Mortimer PS. Lymphatic and venous function in lipoedema. Br J Dermatol. 1996;134(1):1–6. https://doi.org/10.1111/j.1365-2133.1996.tb07831.x. PMid:8745878.

Child AH, Gordon KD, Sharpe P, et al. (2010) Lipedema: an inherited condition. Am J Medical Genetics Part A 152A: 970–76. https://www.ncbi.nlm.nih.gov/pubmed/20358611

Földi E, Földi M. Lipedema. In: Földi E, Földi M, (eds) (2006) Textbook of lymphology. Elsevier: 417–27. https://www.elsevier.com/books/foldis-textbook-of-lymphology/foldi/978-0-7234-3646-1

Szél E, Kemény L, Groma G, Szolnoky G (2014) Pathophysiological dilemmas of lipedema. Medical Hypotheses 83(5): 599–606. https://www.ncbi.nlm.nih.gov/pubmed/25200646

Anatomy

Lipedema is a pathologically progressive condition delineated by symmetrical adipose tissue buildup in the lower limbs, precipitating pain, ecchymosis, and mobility challenges. Notwithstanding its profound impact on individuals' daily lives, it is often overlooked, leading to diagnostic and therapeutic delays. This text elucidates its epidemiology and demographic patterns, which are instrumental for clinicians, researchers, and those afflicted.

The disease's exact prevalence remains elusive due to nonuniform diagnostic criteria and varying levels of recognition among health practitioners. Nonetheless, it is posited to affect a significant segment of the female populace, with prevalence estimates ranging between 10% and 15%. Notably, lipedema's emergence aligns with hormonal flux, such as during puberty, pregnancy, or menopause, suggesting hormonal influences on its trajectory.

Predominantly impacting females with sparse male incidence suggests a gender-specific predisposition, potentially linked to hormonal and genetic influences. Although it can present at any age, its onset is typically noted at adolescence, aligning with major hormonal events. The condition transcends ethnic and regional boundaries, though disparities in disease recognition and access to healthcare may skew prevalence data.

A genetic undercurrent is suggested by familial recurrence, with research efforts aimed at pinpointing genetic markers and pathways that could redefine lipedema's understanding and intervention.

Distinguished by a pattern of fat distribution (Fig. 1) divergent from normative adiposity and other related disorders, lipedema is marked by symmetrical adipose accumulation, often extending from the hips to the ankles, sparing the feet, and resulting in a "pear-shaped" silhouette. This fat is characteristically soft, indentable, and painful, contrasting the firmer consistency of normal fat deposits (Fig. 2). Microscopically, lipedema adipose tissue exhibits fibrosis, angiogenesis, and inflammation not seen in healthy tissue, necessitating a nuanced diagnosis to differentiate it from obesity or lymphedema, which require divergent management strategies.

G. Laur, *Lipoedema*, https://doi.org/10.1007/978-981-96-8939-2_3

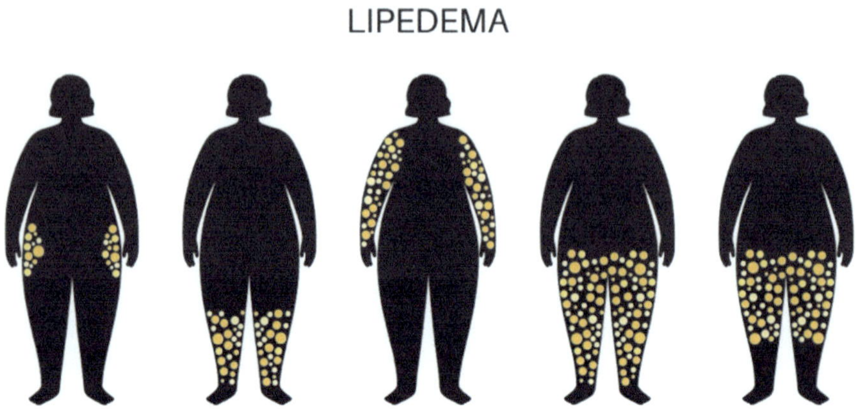

Fig. 1 The most common sites of fat deposition in lipedema

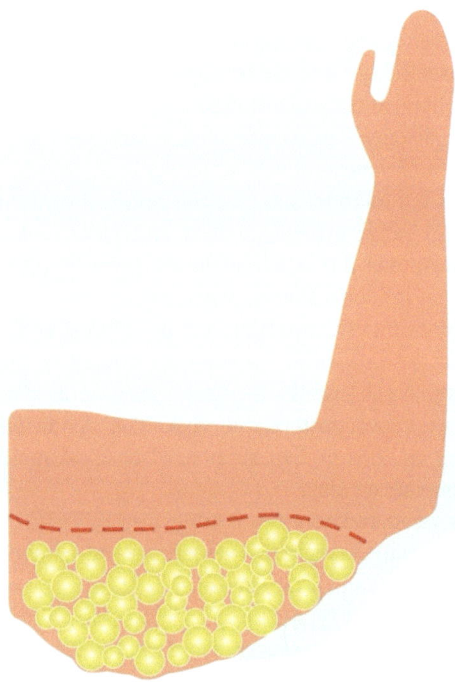

Fig. 2 The most common site of fat deposition in lipedema in the arm

The lymphatic system's anatomy is central to discerning lipedema's pathophysiology and its distinction from lymphedema. This system, tasked with fluid homeostasis and immune function, encounters dysfunction in lipedema, potentially contributing to progressive fat and fluid accumulation. Lipedema features symmetrical fat buildup, whereas lymphedema is characterized by asymmetric swelling due to lymphatic dysfunction, necessitating differentiated management strategies.

Vascular health in lipedema is significantly compromised due to the undue strain placed on the venous network by excessive fat. This strain can lead to venous insufficiency and stasis and potentially increase the risk for venous thromboembolic events. The chronic exertion on vascular structures may culminate in varicosities and a heightened risk of secondary lymphedema, emphasizing the need for a comprehensive vascular evaluation in management plans.

Lipedema also involves substantial changes in connective tissue and the extracellular matrix (ECM), fundamental to the body's structural and functional integrity. The disease is accompanied by increased fibrous tissue and ECM alterations, potentially disrupting lymphatic flow due to fibrosis around the lymph vessels. These changes manifest as palpable nodularity and reduced skin and tissue elasticity, exacerbating the sensation of heaviness and pain and impeding normal lymphatic drainage and venous return. Comprehending these alterations is critical for devising therapeutic interventions aimed at restoring tissue structure and function.

Cutaneous and dermatological alterations significantly burden patients with lipedema, evident in the skin's altered texture and increased thickness. The skin's predisposition to bruising and compromised wound healing, attributable to capillary fragility and vascular and lymphatic insufficiencies, differentiates lipedema from other conditions. These dermatological challenges, coupled with potential secondary conditions like cellulitis, demand a comprehensive management approach that considers the psychological impacts of the disease.

Musculoskeletal complications in lipedema have a profound impact on life quality, manifested in joint stress, diminished mobility, muscular changes, and gait and postural alterations. The abnormal fat distribution necessitates compensatory postural adjustments, wider stances, and altered stride lengths, which may increase fall and injury risks. A thorough management strategy encompassing physical therapy and assistive mobility devices is paramount for enhancing functional capacity and reducing discomfort.

Neurological considerations, particularly pain sensation and management, alongside sensory alterations, are critical dimensions of lipedema. Pain is hypothesized to arise from increased nociceptor pressure, inflammation, and fibrosis and may include neuropathic elements due to peripheral and central nervous system alterations. Management involves a multidisciplinary approach, emphasizing the importance of psychological support in comprehensive care.

Endocrine influences in lipedema, particularly hormonal factors, underscore its progression. The condition's exacerbation linked to hormonal changes and the menstrual cycle, along with metabolic disturbances like insulin resistance and thyroid dysfunctions, highlights the necessity for a thorough evaluation of hormonal and metabolic status in patients. This endocrine understanding is integral to personalized management plans and targeted interventions.

Genetic and molecular insights into lipedema have been invaluable, indicating a hereditary propensity. Research is targeting genetic markers and molecular mechanisms, including aberrant signaling pathways and external factors like diet and physical activity, which modulate gene expression. This integration of genetic and molecular research is vital for unveiling lipedema's root causes and developing personalized medicine approaches.

Accurate identification and management of lipedema depend on establishing solid diagnostic criteria and clinical assessment protocols. Diagnosis relies on comprehensive physical examinations, history documentation, and imaging tests to differentiate lipedema from related conditions. A multidisciplinary diagnostic approach ensures tailored management plans, optimizing patient outcomes and care quality.

In summary, lipedema is characterized by disproportionate fat accumulation in the lower extremities, associated with pain and mobility issues. Its recognition, underpinned by clinical presentation, veno-lymphatic system involvement, and suspected endocrine, genetic, and inflammatory influences, is crucial. Current diagnostic methods are complemented by ongoing research into genetic and molecular aspects, and the development of multidisciplinary treatment strategies is vital. As awareness and technology progress, so do the prospects for managing lipedema, with interdisciplinary research efforts and clinical collaborations shaping a future of prompt recognition and effective treatment.

Suggested Reading

Allen EV, Hines EA. Lipedema of the legs: a syndrome characterized by fat legs and orthostatic edema. Proc Staff Meet Mayo Clinic. 1940;15:184–187. https://lipedemaproject.org/wp-content/uploads/2016/02/1940_Allen_Lipedema-of-the-Legs.pdf.

Blum KS, Karaman S, Proulx ST, et al. Chronic high-fat diet impairs collecting lymphatic vessel function in mice. PLoS One. 2014;9:e94713. doi: https://doi.org/10.1371/journal.pone.0094713.

Escobedo N, Proulx ST, Karaman S, et al. Restoration of lymphatic function rescues obesity in Prox1-haploinsufficient mice. JCI Insight. 2016;1:e85096. doi: https://doi.org/10.1172/jci.insight.85096..

Al-Ghadban S, Cromer W, Allen M, et al. Dilated blood and lymphatic microvessels, angiogenesis, increased macrophages, and adipocyte hypertrophy in lipedema thigh skin and fat tissue. J Obes. 2019;2019:8747461. doi: https://doi.org/10.1155/2019/8747461.

Vandanmagsar B, Youm Y-H, Ravussin A, et al. The NLRP3 inflammasome instigates obesity-induced inflammation and insulin resistance. Nat Med. 2011;17:179–188.

Aldrich MB, Sevick-Muraca EM. Cytokines are systemic effectors of lymphatic function in acute inflammation. Cytokine. 2013;64:362–369

Felmerer G, Stylianaki A, Hollmén M, et al. Increased levels of VEGF-C and macrophage infiltration in lipedema patients without changes in lymphatic vascular morphology. Sci Rep. 2020;10:10947. doi: https://doi.org/10.1038/s41598-020-67987-3.

Rasmussen JC, Tan IC, Marshall MV, et al. Human lymphatic architecture and dynamic transport imaged using near-infrared fluorescence. Transl Oncol. 2010;3:362–372.

Aldrich M, Guilliod R, Fife CE, et al. Lymphatic abnormalities in the normal contralateral arms of subjects with breast cancer-related lymphedema as assessed by near-infrared fluorescent imaging. Biomed Opt Express. 2012;3:1256–1265.

el-Shahaly HA, el-Sherif AK. Is the benign joint hypermobility syndrome benign? Clin Rheumatol. 1991;10:302–307

Lymphatic Dysfunction

The lymphatic system (Fig. 1) is an essential component of the circulatory and immune systems, comprising a network of lymphatic vessels that permeate nearly all tissues and organs. This system functions primarily to transport lymph, a clear fluid containing white blood cells and waste products, from tissues into the circulatory system, while also serving as a key player in immune surveillance and response. Lymphatic vessels, alongside lymph nodes and organs such as the spleen and thymus, collaborate to filter pathogens, distribute lymphocytes, and maintain fluid homeostasis.

In the context of lipedema, the intersection with lymphatic dysfunction is particularly pronounced. Lipedema is characterized by the pathological accumulation of subcutaneous fat, most commonly in the legs and arms, which is often mistaken for simple obesity.

However, the condition also involves a component of lymphatic disturbance, which may not be immediately apparent. The expansion of adipose tissue in lipedema can physically obstruct lymphatic pathways, leading to compromised lymph drainage. This impairment can exacerbate the accumulation of fluid in interstitial spaces, further stressing the lymphatic system and perpetuating a cycle of inflammation, fat deposition, and fibrosis. Such dysfunction at the crossroads of the lymphatic system and adipose tissue contributes to the progressive nature of lipedema, and understanding this relationship is vital for developing effective management strategies for patients suffering from this chronic condition.

Lymphatic vessels (Fig. 2) are integral components of the lymphatic system, serving as conduits for lymph, a fluid that originates from interstitial fluid. These vessels are structured in a network that parallels the circulatory system, but, unlike blood vessels, they form a unidirectional pathway from the peripheral tissues to the subclavian veins at the base of the neck. Beginning as microscopic, blind-ended capillaries in the interstitial spaces, lymphatic vessels absorb protein-rich fluid, cellular debris, and immune cells. The lymph then travels through progressively larger and more structurally complex vessels, including the precollectors and collectors

G. Laur, *Lipoedema*, https://doi.org/10.1007/978-981-96-8939-2_4

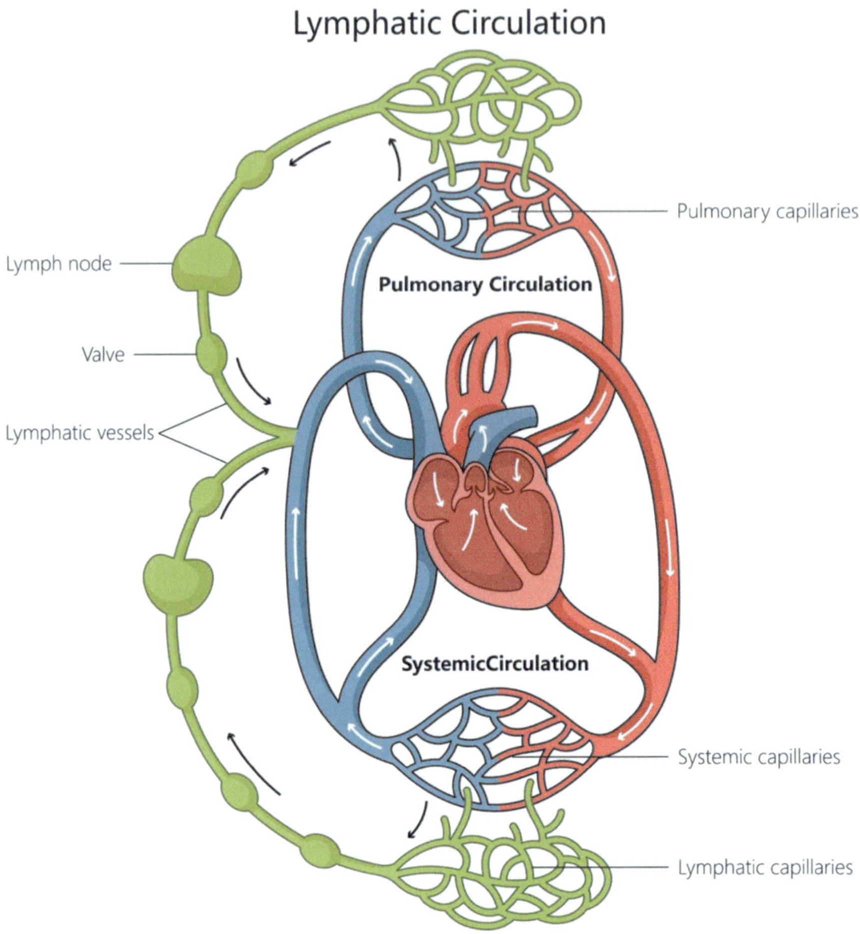

Fig. 1 Interaction between the lymphatic circulation and cardiovascular circulation

that contain valves to prevent backflow and facilitate lymph movement toward the lymph nodes.

Within lymph nodes (Fig. 3), lymph is filtered, and immune responses can be initiated before the lymph is eventually returned to the bloodstream. Lymphatic vessels are unique in their endothelial lining, which is especially adapted with anchoring filaments and intercellular openings known as "button junctions," allowing for efficient fluid uptake and transport under varying pressure conditions.

Additionally, smooth muscle cells in the walls of larger lymphatic vessels, along with external compression from surrounding tissues and organs, aid in propelling lymph forward through rhythmic contractions, a process known as the lymphatic pump mechanism. This system's proper function is critical for maintaining fluid balance, facilitating dietary fat absorption, and immune function, highlighting its multifaceted role in human health.

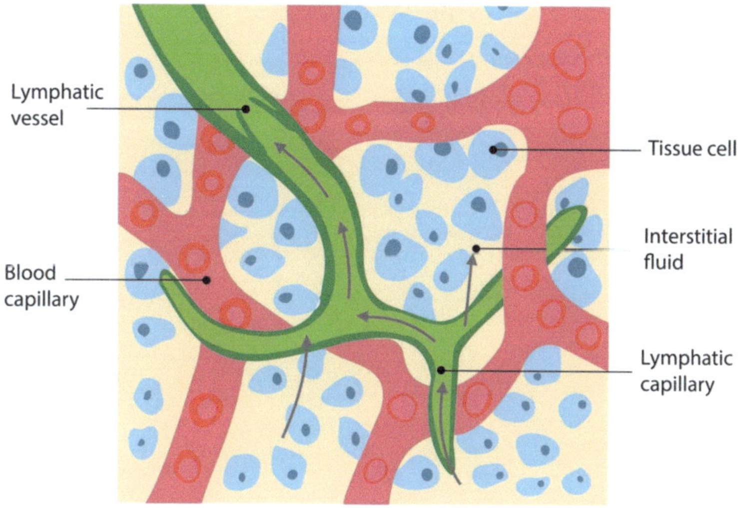

Fig. 2 Lymphatic-capillary interaction at the microvascular level

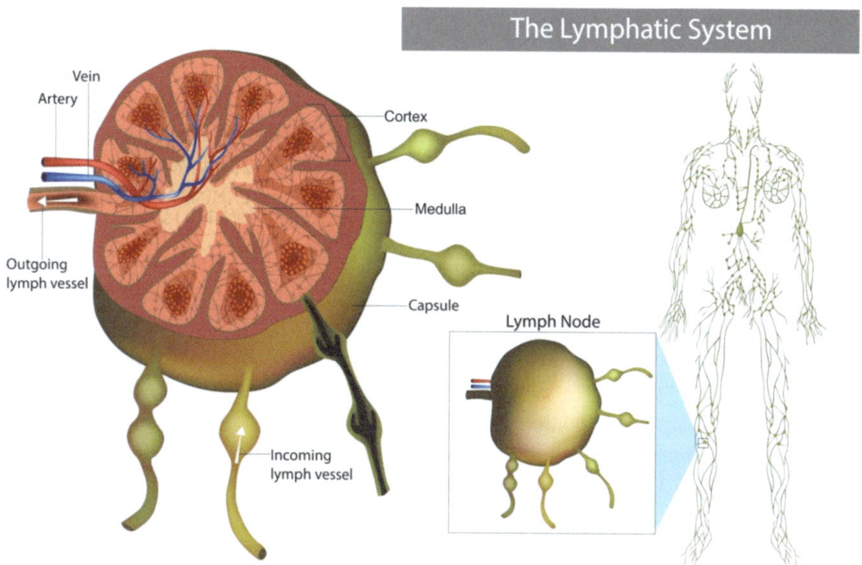

Fig. 3 Lymph nodes and the lymphatic system anatomy

Lymph nodes are integral components of the lymphatic system, serving as biological filters that purify lymphatic fluid before it is returned to the circulatory system. Structurally, lymph nodes are small, bean-shaped organs distributed throughout the body, interconnected by a network of lymphatic vessels. These vessels transport lymph—a fluid containing immune cells, proteins, and waste products—toward the

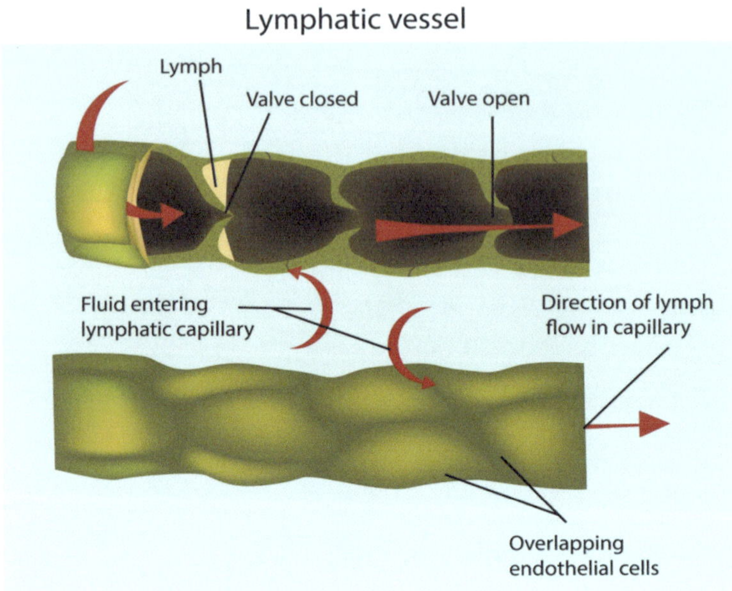

Fig. 4 The valve system on lymphatic capillaries

nodes. Within the nodes, lymph is exposed to a series of specialized compartments enriched with lymphocytes and macrophages. These immune cells scrutinize the lymph for foreign antigens and initiate an immune response when necessary, including the production of antibodies. The nodes also act as a site for the proliferation of lymphocytes, which are crucial for adaptive immunity.

Lymphatic circulation begins in the peripheral tissues with the uptake of interstitial fluid by lymphatic capillaries. This fluid, now called lymph, passes through a series of vessels, each increasing in size, and is filtered through one or more lymph nodes. Valves within these vessels prevent backflow, ensuring unidirectional movement toward the thoracic region, where the lymphatic vessels converge into the thoracic duct or right lymphatic duct. These ducts then empty the lymph into the venous blood circulation via the subclavian veins. This circulation is essential for maintaining fluid balance, for the transport of dietary lipids, and for immune surveillance.

Dysfunctions in lymphatic circulation (Fig. 4) can lead to lymphedema, characterized by swelling due to lymph accumulation, and can contribute to various immune-related diseases. Understanding the architecture and function of lymph nodes and lymphatic circulation is necessary in medical disciplines, from oncology to the treatment of immune and inflammatory disorders.

The lymphatic system in common lipedema-affected areas, such as the legs, arms, and hips, functions to maintain fluid balance and facilitate immune responses. However, in lipedema, this system exhibits compromised efficiency. Lipedema-associated lymphatic dysfunction is characterized by a reduced transport capacity of the lymphatic vessels, which may result from either a primary malformation or secondary impairment due to the burden of excess adipose tissue. Lymphatic vessels in these areas are responsible for draining protein-rich lymph fluid from the interstitial spaces, and their inadequate function can lead to the characteristic edema of lipedema. Histological studies often reveal hyperplasia of the adipocytes and fibrotic changes in the connective tissue that can physically obstruct the lymphatic flow. Moreover, the increased tissue pressure from expanded fat cells may collapse the initial lymphatic capillaries, impeding the uptake of lymph. The dysfunctional lymphatic circulation contributes to a chronic inflammatory state within the adipose tissue, exacerbating the pathological deposition of fat and fibrosis. This creates a vicious cycle, where the progression of lipedema further taxes the lymphatic system, thereby intensifying the clinical manifestations of the disease. Understanding the specifics of lymphatic system dysfunction in lipedema-affected areas is crucial for targeted therapeutic interventions aimed at alleviating symptoms and slowing down disease progression.

In lipedema, notable changes occur within the lymphatic system, impacting its vital functions. This system, integral to maintaining fluid balance and immune defense, becomes compromised due to the pathological expansion of adipose tissue characteristic of lipedema. The architecture of lymphatic vessels, normally a complex network designed to facilitate the drainage of lymph fluid, becomes distorted. This distortion hinders the efficient transport of lymph, leading to the accumulation of fluid within the interstitial spaces. The resulting lymph stasis contributes to the chronic inflammatory state observed in lipedema, further exacerbating tissue swelling and fibrosis. The dysfunction is often progressive, with early stages marked by a pitting edema that eventually gives way to non-pitting edema as fibrotic changes ensue. This alteration in lymphatic function is not merely a consequence of lipedema but also a perpetuating factor, as the impaired lymph drainage facilitates ongoing cycles of inflammation, adipose tissue hypertrophy, and fibrosis. Recognizing and addressing the changes in lymphatic function are therefore crucial components in the management of lipedema, with therapeutic strategies often focusing on enhancing lymphatic drainage and mitigating secondary tissue changes.

Lymphatic dysfunction (Fig. 5) arises from a disruption in the normal operation and structure of the lymphatic system, which can be triggered by a variety of mechanisms. One primary cause is genetic predisposition, where mutations in genes responsible for lymphatic development and function lead to congenital malformations or deficiencies in the lymphatic vessels.

Additionally, inflammation can be both a cause and a consequence of lymphatic dysfunction. Chronic inflammation can damage lymphatic vessels, reducing their ability to transport lymph efficiently, while the resulting accumulation of lymph can further perpetuate the inflammatory response. Infections can also directly damage lymphatic tissues or lead to the formation of scar tissue that obstructs lymph flow. Moreover, mechanical obstruction due to tumors or surgical removal of lymph nodes can impede lymphatic circulation, leading to secondary lymphedema. Metabolic diseases, such as obesity and diabetes, can induce changes in the extracellular matrix that surrounds lymphatic vessels, affecting their patency and

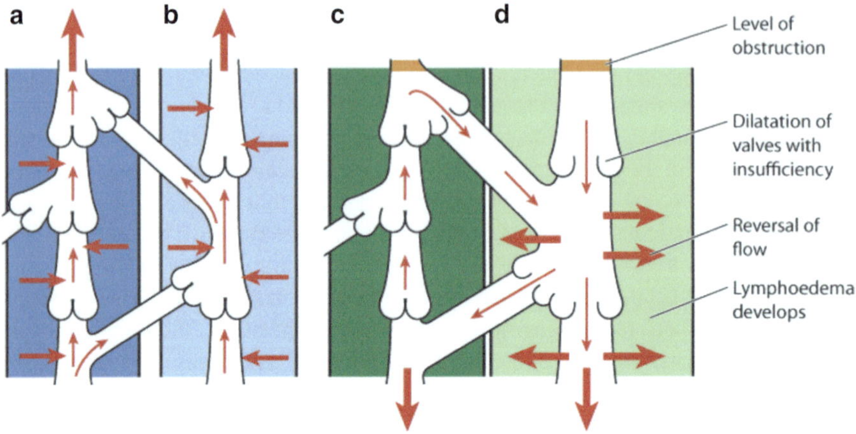

Fig. 5 Flow pattern in lymphatic capillaries with and without obstruction

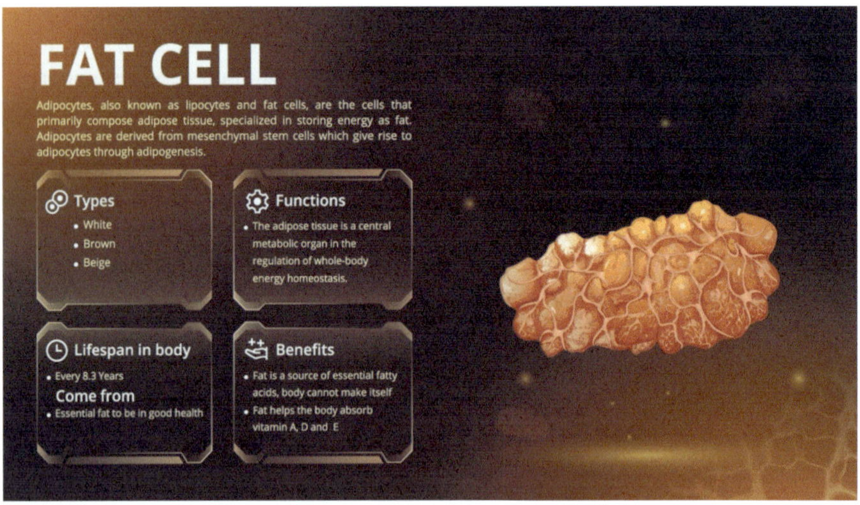

Fig. 6 Key features of adipocytes

contractility. Finally, certain lifestyle factors, including limited physical activity and a high-sodium diet, can exacerbate lymphatic dysfunction by increasing lymphatic load and vascular permeability. Understanding these mechanisms is crucial for the prevention and treatment of lymphatic diseases and for improving the management of related conditions such as lipedema.

Localized subcutaneous fat accumulation (Fig. 6) deposition, particularly in adipose tissue-rich regions, can significantly impact lymphatic flow by mechanically altering the architecture and function of the lymphatic system. The expansion of adipose tissue associated with obesity or conditions like lipedema can physically compress lymphatic vessels, impeding the normal propulsion of lymph through these channels. This compression may lead to lymphatic vessel insufficiency and subsequent lymph stasis, whereby the transport capacity of the lymphatic system is overwhelmed by the increased fluid volume that needs to be drained. Additionally, the hyperplasia and hypertrophy of adipocytes in obesity can result in a heightened inflammatory state. The secretion of pro-inflammatory cytokines and adipokines can further exacerbate lymphatic endothelial cell dysfunction, disrupting the integrity of the lymphatic vessels and their valves, leading to reflux and impaired lymph clearance. Moreover, excess fat and the resulting inflammation can promote fibrosis of the lymphatic vessels, reducing their elasticity and contractility, which are essential for effective lymph movement. Collectively, these alterations not only compromise lymphatic flow but also contribute to the progressive nature of lymph-related disorders, highlighting the importance of maintaining a healthy body weight and addressing adiposity to preserve lymphatic function.

Symptoms and signs of impaired lymphatic flow can be both varied and debilitating, as the lymphatic system is integral to fluid balance, immune response, and fat metabolism. Clinical manifestations typically begin with edema, characterized by swelling due to fluid accumulation, often presenting in the extremities. This swelling may initially be soft and pitting but can become non-pitting as fibrotic changes occur over time. Patients may also report feelings of heaviness or fullness, aching pain, and reduced mobility in the affected limbs. As the condition progresses, recurrent infections, such as cellulitis, can occur due to compromised immune surveillance. Skin changes are also common and can include thickening, hyperpigmentation, and, in advanced cases, the development of papillomatosis or lymphostatic verrucosis. Additionally, lymphorrhea, the leakage of lymph fluid through the skin, can be observed in severe cases, indicating profound lymphatic failure. These symptoms can significantly impact quality of life and may be exacerbated by factors such as prolonged standing, heat, or physical strain. Early recognition and management of these symptoms are critical in preventing progression and improving patient outcomes in lymphatic disorders.

Differentiating lipedema from lymphedema is crucial for appropriate management, as both conditions present with limb enlargement but have distinct pathophysiological mechanisms and clinical courses. Lipedema is primarily characterized by the bilateral and symmetrical deposition of adipose tissue in the extremities, sparing the feet, and is often painful with a tendency to bruise easily. It commonly arises during hormonal changes such as puberty, pregnancy, or menopause, suggesting a hormonal component to its etiology. Unlike lymphedema, lipedema does not typically present with pitting edema, and the skin remains pliable rather than thickened.

Lipedema progresses through several stages, starting with stage 1, where the skin surface remains smooth but the subcutaneous fat begins to increase. In stage 2, the skin surface becomes uneven or nodular, resembling a mattress in appearance, due to the increasing size of the fat lobules.

Stage 3 is marked by large extrusions of the skin and fat, leading to significant deformity. Some practitioners also recognize a stage 4, characterized by the

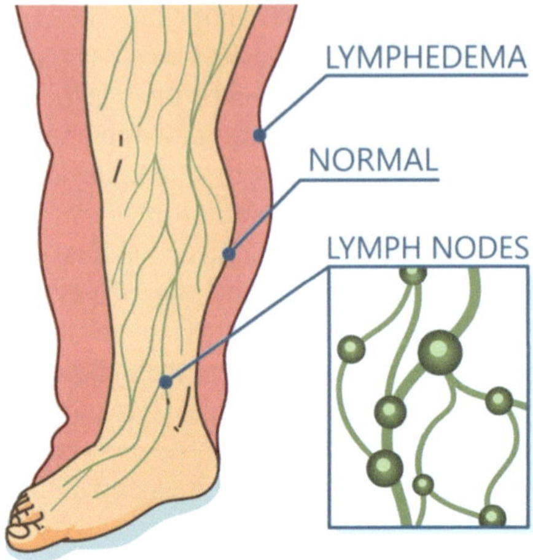

Fig. 7 Effect of lymphatic dysfunction on leg girth

development of lymphedema, termed lipolymphedema, due to the severe and prolonged impairment of lymphatic function secondary to the increased fat mass.

Staging of lipedema is important as it guides the therapeutic approach and prognosis. Early stages may respond to conservative measures such as compression therapy and weight management, while advanced stages may require more invasive interventions like liposuction to remove dysfunctional adipose tissue. Accurate diagnosis and staging are therefore essential for effective treatment and mitigation of progression.

Lymphatic dysfunction in lipedema can lead to a cascade of complications that exacerbate the patient's condition and impact their quality of life. The impaired lymphatic drainage associated with lipedema contributes to an increase in interstitial fluid, which can lead to chronic swelling and discomfort. Over time, the persistent excess fluid may result in fibrosis of the surrounding tissue, which further impedes the efficiency of lymphatic flow and reduces the elasticity of the skin and subcutaneous tissue. The chronicity of this process can also foster an environment conducive to recurrent infections, such as cellulitis, due to the impaired immune function inherent in a stagnant lymphatic system. Moreover, the constant strain on the lymphatic vessels can cause them to become dilated and dysfunctional, a condition known as lymphangiectasia, which may allow protein-rich lymph to seep into the surrounding tissue, promoting additional fibrosis and fat deposition. In advanced cases, the ongoing stress on the lymphatic system can lead to the development of secondary lymphedema, further compounding limb volume and increasing the risk of complications. The interplay between lipedema and lymphatic dysfunction highlights the importance of early intervention to manage symptoms and prevent the progression to these severe complications.

Secondary lymphedema (Fig. 7) represents a significant risk in the clinical progression of lipedema due to the cumulative impact of chronic adipose tissue accumulation on the lymphatic system. In individuals with lipedema, the excessive and pathological fat deposition, particularly in the lower extremities, can exert undue pressure on the lymphatic vessels, thereby impeding the normal flow of lymph. This sustained pressure can cause mechanical obstruction and functional impairment of the lymphatic vessels, leading to their insufficiency and the eventual development of secondary lymphedema, termed as lipolymphedema. This condition is marked by a further increase in limb volume, non-pitting edema, and a higher propensity for fibrotic changes and infection due to the impaired immune surveillance and fluid stasis. The risk of secondary lymphedema in patients with lipedema underscores the importance of early diagnosis and intervention, including weight management, physical therapy, and potentially surgical options to alleviate the lymphatic load and prevent the progressive deterioration of lymphatic function that characterizes this complex interrelated condition.

Infections and skin changes are notable complications of lipedema that arise due to altered lymphatic drainage and adipose tissue architecture. The compromised lymphatic system often seen in lipedema can lead to a localized immune deficiency, rendering the skin and subcutaneous tissues more susceptible to infections such as cellulitis. These infections can be recurrent and may exacerbate the lymphatic impairment, creating a vicious cycle of inflammation and infection. Skin changes in lipedema are characterized by a thickening and hardening of the skin and underlying tissues, known as fibrosis, which results from chronic inflammation and the accumulation of extracellular matrix components. Additionally, the skin may appear dimpled, similar to the texture of an orange peel, which is referred to as peau d'orange. Over time, the continual expansion of adipose tissue can lead to further dermal and epidermal changes, including the development of stretch marks (striae distensae) and hyperpigmentation due to hemosiderin deposition from micro-hemorrhages. These dermatological manifestations not only have physical implications but can also significantly impact the psychological and social well-being of individuals with lipedema, making comprehensive care, including infection prevention and skin treatment, an essential component of lipedema management.

The co-occurrence of lipedema and lymphedema can profoundly affect patient mobility and quality of life. The dual burden of excess fat accumulation and fluid retention significantly increases limb volume, which can lead to a restriction in the range of motion and difficulties with ambulation. The physical discomfort, combined with the visible disfigurement, often results in psychosocial distress, including body image issues, anxiety, and depression. The increased weight of the limbs can cause joint pain, particularly in the knees, hips, and ankles, exacerbating the risk of osteoarthritis and further limiting mobility. The combined impact of lipedema and lymphedema may also make it challenging for patients to find appropriate clothing and footwear, engage in physical activity, and maintain social interactions, which are essential for a good quality of life. Moreover, the chronic nature of these conditions and the need for ongoing self-care, including compression therapy and lymphatic drainage massages, can impose a significant time and financial burden on individuals.

Consequently, the management of lipedema with coexisting lymphedema requires a comprehensive approach that not only addresses the physical symptoms but also provides psychosocial support to improve overall quality of life for affected patients.

In conclusion, lymphatic dysfunction plays a role in the pathophysiology of lipedema, with profound implications for the progression of the disease and the patient's quality of life. The obstruction and impairment of lymphatic vessels due to excess adipose tissue can lead to a range of complications, including secondary lymphedema, increased susceptibility to infections, and chronic inflammation. These complications not only exacerbate the physical symptoms of lipedema but also impose significant psychosocial burdens, affecting mobility, self-image, and overall well-being. Early and accurate diagnosis of lipedema is crucial, as it allows for the implementation of timely and effective management strategies aimed at alleviating lymphatic dysfunction and preventing its complications. A holistic approach to treatment, encompassing dietary modifications, physical therapy, compression garments, and, where necessary, surgical interventions, is essential for improving clinical outcomes. Furthermore, education and support for patients are integral to ensure adherence to management plans and to foster coping strategies for living with this chronic condition. Ultimately, an integrated model of care that addresses both the physical and emotional facets of lipedema is imperative for enhancing the quality of life for those affected by this multifaceted disorder.

Suggested Reading

Herbst K.L., Kahn L.A., Iker E., Ehrlich C., Wright T., McHutchison L., Schwartz J., Sleigh M., MC Donahue P. , Lisson K.H., et al. Standard of care for lipedema in the United States. *Phlebol. Phlebol.* 2021;36:779–796. https://doi.org/10.1177/02683555211015887.

Kamali P., Lin S.J. Lymphedema: Presentation, Diagnosis, and Treatment. *Plast. Reconstr. Surg.* 2016;137:1654–1655. doi: https://doi.org/10.1097/PRS.0000000000002136.

Greene A.K., Grant F.D., Slavin S.A. Lower-Extremity Lymphedema and Elevated Body-Mass Index. *N. Engl. J. Med.* 2012;366:2136–2137. https://doi.org/10.1056/NEJMc1201684.

Rockson S.G. Current concepts and future directions in the diagnosis and management of lymphatic vascular disease. *Vasc. Med.* 2010;15:223–231. https://doi.org/10.1177/1358863X10364553.

Cormier J.N., Askew R.L., Mungovan K.S., Xing Y., Ross M.I., Armer J.M. Lymphedema beyond breast cancer: A systematic review and meta-analysis of cancer-related secondary lymphedema. *Cancer.* 2010;116:5138–5149. https://doi.org/10.1002/cncr.25458.

Fu M.R., Deng J., Armer J.M. Putting Evidence into Practice: Cancer-Related Lymphedema. *Clin. J. Oncol. Nurs.* 2014;18:68–79. https://doi.org/10.1188/14.CJON.S3.68-79.

Rockson S.G., Keeley V., Kilbreath S., Szuba A., Towers A. Cancer-associated secondary lymphoedema. *Nat. Rev. Dis. Prim.* 2019;5:22. https://doi.org/10.1038/s41572-019-0072-5.

Goss J.A., Greene A.K. Diagnosis and Staging of Lymphedema. *Semin. Plast. Surg.* 2018;32:12–16. doi: https://doi.org/10.1055/s-0038-1635117.

Stemmer R. Stemmer's sign—Possibilities and limits of clinical diagnosis of lymphedema. *Wien. Med. Wochenschr.* 1999;149:85–86.

Suehiro K., Mizumoto Y., Morikage N., Harada T., Samura M., Nagase T., Takeuchi Y., Mizoguchi T., Suzuki R., Kurazumi H., et al. Hardness Sensed by Skin Palpation in Legs with Lymphedema Is Predominantly Correlated with Dermal Thickening. *Lymphat. Res. Biol.* 2021 https://doi.org/10.1089/lrb.2020.0133.

Grada A.A., Phillips T.J. Lymphedema: Diagnostic workup and management. *J. Am. Acad. Dermatol.* 2017;77:995–1006. doi: https://doi.org/10.1016/j.jaad.2017.03.021.

Zhang J., Hoffner M., Brorson H. Adipocytes are larger in lymphedematous extremities than in controls. *J. Plast. Surg. Hand Surg.* 2021:1–8. https://doi.org/10.1080/2000656X.2021.1953042.

Crescenzi R., Donahue P.M.C., Garza M., Lee C.A., Patel N.J., Gonzalez V., Jones R.S., Donahue M.J. Elevated magnetic resonance imaging measures of adipose tissue deposition in women with breast cancer treatment-related lymphedema. *Breast Cancer Res. Treat.* 2021;191:115–124. https://doi.org/10.1007/s10549-021-06419-w.

Mortimer P.S., Rockson S.G. New developments in clinical aspects of lymphatic disease. *J. Clin. Investig.* 2014;124:915–921. https://doi.org/10.1172/JCI71608.

Fat Metabolism and Dysfunction in Lipedema

Fat metabolism (Fig. 1), also known as lipid metabolism, is a crucial biological process that involves the breakdown, synthesis, and distribution of fats in the body. It plays a significant role in energy storage and production, cell membrane structure, and the synthesis of important biomolecules. The process begins with lipolysis, wherein triglycerides are broken down into glycerol and free fatty acids (FFAs) by enzymes called lipases. These FFAs can then enter the mitochondria, where they undergo beta-oxidation, converting them into acetyl-CoA molecules. Acetyl-CoA enters the citric acid cycle, leading to the production of adenosine triphosphate (ATP), which is the cell's energy currency. Additionally, fat metabolism is closely regulated by hormones such as insulin and glucagon, which respond to the body's energy needs, ensuring a balance between fat storage and utilization.

The relevance of metabolic dysfunction in lipedema is increasingly recognized in the medical community. Lipedema is a chronic condition characterized by the abnormal accumulation of adipose tissue, primarily in the legs and arms, leading to pain, swelling, and mobility issues. This disorder is distinct from obesity, as the fat deposition in lipedema is resistant to traditional weight loss methods. Emerging research suggests that individuals with lipedema may have underlying metabolic dysfunctions, including impaired fat metabolism and altered lymphatic function. These metabolic anomalies can exacerbate the accumulation of lipedema fat and contribute to the progression of the disease. Understanding the metabolic underpinnings of lipedema is crucial for developing targeted treatments that address not only the symptoms but also the root causes of the condition, potentially improving outcomes for those affected.

Adipose tissue, commonly known as body fat, plays a crucial role in energy storage, insulation, and regulation of body temperature. It is primarily categorized into three types, i.e., white, brown, and beige fat, each with distinct functions and physiological roles. White adipose tissue (WAT) is the most abundant type, serving as the main energy reservoir through the storage of triglycerides and release of fatty acids during periods of energy deficit. WAT also plays a significant role in hormone production, including leptin, which regulates appetite and energy balance. Brown

G. Laur, *Lipoedema*, https://doi.org/10.1007/978-981-96-8939-2_5

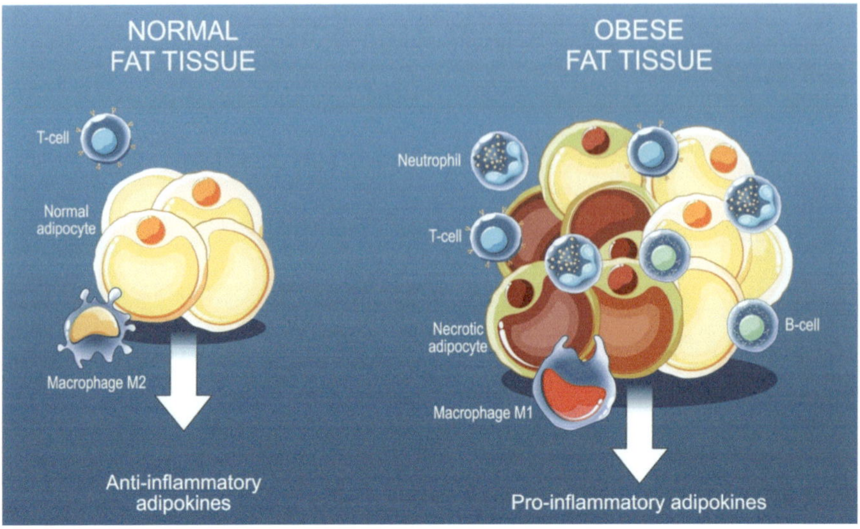

Fig. 1 Key features between normal fat tissue and obese fat tissue

adipose tissue (BAT), in contrast, is specialized in energy expenditure and heat production, a process known as thermogenesis. BAT's unique ability to burn calories and produce heat is attributed to the presence of a large number of mitochondria containing uncoupling protein 1 (UCP1), which allows the release of energy as heat. Beige adipose tissue, or beige fat, is a relatively recent discovery and is characterized by its ability to convert from white fat cells in response to certain stimuli like cold exposure or exercise. Beige fat shares similarities with brown fat in terms of thermogenic capacity and energy expenditure, making it a potential target for obesity and metabolic disease therapies. The differentiation between these types of adipose tissue underscores the complexity of fat metabolism and its impact on overall metabolic health.

Adipocytes, or fat cells, are specialized cells primarily involved in energy storage and homeostasis, playing a crucial role in the body's metabolic activity. These cells store energy in the form of lipids within large intracellular droplets, which can be mobilized and utilized as fuel during periods of energy deficit.

Adipocytes are not merely passive storage depots but actively participate in metabolic regulation by secreting a variety of signaling molecules, including adipokines such as leptin, adiponectin, and resistin. These adipokines influence a wide range of physiological processes, including appetite regulation, insulin sensitivity, inflammation, and lipid metabolism. Furthermore, adipocytes are involved in the modulation of systemic energy balance and the metabolic integration between various organs, such as the liver, muscle, and brain. The biology of adipocytes extends beyond their metabolic activities, as they also play roles in thermogenesis, particularly through the action of brown and beige adipocytes, which convert energy from lipids into heat, contributing to the regulation of body temperature and energy expenditure. Understanding adipocyte biology and metabolic activity is therefore essential for elucidating the complex mechanisms underlying metabolic health and disease.

Adipose tissue in lipedema-affected areas exhibits distinct pathological and physiological characteristics that differentiate it from normal adipose tissue. Lipedema is a chronic condition characterized by the symmetric enlargement of the legs and arms due to the deposition of adipose tissue, leading to pain, tenderness, and easy bruising in the affected areas. The adipose tissue in lipedema is fibrotic, with an increased number of adipocytes that are larger and more irregularly shaped compared to those in healthy individuals. These changes contribute to impaired lymphatic drainage and increased fluid accumulation, exacerbating the swelling and discomfort experienced by patients. Furthermore, the adipose tissue in lipedema is resistant to traditional weight loss methods, suggesting a metabolic dysfunction that prevents the effective mobilization and utilization of stored lipids. Recent research has indicated that the adipose tissue in lipedema may have altered expression of adipokines and inflammatory markers, contributing to an inflammatory microenvironment that can further disrupt normal adipose tissue function and exacerbate the condition. Understanding the unique properties of adipose tissue in lipedema is crucial for developing targeted therapeutic strategies that can address the underlying pathophysiology of the disease.

Altered lipogenesis and lipolysis are hallmark metabolic disturbances observed in lipedema, a chronic disorder characterized by the abnormal accumulation of adipose tissue, particularly in the lower extremities. In lipedema, lipogenesis—the process by which acetyl-CoA is converted into triglycerides for storage in adipocytes—is often upregulated, leading to an increase in fat deposition. Conversely, lipolysis—the catabolic process involving the hydrolysis of triglycerides into free fatty acids and glycerol—appears to be impaired or resistant to normal regulatory mechanisms such as hormonal signals. This dysfunctional metabolic scenario contributes to the disproportionate and often painful fat accumulation seen in patients with lipedema, which is typically refractory to lifestyle interventions such as diet and exercise. Research suggests that this altered adipose tissue metabolism may be due to intrinsic defects in adipocyte function, aberrant expression of enzymes involved in lipid metabolism, or dysregulated adipokine secretion. Such insights into the pathophysiology of lipedema underscore the necessity for targeted therapeutic strategies that can correct the underlying metabolic imbalances specific to this condition.

The hormonal regulation of adipose tissue metabolism is complex and involves a multitude of hormones such as insulin, catecholamines, and sex hormones, among others. These hormones traditionally modulate lipogenesis and lipolysis, ensuring a balance between energy storage and release. In the context of lipedema, hormonal dysregulation plays a significant role in the pathophysiology of the disease. Insulin (Fig. 2), for instance, which promotes lipogenesis and inhibits lipolysis, may have an altered effect in the adipocytes of patients with lipedema, contributing to excessive fat accumulation.

Similarly, catecholamines, which normally stimulate fat breakdown, may be less effective in triggering lipolysis in lipedema. This could be due to a downregulation

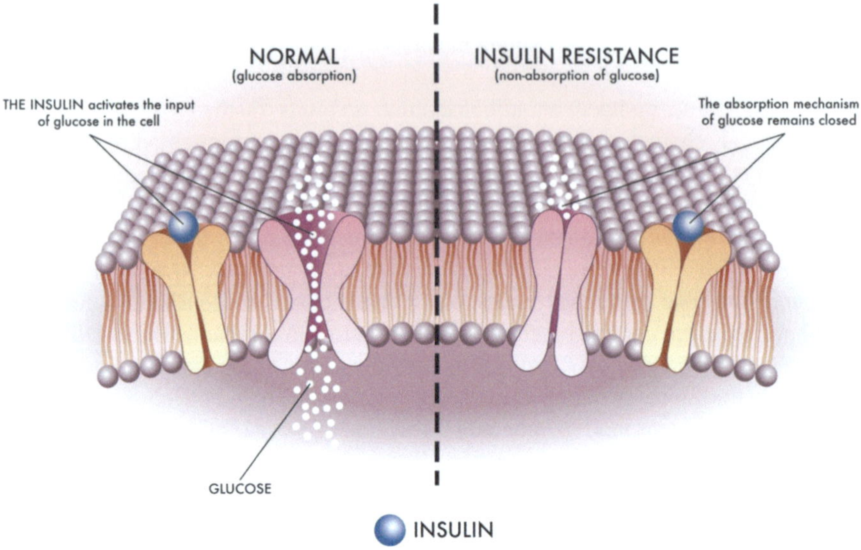

Fig. 2 Insulin resistance mechanism at the cell membrane level

of beta-adrenergic receptors or alterations in the signaling pathways downstream of these receptors. Additionally, the influence of sex hormones is evident as lipedema predominantly affects women and often exacerbates during hormonal fluctuations such as puberty, pregnancy, and menopause. Estrogen, in particular, is known to affect adipose tissue distribution and function, and its role in lipedema fat metabolism is a subject of ongoing research. The interplay of these hormones and their receptors, and the resultant dysfunction, is a key area of interest in understanding the etiology of lipedema and in developing targeted treatments that address the hormonal imbalances contributing to the disease.

Insulin resistance is a pathophysiological condition where cells fail to respond to the normal actions of the hormone insulin, resulting in impaired glucose uptake, hyperglycemia, and increased lipogenesis. Its role in lipedema is particularly intriguing, as insulin is a key regulator of adipose tissue function. In individuals with lipedema, insulin resistance may contribute to the disproportionate accumulation of fat in the affected areas. This condition is exacerbated by the fact that insulin resistance promotes the storage of triglycerides in adipocytes, while simultaneously inhibiting lipolysis, the breakdown of these stored fats. Consequently, the adipose tissue expands due to both increased fatty acid influx and decreased mobilization. The exact mechanism by which insulin resistance develops in lipedema is not fully understood, but it is hypothesized to involve a combination of genetic predisposition, hormonal imbalances, and possibly the low-grade inflammation often observed in adipose tissue. Moreover, insulin resistance in lipedema can have systemic effects, potentially contributing to the development of comorbid conditions such as type 2 diabetes, dyslipidemia, and cardiovascular disease.

Therefore, understanding the role of insulin resistance in lipedema is critical for the development of comprehensive treatment strategies that address both local adipose tissue dysfunction and associated systemic metabolic risks.

The composition of lipedema fat is distinctive and contributes to the pathological features of the condition. Lipedema fat often has a higher proportion of fibrous tissue compared to normal adipose tissue, which is believed to contribute to the pain and tenderness experienced by individuals with the condition. The extracellular matrix within lipedema fat is typically altered, with an increase in collagen and other connective tissue proteins that can lead to reduced blood flow and lymphatic drainage, exacerbating fluid retention and tissue swelling. Moreover, the lipid profile within lipedema fat may differ, potentially displaying an atypical distribution of fatty acid chains, which might affect the function and metabolism of the adipocytes. The adipocytes themselves are frequently found to be hypertrophic, or enlarged, which can affect their function and the secretion of adipokines, the signaling molecules that regulate inflammation and metabolic processes. This altered adipokine profile can contribute to systemic metabolic dysfunction. The unique composition of lipedema fat, with its complex interplay of fibrosis, altered lipid profile, and adipokine dysregulation, underpins the clinical manifestations of lipedema and poses challenges for treatment, emphasizing the need for further research into the molecular underpinnings of this tissue pathology.

Structural and functional differences between lipedema adipose tissue and normal adipose tissue are essential in understanding the pathology of lipedema. Structurally, lipedema adipose tissue is characterized by an increased number of adipocytes, which are often hypertrophic, and a dense fibrous network, distinguishing it from the more vascularized and less fibrotic normal adipose tissue. Functionally, these adipocytes demonstrate an abnormal metabolic profile, with a propensity for lipogenesis and an impaired lipolytic response to catecholamines, which may contribute to the progressive nature of fat accumulation in lipedema. Additionally, the hypertrophic adipocytes in lipedema tissue can secrete an altered profile of adipokines, leading to a pro-inflammatory state that can exacerbate the dysfunction of lymphatic vessels, impairing fluid clearance and promoting edema. The presence of excess fibrous tissue also contributes to the reduced oxygenation and potential hypoxia within the tissue, further impairing adipocyte metabolism and promoting the accumulation of lipids. The combined structural and functional abnormalities of lipedema adipose tissue underscore the complexity of the disease and highlight the need for targeted therapeutic strategies that address both the abnormal adipocyte metabolism and the altered tissue architecture.

Pain and sensitivity in lipedema adipose tissue are defining characteristics of this chronic condition, setting it apart from other forms of obesity or lymphedema. The adipose tissue of patients with lipedema is often tender to the touch, and this hypersensitivity is believed to arise from a confluence of factors. Histological analysis reveals a proliferation of fibrous connective tissue, which can entrap nerves and lead to a heightened pain response. Additionally, the expanded adipocytes may exert pressure on local structures, including nerve endings, exacerbating the sensation of pain. The pain in lipedema is also associated with inflammation, as inflammatory mediators are elevated in the tissue, further sensitizing nerve endings. Moreover, the vascular anomalies present in lipedema—such as increased capillary fragility and lymphatic dysfunction—contribute to edema, which can provoke an aching sensation and contribute to the characteristic pain profile of the disease.

The complex interaction between these structural and biochemical changes in lipedema adipose tissue underscores the need for a multidisciplinary approach to pain management in affected individuals, including both pharmacological and non-pharmacological interventions to address the unique aspects of lipedema-associated pain.

Diet plays a fundamental role in fat metabolism, serving as a modifiable factor that can influence the balance between lipogenesis and lipolysis, thereby affecting overall energy homeostasis. The quality and quantity of dietary intake directly affect the enzymatic processes involved in the synthesis and breakdown of adipose tissue. High intakes of simple carbohydrates can lead to increased insulin secretion, promoting lipogenesis and the storage of fat, particularly in visceral adipose tissue. Conversely, diets rich in monounsaturated and polyunsaturated fatty acids, such as those found in fish, nuts, and certain plant oils, can enhance lipid oxidation and have been associated with a more favorable adipose tissue distribution. Moreover, caloric restriction is known to induce lipolysis, resulting in the mobilization of fatty acids from adipose stores. The balance of macronutrients, along with the timing and pattern of eating, also influences circadian rhythms in metabolic processes. For instance, intermittent fasting regimens have been shown to affect circadian biology and may have beneficial effects on fat metabolism by enhancing diurnal patterns of hormone release that favor lipolysis over lipogenesis. Therefore, dietary interventions remain a critical component in the management of metabolic health, with the potential to alter the trajectory of metabolic diseases through their impact on adipose tissue metabolism.

Obesity and dietary habits play a significant role in the progression of lipedema, a condition characterized by the abnormal accumulation of fat in the lower body. While the etiology of lipedema is not fully understood and is distinct from common obesity, excess weight can exacerbate the condition. Adipose tissue in lipedema is thought to be resistant to the effects of dieting and exercise, often not responding to general weight loss strategies. This resistance may be due in part to the pathophysiological mechanisms underlying lipedema, which include atypical adipocyte proliferation, altered lymphatic function, and potential hormonal imbalances. Nevertheless, obesity can worsen lipedema symptoms by increasing the load on already compromised lymphatic vessels, thereby intensifying edema and inflammation. Diet, particularly a high intake of processed foods and refined carbohydrates, may contribute to systemic inflammation and exacerbate the accumulation of lipedema fat. Moreover, certain diets that are rich in anti-inflammatory components and are low in refined sugars and fats may help manage the progression of lipedema by reducing inflammation and potentially influencing the profile of adipokines and other signaling molecules involved in fat metabolism. It is crucial to understand the complex interplay between obesity, diet, and lipedema progression to inform nutritional guidance and therapeutic strategies for individuals with this condition.

The interaction between lymphatic dysfunction and fat metabolism plays a role in the pathogenesis of lipedema, a condition characterized by the disproportionate accumulation of adipose tissue in the extremities. Lipedema adipose tissue often presents with a compromised lymphatic system, which is responsible for the transport and removal of interstitial fluids, including the products of lipolysis. When the lymphatic system is dysfunctional, as often observed in lipedema, there is an impediment to efficient lipid mobilization and removal, leading to local lipid accumulation and adipose tissue hypertrophy. This lymphatic insufficiency may also contribute to chronic inflammation within the adipose tissue, further disrupting normal adipocyte function and signaling pathways involved in lipid metabolism. The resulting adipose tissue fibrosis can create a self-perpetuating cycle, where impaired lymphatic function exacerbates fat deposition, and the expanded adipose tissue further hinders lymphatic flow. The delicate balance between lymphatic function and fat metabolism is thus central to understanding lipedema and emphasizes the need for therapeutic approaches that address both the lymphatic abnormalities and the metabolic dysfunction to effectively manage and treat lipedema.

Impaired lymph drainage has profound effects on adipose tissue, particularly in the context of lipedema, a condition marked by abnormal fat accumulation. The lymphatic system plays a crucial role in maintaining tissue fluid homeostasis, and its dysfunction can lead to the accumulation of interstitial fluid, exacerbating the formation of fibrotic adipose tissue. In lipedema, the impaired drainage is believed to cause a chronic inflammatory response within the adipose tissue, which may alter the normal function of adipocytes and promote the proliferation of connective tissue. This inflammatory milieu can disrupt adipokine secretion, leading to altered metabolic signaling and contributing to the expansion and fibrosis of adipose tissue.

Furthermore, the excess interstitial fluid (Fig. 3) may increase tissue turgor, placing mechanical stress on the adipocytes and the extracellular matrix, potentially inducing hypoxia and further promoting fibrosis. The impact of impaired lymph drainage on adipose tissue is a critical factor in the progression of lipedema, as it not only influences the characteristic pathological changes but also poses challenges for effective treatment, emphasizing the importance of therapeutic strategies aimed at restoring lymphatic function and addressing the consequent adipose tissue alterations.

Genetic predisposition plays a significant role in the manifestation of altered fat metabolism, which is a central feature in various metabolic disorders. The heritability of traits such as obesity, insulin resistance, and lipid profile variations is well-documented, with numerous genetic loci identified that contribute to these conditions. Genes involved in the regulation of adipocyte differentiation, fatty acid uptake, synthesis, storage, and lipolysis are all potential contributors to an individual's propensity for altered fat metabolism. Single-nucleotide polymorphisms (SNPs) in genes such as fat mass and obesity-associated gene (FTO), peroxisome proliferator-activated receptor-γ (PPARγ), lipoprotein lipase (LPL), and leptin have been linked to obesity and metabolic syndrome. Additionally, genetic syndromes such as lipodystrophy, characterized by the abnormal distribution of adipose tissue, further illustrate the role of genetics in fat metabolism. Epigenetic factors, including

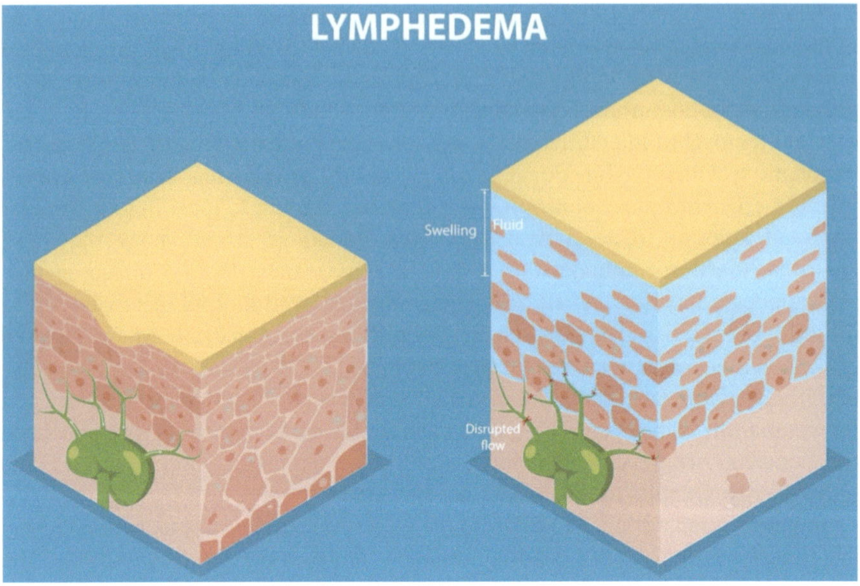

Fig. 3 Effect of lymphedema on the level of interstitial fluid

DNA methylation and histone modification, also influence gene expression related to adipogenesis and lipid turnover, and they can be modulated by environmental factors, creating a complex interplay between genetics and lifestyle. Understanding the genetic basis of altered fat metabolism is critical for identifying at-risk individuals and developing personalized interventions that could modify the course of metabolic diseases.

Hormonal imbalances can have profound effects on adipose tissue, influencing its distribution, function, and overall metabolic activity. Hormones, such as insulin, glucocorticoids, sex hormones (estrogens and androgens), and thyroid hormones, play crucial roles in adipogenesis, the process by which preadipocytes differentiate into mature adipocytes. They also regulate lipolysis and lipogenesis—the breakdown and synthesis of fats, respectively. For instance, insulin typically acts to promote glucose uptake and lipid storage in adipose tissue, inhibiting lipolysis. Conversely, cortisol can stimulate lipolysis but also favors visceral fat deposition. Estrogens are known to have a protective effect against the development of central obesity, while androgens tend to promote the accumulation of visceral fat. Thyroid hormones stimulate fat mobilization, increasing the basal metabolic rate and enhancing lipolysis. An imbalance in any of these hormonal axes can lead to altered adipose tissue metabolism, contributing to conditions such as obesity, metabolic syndrome, and lipodystrophy. For example, insulin resistance, a state of diminished response to insulin, is a common feature of metabolic syndrome and can lead to increased fat storage and hyperglycemia. Furthermore, hormonal imbalances can modulate the secretion of adipokines, which are cytokines released by adipose tissue, thus affecting systemic inflammation and insulin sensitivity. Therefore, maintaining hormonal homeostasis is vital for the proper functioning of adipose tissue and overall metabolic health.

Evaluating fat metabolism dysfunction in lipedema is a critical aspect of understanding and managing the disease. Lipedema is characterized by the pathological accumulation of adipose tissue, primarily in the lower limbs, which does not respond to conventional weight loss strategies. This condition suggests an inherent dysfunction in the metabolic processing of fat. Clinically, lipedema fat metabolism can be evaluated through a combination of patient history, physical examination, and diagnostic tests.

Patients typically present with a disproportionate distribution of subcutaneous fat, which is often painful and tender to the touch. Biochemical assessments may reveal altered profiles of circulating lipids, adipokines, and inflammatory markers. Imaging studies such as MRI and DEXA scans can provide insights into the distribution and density of lipedema fat. Metabolic dysfunction in lipedema may be further elucidated through the examination of adipocyte function, including the capacity for lipogenesis and lipolysis, which are often impaired in lipedema tissues. Functional assessments of the lymphatic system, which can be compromised in lipedema, also contribute to the overall evaluation of fat metabolism dysfunction. Understanding the nuances of fat metabolism in lipedema is essential for the development of targeted therapies that can alleviate symptoms and prevent disease progression.

The role of fat metabolism in lipedema is central to both the pathology and the comprehensive management of the condition. Lipedema is characterized by abnormal and excessive fat deposition in the lower extremities, which is resistant to conventional weight loss strategies. This resistance suggests a fundamental difference in the way lipedema fat metabolizes, stores, and mobilizes lipids. Fat metabolism in lipedema is marked by an impaired lipolytic response, the process by which stored fat is broken down into free fatty acids. Moreover, there appears to be an alteration in adipocyte function, with a potential shift toward lipogenesis over lipolysis, contributing to the accumulation of fatty tissue. The dysfunctional fat metabolism is often accompanied by lymphatic dysfunction, exacerbating fluid retention and tissue swelling. Inflammatory processes also play a role, as adipose tissue in lipedema tends to exhibit an inflammatory profile with increased fibrosis, which can further disrupt metabolic function. Evaluating and understanding these metabolic alterations is crucial for developing targeted treatments. Comprehensive management of lipedema, therefore, involves a multimodal approach that includes dietary modifications, pharmacological interventions aimed at improving lymphatic flow and reducing inflammation, and potentially surgical options to remove dysfunctional adipose tissue. Integrating knowledge of fat metabolism with clinical strategies can help mitigate symptoms and improve the quality of life for individuals with lipedema.

Suggested Reading

Herbst KL, Kahn LA, Iker E, Ehrlich C, Wright T, McHutchison L, et al.. Standard of care for lipedema in the united states. *Phlebology* (2021) 36(10):779–96. https://doi.org/10.1177/02683555211015887

Herbst KL. Rare adipose disorders (RADs) masquerading as obesity. *Acta Pharmacol Sin* (2012) 33(2):155–72. https://doi.org/10.1038/aps.2011.153.

Child AH, Gordon KD, Sharpe P, Brice G, Ostergaard P, Jeffery S, et al.. Lipedema: an inherited condition. *Am J Med Genet A* (2010) 152A(4):970–6. https://doi.org/10.1002/ajmg.a.33313.

Torre YS, Wadeea R, Rosas V, Herbst KL. Lipedema: friend and foe. *Horm Mol Biol Clin Investig* (2018) 33(1):1–15. https://doi.org/10.1515/hmbci-2017-0076.

Chen GC, Arthur R, Iyengar NM, Kamensky V, Xue X, Wassertheil-Smoller S, et al.. Association between regional body fat and cardiovascular disease risk among postmenopausal women with normal body mass index. *Eur Heart J* (2019) 40(34):2849–55. https://doi.org/10.1093/eurheartj/ehz391

Beltran K, Herbst KL. Differentiating lipedema and dercum's disease. *Int J Obes (Lond)* (2017) 41(2):240–5. https://doi.org/10.1038/ijo.2016.205.

AL-Ghadban S, Cromer W, Allen M, Ussery C, Badowski M, Harris D, et al.. Dilated blood and lymphatic microvessels, angiogenesis, increased macrophages, and adipocyte hypertrophy in lipedema thigh skin and fat tissue. *J Obes* (2019) 2019:10. https://doi.org/10.1155/2019/8747461.

Allen M, Schwartz M, Herbst KL. Interstitial fluid in lipedema and control skin. *Women's Health Rep* (2020) 1(1):480–7. https://doi.org/10.1089/whr.2020.0086.

Suga H, Araki J, Aoi N, Kato H, Higashino T, Yoshimura K. Adipose tissue remodeling in lipedema: adipocyte death and concurrent regeneration. *J cutaneous pathology.* (2009) 36(12):1293–8. https://doi.org/10.1111/j.1600-0560.2009.01256.x.

Wolf S, Deuel JW, Hollmén M, Felmerer G, Kim B-S, Vasella M, et al.. A distinct cytokine profile and stromal vascular fraction metabolic status without significant changes in the lipid composition characterizes lipedema. *Int J Mol Sci* (2021) 22(7):3313. https://doi.org/10.3390/ijms22073313.

Felmerer G, Stylianaki A, Hägerling R, Wang A, Ströbel P, Hollmén M, et al.. Adipose tissue hypertrophy, an aberrant biochemical profile and distinct gene expression in lipedema. *J Surg Res* (2020) 253:294–303. https://doi.org/10.1016/j.jss.2020.03.055.

Koyama H, Tanaka T, Imaeda K. Suspected case of lipoedema in Japanese woman with a characteristic histology in skin biopsy. *BMJ Case Rep* (2017) 2017:bcr–2017-221049. https://doi.org/10.1136/bcr-2017-221049.

Felmerer G, Stylianaki A, Hollmén M, Ströbel P, Stepniewski A, Wang A, et al.. Increased levels of VEGF-C and macrophage infiltration in lipedema patients without changes in lymphatic vascular morphology. *Sci Rep* (2020) 10(1):10947. https://doi.org/10.1038/s41598-020-67987-3.

Taylor NE, Foster WC, Wick MR, Patterson JW. Tumefactive lipedema with pseudoxanthoma elasticum-like microscopic changes. *J Cutaneous Pathol.* (2004) 31(2):205–9. https://doi.org/10.1111/j.0303-6987.2004.00168.x.

Kaiserling E. Zur histologie des lipödems. In: Strößenreuther R, editor. *Lipödem und Cellulitis sowie andere Erkrankungen des Fettgewebes*. Köln: Viavital-Verlag; (2001). p. 90–9.

Al-Ghadban S, Bunnell BA. Characterization of adipose tissue and adipose tissue derived stem cells in Lipedema. *Cell Mol Biol* (2021). Available at: https://unthsc-ir.tdl.org/handle/20.500.12503/30514.

Strößenreuther R. Das lipödem. In: *Lipödem und Cellulitis sowie andere Erkrankungen des Fettgewebes*. Köln: Viavital-Verlag; (2001). p. 41–54.

Foundation L. FIRST LOOK: *Learning by Listening - Early findings from the Lipedema Foundation Registry survey 2022*. Available at: https://www.lipedema.org/s/LF_First-Look-Registry-Report.pdf.

Cena H., Calder P. C. Defining a healthy diet: evidence for the role of contemporary dietary patterns in health and disease. *Nutrients*. 2020;12:334. https://doi.org/10.3390/nu12020334.

Chaudhury A., Duvoor C., Reddy Dendi V.S., Kraleti S., Chada A., Ravilla R., Marco A., Shekhawat N. S., Montales M. T., Kuriakose K., Sasapu A., Beebe A., Patil N., Musham C. K., Lohani G. P., Mirza W. Clinical review of antidiabetic drugs: implications for type 2 diabetes mellitus management. *Front. Endocrinol.* 2017;8:6. https://doi.org/10.3389/fendo.2017.00006.

Church C., Horowitz M., Rodeheffer M. WAT is a functional adipocyte? *Adipocyte*. 2012;1:38–45. https://doi.org/10.4161/adip.19132.

Coppens I., Asai T., Tomavo S. Chapter 8 – Biochemistry and metabolism of Toxoplasma gondii: carbohydrates, lipids and nucleotides. In: Weiss L. M., Kim K., editors. *Toxoplasma Gondii*. 2nd ed. Academic; 2014. pp. 257–295.

Denisenko Y. K., Kytikova O. Y., Novgorodtseva T. P., Antonyuk M. V., Gvozdenko T. A., Kantur T. A. Lipid-induced mechanisms of metabolic syndrome. *J. Obes.* 2020;2020:5762395. https://doi.org/10.1155/2020/5762395.

Di Mauro S., Trevisan C., Hays A. Disorders of lipid metabolism in muscle. *Muscle Nerve*. 1980;3:369–388. https://doi.org/10.1002/mus.880030502.

Dias S., Paredes S., Ribeiro L. Drugs involved in dyslipidemia and obesity treatment: focus on adipose tissue. *Int. J. Endocrinol.* 2018;4:2637418. https://doi.org/10.1155/2018/2637418.

Kalra SP, Dube MG, Pu S, Xu B, Horvath TL, Kalra PS. Interacting appetite-regulating pathways in the hypothalamic regulation of body weight. Endocr Rev. 1999;20:68–100.

Stanley BG, Kyrkouli SE, Lampert S, Leibowitz SF. Neuropeptide Y chronically injected into the hypothalamus: a powerful neurochemical inducer of hyperphagia and obesity. Peptides. 1986;7:1189–1192.

Zarjevski N, Cusin I, Vettor R, Rohner-Jeanrenaud F, Jeanrenaud B. Chronic intracerebroventricular neuropeptide-Y administration to normal rats mimics hormonal and metabolic changes of obesity. Endocrinology. 1993;133:1753–1758.

Leibowitz SF. Brain peptides and obesity: pharmacologic treatment. Obes Res. 2002;3:573S–589S.

Wilding JP, Gilbey SG, Bailey CJ, Batt RA, Williams G, Ghatei MA, Bloom SR. Increased neuropeptide-Y messenger ribonucleic acid (mRNA) and decreased neurotensin mRNA in the hypothalamus of the obese (ob/ob) mouse. Endocrinology. 1993;132:1939–1944.

Schwartz MW, Baskin DG, Bukowski TR, Kuijper JL, Foster D, Lasser G, Prunkard DE, Porte D Jr., Woods SC, Seeley RJ, et al. Specificity of leptin action on elevated blood glucose levels and hypothalamic neuropeptide Y gene expression in ob/ob mice. Diabetes. 1996;45:531–535.

Cowley MA, Grove KL. Ghrelin-satisfying a hunger for the mechanism. Endocrinology. 2004;145:2604–2606.

Gilg S, Lutz TA. The orexigenic effect of peripheral ghrelin differs between rats of different age and with different baseline food intake, and it may in part be mediated by the area postrema. Physiol Behav. 2006;87:353–359.

Tschop M, Smiley DL, Heiman ML. Ghrelin induces adiposity in rodents. Nature. 2000;407:908–913.

Parati G, Lombardi C, Narkiewicz K. Sleep apnea: epidemiology, pathophysiology, and relation to cardiovascular risk. Am J Physiol Regul Integr Comp Physiol. 2007;293:R1671–R1683.

Havel PJ. Update on adipocyte hormones: regulation of energy balance and carbohydrate/lipid metabolism. Diabetes. 2004;53 Suppl 1:S143–S151.

Ukkola O. Endocrinological activities of ghrelin: new insights. Eur J Intern Med. 2003;14:351–356.

Maeda K, Okubo K, Shimomura I, Mizuno K, Matsuzawa Y, Matsubara K. Analysis of an expression profile of genes in the human adipose tissue. Gene. 1997;190:227–235.

Koerner A, Kratzsch J, Kiess W. Adipocytokines: leptin.the classical, resistin.the controversical, adiponectin.the promising, and more to come. Best Pract Res Clin Endocrinol Metab. 2005;19:525–546.

Brzozowski T, Konturek PC, Konturek SJ, Brzozowska I, Pawlik T. Role of prostaglandins in gastroprotection and gastric adaptation. J Physiol Pharmacol. 2005;56 Suppl 5:33–55.

Nawrot-Porabka K, Jaworek J, Leja-Szpak A, Palonek M, Szklarczyk J, Konturek SJ, Pawlik WW. Leptin is able to stimulate pancreatic enzyme secretion via activation of duodeno-pancreatic reflex and CCK release. J Physiol Pharmacol. 2004;55 Suppl 2:47–57.

Singla P, Bardoloi A, Parkash AA. Metabolic effects of obesity: A review. World J Diabetes. 2010 Jul 15;1(3):76-88. https://doi.org/10.4239/wjd.v1.i3.76. PMID: 21537431; PMCID: PMC3083889.

Inflammatory Processes and Cellular Mechanisms

While the etiology of lipedema remains multifaceted and not fully elucidated, growing evidence suggests that inflammatory processes and cellular mechanisms play a role in its pathogenesis. Understanding inflammatory pathways in lipedema is crucial for several reasons, including understanding the disease mechanism, developing targeted treatments, preventing progression, distinguishing it from obesity or lymphedema, managing pain and other symptoms, reducing the risk of comorbidities, and promoting personalized medicine approaches. Lipedema is a complex condition characterized by painful fat accumulation in the legs, and understanding the specific inflammatory pathways involved can provide insights into the underlying mechanisms of the disorder. Current treatment options often focus on symptom management rather than addressing the root cause. Understanding the specific inflammatory pathways involved in lipedema can lead to more effective treatments, potentially including pharmacological interventions that target these pathways to reduce inflammation and its effects.

Preventing progression of lipedema, a more severe form, can be achieved by developing strategies to prevent or slow this progression. Despite the multiple differential diagnosis, lipedema is frequently misdiagnosed due to its overlapping symptoms with other conditions. However, a deeper understanding of its distinct inflammatory signatures may improve diagnostic accuracy and timeliness.

Unlike typical obesity, where adipose tissue inflammation is primarily associated with visceral fat, lipedema is characterized by inflammation in the subcutaneous adipose tissue. Studies have demonstrated increased levels of pro-inflammatory cytokines, such as tumor necrosis factor-alpha (TNF-α), IL-6, and MCP-1 (Fig. 1), within the affected regions. Adipose tissue inflammation, especially in the setting of diseases such as lipedema, obesity, and metabolic syndrome, is an intricate process that involves multiple cellular and molecular pathways.

In circumstances such as obesity, adipocytes (fat cells) undergo enlargement (hypertrophy) and multiplication (hyperplasia) in response to an increase in the size and quantity of fat cells. This enlargement can result in cellular stress and malfunction. When adipocytes increase in size, the blood flow to each cell may not be

G. Laur, *Lipoedema*, https://doi.org/10.1007/978-981-96-8939-2_6

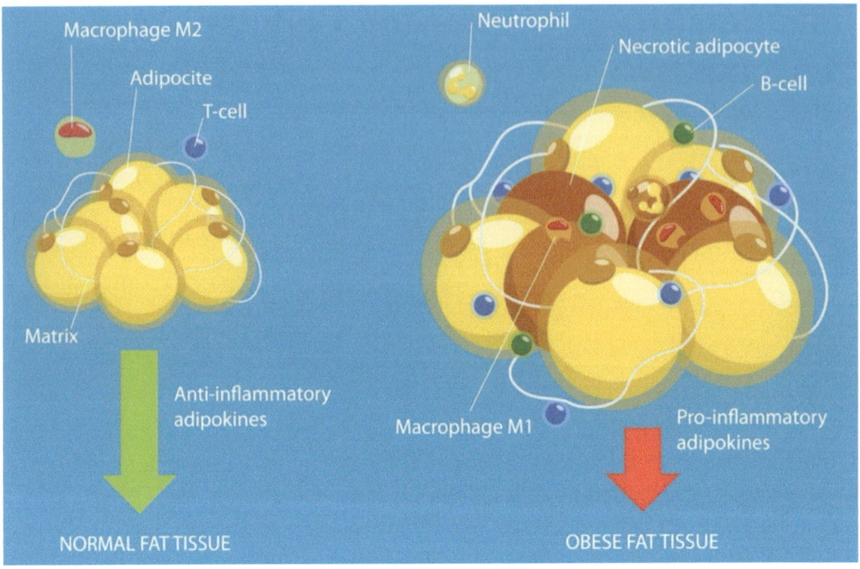

Fig. 1 Lymphocytic population difference between normal and obese fat tissue

enough, resulting in hypoxia, which is a condition characterized by a deficiency of oxygen. Hypoxia is a crucial stimulus that initiates inflammation in fat tissue. Immune cells, specifically macrophages, enter the adipose tissue as a reaction to cellular stress and lack of oxygen. At first, these cells strive to uphold the proper functioning of the tissue, but as time goes on, the continuous presence of immune cells leads to long-lasting inflammation. Adipocytes and immune cells present in the adipose tissue secrete pro-inflammatory cytokines (such as TNF-α, IL-6) and chemokines. These chemicals enhance the recruitment of more immune cells and intensify the inflammatory response. Adipocytes undergo endoplasmic reticulum (ER) stress when exposed to situations such as excessive dietary intake or hormonal abnormalities. This stress can also lead to the initiation of inflammatory processes. Oxidative stress occurs when there is an imbalance between free radicals and antioxidants in the body. This imbalance can cause damage to cells and tissues, including adipose tissue, and can also contribute to inflammation. Adipocytes that have increased in size have a tendency to release a greater amount of free fatty acids. These fatty acids have the ability to cause insulin resistance and are also recognized for their ability to trigger inflammatory pathways.

Obesity and lipedema cause structural changes in the extracellular matrix of adipose tissue. This process can result in fibrosis, a condition characterized by the thickening and scarring of connective tissue. Fibrosis, in turn, exacerbates tissue dysfunction and inflammation. Adipose tissue inflammation can be both influenced by and contribute to malfunctions in additional organ systems, such as the liver, muscles, and pancreas. This systemic interaction can worsen the inflammatory condition. Genetic predispositions may contribute to the development of lipedema in certain cases, along with hormonal influences. Disruptions in hormonal levels, namely, estrogen, can also play a role in the emergence and worsening of inflammation in adipose tissue.

At first, the inflammation may be limited to the fat tissue, but eventually, it might affect the entire body. This is especially apparent in chronic situations, where long-lasting inflammation in adipose tissue contributes to systemic metabolic disruptions, such as insulin resistance and cardiovascular illnesses.

Within the realm of lipedema, the phenomenon of adipose tissue inflammation has distinctive attributes, potentially linked to hormonal susceptibility, hereditary elements, and specific patterns of adipose tissue arrangement and enlargement. Gaining a comprehensive understanding of these mechanisms is of utmost importance in order to create precise treatments and effective management strategies for illnesses linked to inflammation of adipose tissue.

The infiltration of macrophages into adipose tissue is a hallmark of lipedema. These immune cells play a critical role in the maintenance of chronic inflammation and can adopt pro-inflammatory phenotypes, contributing to the perpetuation of adipose tissue dysfunction. Studies have provided significant insights into the role of macrophages in lipedema, particularly focusing on their impact on adipogenic differentiation and the potential for therapeutic targeting. Lipedema is marked by a unique type of macrophage infiltration, primarily consisting of immunosuppressive M2 macrophages. These M2 macrophages, identified as CD206+CD163+Clever-1+, play a crucial role in influencing the adipogenic differentiation of adipose-derived stem cells (ADSCs). Repolarization of these lipedema macrophages normalizes adipogenic differentiation, aligning it with levels seen in non-lipedema (control) groups. Macrophages can shift between pro-inflammatory M1 and anti-inflammatory M2 phenotypes, with M2 being predominant in lipedema. The study's cytometry by time-of-fligh (CyTOF) analysis and RNA sequencing reveal a pronounced M2 phenotype in lipedema macrophages, characterized by upregulation of M2 markers and downregulation of M1 inflammatory markers. The presence of M2 macrophages contributes to an immunosuppressive environment within the adipose tissue. M2 macrophages in lipedema adipose tissue inhibit the proliferation of adipocyte progenitors, impacting adipogenic differentiation. Treatment with PI3Kγ inhibitor IPI-549, which reduces CD163 expression on macrophages, showed a normalization of adipogenic differentiation in ADSCs. This suggests a potential therapeutic pathway by targeting macrophage polarization.

Studies highlight the importance of macrophage polarization in lipedema pathophysiology, distinct from other conditions like obesity where M1 macrophages predominate.

CD163+ macrophages, associated with anti-inflammatory functions, are identified as a key feature in lipedema. This is in contrast to their role in other inflammatory diseases and tumor environments, where they support inflammation and tumor growth. The Toll-like receptor (TLR) pathway (Fig. 2) may play a role in the chronic inflammation and immune dysregulation observed in affected tissues. TLRs, particularly TLR4, are part of the innate immune system and recognize pathogen-associated and damage-associated molecular patterns (PAMPs and DAMPs),

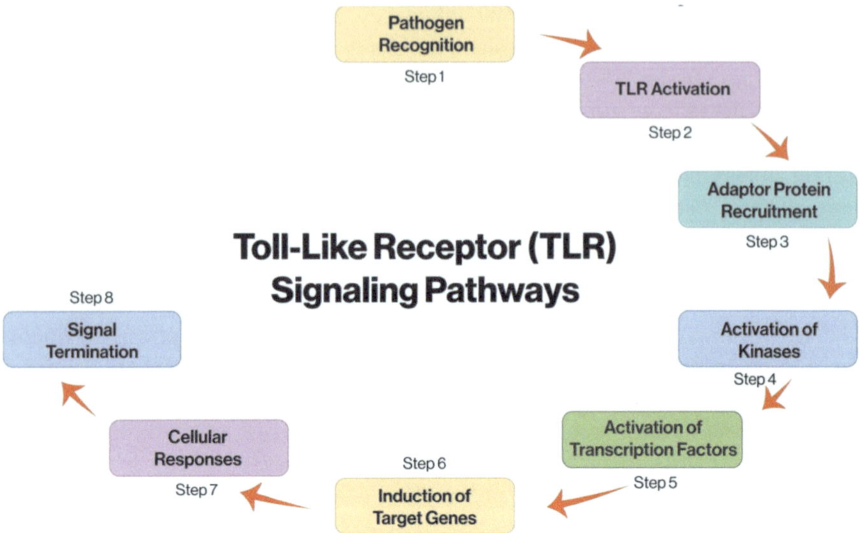

Fig. 2 Diagram of the Toll-like receptor signaling pathway

triggering inflammatory cascades. In lipedema, there is evidence of low-grade, persistent inflammation in subcutaneous adipose tissue, with increased macrophage infiltration and cytokine release. Activation of TLR pathways in adipocytes and immune cells may contribute to this inflammatory environment by promoting the release of pro-inflammatory mediators such as TNF-α and IL-6. This inflammation can drive tissue remodeling, vascular changes, and pain sensitization seen in lipedema.

Lymphatic impairment is a common feature of lipedema. Lymphatic vessels within affected areas often exhibit structural abnormalities and impaired function. This lymphatic dysfunction can lead to the accumulation of inflammatory cells and molecules in the interstitial spaces.

Early-stage patients with lipedema exhibit abnormal lymphatic anatomy, including segmented, tortuous, and/or dilated vessels, and interstitial accumulation. These abnormalities are not exclusive to lipedema and are not definitive for diagnosis. Despite these findings, no individuals with lipedema showed dermal backflow in the legs, a common feature in acquired lymphedema. Unlike lymphedema, individuals with stage 1 and 2 lipedema exhibit dilated lymphatic vessels in the lower extremities, showing greater lymphatic pumping rates compared to control individuals. Despite this, these patients do not show dermal backflow, indicating adequate functioning to prevent backflow into the dermal layers. These findings challenge the conventional understanding of lymphatic dysfunction and highlight the need for further research to understand the relationship between these structural changes and lipedema. The study also suggests a potential link between cytokine activity, capillary permeability, and lymphatic function in lipedema. Challenges in lymphatic imaging and quantifying lymphatic abnormalities highlight the complexity of diagnosing lymphatic changes in lipedema and the need for more refined metrics and techniques. The findings suggest that therapies aiding lymphatic transport could be beneficial in managing early-stage lipedema, potentially maintaining fluid homeostasis and preventing progression toward lipolymphedema.

In contrast, those with stage 1 and 2 lipedema demonstrated higher lymphatic pumping rates, possibly due to lymphatic preload from enhanced capillary permeability. Despite vessel dilation, there was no reduction in lymphatic pumping in individuals with lipedema, a surprising contrast to other conditions with acute inflammation.

Studies suggest that early-stage lipedema may initially show enhanced lymphatic pumping, but disease progression could lead to a state where the lymphatic load exceeds the pumping capacity, potentially transitioning to lipolymphedema. Treatments like complete decongestive therapy or intermittent pneumatic compression may assist lymphatic transport, potentially mitigating progression to lipolymphedema.

Inflammation plays a role in this process, contributing to chronic lymphatic insufficiency. Lymphatic abnormalities in lipedema were more prevalent in the lower extremities, possibly due to the greater demands on lymphatics in these areas to propel lymph against gravity. Diagnostic challenges include the presence of apparent dilated lymphatics, especially in the medial ankles and legs, but histological examinations revealed non-dilated lymphatic vessels, highlighting the complexity of accurately diagnosing and understanding lymphatic abnormalities in lipedema.

The relationship between lymphatic dysfunction and inflammatory processes is a complex and dynamic one that is crucial to understand in various pathological conditions, including lipedema, lymphedema, and other inflammatory diseases. Lymphatic dysfunction involves impaired lymphatic flow, reduced lymphatic uptake, dilated or tortuous lymphatic vessels, and, in some cases, dermal backflow. This dysfunction can lead to fluid accumulation (edema) and altered immune cell trafficking. Inflammation is the body's response to injury or infection, involving immune cells, blood vessels, and molecular mediators. Chronic inflammation can lead to tissue damage and is a feature of many chronic diseases. The interplay between lymphatic dysfunction and inflammation can create a vicious cycle where lymphatic dysfunction exacerbates inflammation and inflammation, in turn, further impairs lymphatic function. Breaking this cycle is a key therapeutic target in diseases like lipedema.

Inflammatory processes can alter immune cell trafficking, leading to immune cell accumulation in tissues, which can perpetuate inflammation and tissue damage. In lipedema, increased fatty tissue may exert physical pressure on lymphatic vessels, impairing their function. This, combined with potential inflammatory processes within the adipose tissue, can contribute to the development of lipolymphedema, where both adipose tissue pathology and lymphatic dysfunction are present.

Lipedema, a disorder causing painful fat accumulation, primarily affects women and often emerges during hormonal changes such as puberty, pregnancy, and menopause. Growing awareness of lipedema has led to better understanding of its progression through various classification systems. However, the underlying causes of lipedema's pathophysiology remain unclear. Given its prevalence in women during hormonal shifts, estrogen's influence is suspected to play a significant role.

This condition is marked by an unusual increase in fat, especially in the lower body, potentially linked to estrogen's impact on fat storage and metabolism. Estrogen influences the way fat is accumulated and processed in different body regions, contributing to the differences in fat distribution between men and women. For instance, pre-menopausal women typically store fat in the lower body. The interaction of estrogen receptor signaling with adipocyte estrogen production may be a crucial factor in the development of lipedema's associated adipose tissue dysfunction. The role of estrogen receptors ERα and ERβ in lipedema's abnormal fat accumulation remains debated.

We hypothesize that in lipedema, an imbalance in the ERα/ERβ ratio might lead to various metabolic changes, including altered gene expression, changes in fatty acid uptake, and reduced lipolysis. Moreover, an increase in estrogen production within lower body fat cells could further exacerbate these effects, leading to increased adipogenesis and fat accumulation.

Estrogen's role in adipose tissue regulation, particularly through estrogen receptors, is likely crucial in lipedema's pathophysiology. However, it is important to recognize that estrogen synthesis and signaling might be part of a broader set of contributing factors. While estrogen is predominantly produced in female reproductive organs, adipose tissue can also synthesize estrogen, contributing significantly to estrogen levels. The dysregulation in estrogen production and signaling within adipose tissue may play a part in lipedema's characteristic lower body fat accumulation.

Regulating gene transcription through nuclear receptors, including estrogen receptors, involves complex interactions with coregulators. These coregulators are essential for proper estrogen receptor signaling and have been linked to various diseases. Their role in lipedema's excessive fat accumulation warrants investigation. Coregulators influence estrogen receptor activity and can enhance or suppress the transcriptional activity of target genes. The involvement of estrogen receptors in adipose tissue's lipid metabolism is further complicated by their varying expression levels. For instance, ERα tends to be more prevalent than ERβ in certain adipose tissues. This variation might contribute to the differences in fat distribution and metabolism between men and women. Additionally, estrogen's influence on vascular endothelial growth factors (VEGFs) suggests a potential role in adipose tissue growth through angiogenesis. Estrogen also modulates the activity of GLUT4, a key transporter in glucose metabolism, and affects the balance of adrenergic receptors, which regulate lipolysis. The balance between α- and β-adrenergic receptors varies by adipose depot, potentially influencing fat distribution. Estrogen's regulation of these receptors could explain why patients with lipedema struggle to lose fat despite dietary changes.

Lastly, the role of peroxisome proliferator-activated receptor gamma (PPARγ) in lipid metabolism, particularly in its regulation by estrogen receptors, is another area of interest. While studies show conflicting results regarding ERα's influence on

PPARγ activity, it is clear that a regulatory relationship exists. Understanding this relationship is crucial for grasping the complexities of lipedema and devising effective treatments.

Adipocytes in lipedema undergo significant morphological and functional changes. Enlarged adipocytes, altered adipokine secretion patterns, and impaired adipose tissue expandability are observed. These alterations contribute to adipose tissue inflammation and insulin resistance. Through multifaceted analyses of whole lipedema tissue, ADSCs, and adipocytes using omics platforms, the researchers discovered deranged metabolic and lipid profiles, as well as dysregulated signaling pathways driving key biological processes such as adipogenesis, cell cycle, lipid metabolism, and cell proliferation and differentiation. The global molecular profiles in lipedema uniquely distinguish it from normal fat and define it as a distinct disease tissue.

Lipids play important roles in physiological processes such as energy homeostasis, bioenergetics, apoptosis, signal transduction, and cell recognition. Defective lipid catabolic pathways are involved in the pathogenesis of several metabolic diseases. Neutral lipids, such as triglycerides, are less likely to promote metabolic disorders compared to other lipid classes such as sphingolipids and glycerophospholipid (GPLs). Studies found that the adipocyte lipidomics profile is significantly altered in lipedema, particularly in relation to sphingolipid metabolites, suggesting that a disrupted lipid profile in adipocytes could contribute to metabolic dysfunction and pathogenesis in lipedema. The gene expression profiles defined in lipedema whole tissue and ADSCs highlighted potential molecular drivers of lipedema. Over 7820 significantly differentially expressed genes were identified in RNA sequencing (RNA-seq) data from lipedema adipose tissue and ADSCs. The top-ranking signaling pathways and gene ontology (GO)-molecular functions related to cell cycle and mitotic spindle checkpoints were identified. Bub1 was chosen for further study due to its role in proliferation in other diseases, as aberrant Bub1 expression has been shown to promote cell proliferation in several cancers.

The study also investigated the effects of Bub1 inhibition on ADSC proliferation using 2OH-BNPP1. Excitingly, either 2OH-BNPP1 treatment or CRISPR/Cas9-mediated Bub1 gene depletion can dramatically reduce lipedema ADSC proliferation. Treatment of lipedema ADSCs with 2OH-BNPP1 also profoundly inhibited histone H2A phosphorylation, further supporting a key role for Bub1 in enhanced ADSC proliferation and pathological adipogenesis in lipedema.

Lipedema is associated with increased angiogenic activity, characterized by the formation of new blood vessels. This process is thought to be driven by factors like VEGF and fibroblast growth factors (FGF)-2, potentially contributing to the maintenance of the inflammatory milieu. Angiogenesis in lipedema is a condition characterized by increased blood vessel formation and dilation. It highlights the presence of hypertrophic adipocytes in lipedema fat, which is independent of obesity and is present in both nonobese and obese patients. Increased macrophages in the skin and fat of patients with lipedema suggest an inflammatory state, while crown-like structures (CLS) are also found in lipedema fat. Angiogenesis in lipedema tissue is observed, with an increase in blood vessel numbers in dermal skin, particularly in nonobese patients with lipedema. The dilation of capillaries in nonobese lipedema indicates changes in the microvasculature. Elevated levels of vascular endothelial growth factor (VEGF) in patients with lipedema indicate active angiogenesis, which is a key regulator in the formation of new blood vessels. Lymphatic vessel changes in lipedema are more subtle than blood vasculature changes, with an expansion in lymphatic vessels, particularly in obese patients with lipedema, possibly due to increased lymph generation. Angiogenesis in lipedema may be driven by hypoxia in the tissue, potentially due to enlarged adipocyte size or microvascular dysfunction. The observed angiogenesis in lipedema fat is not consistently accompanied by lymphangiogenesis, potentially leading to lymphatic system overload and fluid accumulation. In vitro studies of angiogenic properties in lipedema adipocytes showed increased angiogenic properties in endothelial cells, with a more pronounced response in lipedema adipocytes compared to healthy adipocytes. The association of lipedema with hypermobile joints suggests a connective tissue disorder that might influence angiogenesis and capillary structure. Future research aims to further characterize the cytokines driving angiogenesis in lipedema and develop models for studying vascular remodeling in lipedema tissue.

Progressive fibrosis within lipedematous tissue is a common finding. Fibroblasts become activated, leading to increased collagen deposition and altered extracellular matrix composition. This fibrotic transformation can exacerbate tissue stiffness and hinder lymphatic function. Fibrosis in adipose tissue is a significant contributor to metabolic dysregulation associated with obesity.

This condition is characterized by the excessive accumulation of the extracellular matrix (ECM) during the unhealthy expansion of adipose tissue, often due to overnutrition. In obese adipose tissue, hypoxia activates various pro-fibrotic signaling pathways across different cell types, resulting in the overproduction of ECM components like collagens, non-collagenous proteins, and enzymes involved in ECM synthesis. This leads to local fibrosis, causing mechanical stress, cell necrosis, inflammation in the adipose tissue, and systemic effects such as lipotoxicity and insulin resistance.

Understanding the processes underlying obesity-induced fibrosis is essential for developing therapeutic strategies to mitigate the pathological changes in obese adipose tissue. Recent advances in the field, including newly identified fibrotic factors, contributing cell populations, and novel mechanisms behind fibrosis development, have been discussed. The ECM in adipose tissue consists of various proteins, including collagens and non-collagenous proteins, which are vital for adipogenesis and other functions of adipose tissue. Collagens, the primary ECM component, exhibit diverse distribution patterns in different white adipose tissue depots and are essential for maintaining tissue integrity. Non-collagenous proteins, like fibronectin and thrombospondin, also play crucial roles in the metabolic regulation of adipose tissue during obesity. Abnormal ECM remodeling and fibrosis are driven by hypoxia, which is the starting point for abnormal ECM remodeling. The interplay between various cell types, including adipocytes, endothelial cells, macrophages, and adipose-derived stem cells (ASCs), contributes to fibrosis development. Each cell type plays a distinct role in this process, secreting various collagens, non-collagenous proteins, pro-inflammatory factors, and ECM enzymes. Targeting fibrosis in adipose tissue has emerged as a promising strategy to combat obesity and related metabolic diseases. Potential therapeutic targets include HIF1α, the TGF-β pathway, and novel fibrotic factors like endotrophin. Anti-fibrotic therapies, both as standalone treatments and in combination with lifestyle changes, have been discussed.

Lipedema is a painful and often overlooked condition of adipose tissue, which is characterized by symmetrical swelling of the limbs. This swelling occurs when fat is deposited under the skin in the buttocks, thighs, legs, and arms, while the most distant parts of the limbs are spared. While the exact cause and development of lipedema are not fully understood, past studies have suggested that hormonal and genetic variables may play a role. Individuals afflicted with lipedema experience symptoms such as pain, susceptibility to bruising, soreness, and physical deformity. Lipedema is mostly characterized by pain as its predominant symptom. Given the correlation between pain, depression, and diminished quality of life, the primary therapy strategy focuses on alleviating pain. The pain experienced in lipedema is caused by allodynia, which is an increased sensitivity to pain, as well as excessive signaling from the sympathetic nervous system and the presence of estrogens. While the exact cause of discomfort in lipedema is unclear, successful treatment of lipedema should result in a significant reduction in pain. The effectiveness of conservative treatment is a subject of contention. Microcannular tumescent liposuction is the optimal therapy choice for treating lipedema. There exists a substantial amount of evidence indicating that this technique effectively lowers pain in patients suffering from lipedema.

Patients with lipedema often experience allodynic and neuropathic pain in the afflicted tissues, which is distinct from symptoms associated with obesity or lymphedema [4]. The clinical therapy of lipedema must prioritize the treatment of pain, as more than 90% of patients experience some form of tissue discomfort.

Pain in the lower extremities is a common symptom of lipedema, and the areas affected by the condition tend to expand as the lipedema progresses. The etiology of lipedema discomfort is still unclear, although research is being conducted to examine the disease pathology in affected regions, such as the thighs and abdomen For instance, a study found a correlation between imaging markers and lower-extremity tissue sodium levels in patients with lipedema, which, in turn, was associated with lower-extremity discomfort. The presence of intense pain suggests that neurogenic inflammation—mediated by sensory neurons—may play a significant role in modulating pain in lipedema, potentially through interactions with both the sympathetic and parasympathetic nervous systems. The evaluation of these pathways has not been conducted with strict rigor, and there is still limited comprehension of the pain correlates linked with lipedema. A precise assessment of the severity of lipedema and the identification of factors contributing to lipedema-associated discomfort could provide valuable insights into the mechanisms underlying the development of lipedema.

Lipedema, distinct from general obesity and lower limb lymphedema, remains a condition with largely unknown causes. A key differentiator of lipedema is the intense pain experienced by affected women, distinct from other similar conditions. Our research indicates that patients with lipedema consistently report nociceptive pain, which is objectively confirmed through mechanical allodynia responses. Notably, lipedema dermal tissue shows significant differences in neuronal cell body distribution and neuropeptide levels, which may contribute to neuronal sensitization. Clinically, lipedema is identified in three stages based on physical symptoms and fat distribution. However, the prevalent symptom of pain is not yet factored into these stages. Variations in pain incidence and the subjective nature of existing survey methods have hindered comprehensive pain assessment in lipedema. Presently, tools like the SF-36, encompassing pain and vitality assessments, are used to differentiate lipedema from other conditions. Our study sought to objectively measure pain, including dermal sensitivity, in patients with lipedema. The results, corroborating patients' reports, indicated a significant response to temperature and pressure-induced pain. Surprisingly, we found the strongest mechanical sensitization in the calves and arms, despite more considerable fat expansion in the thighs. The root cause of lipedema's pain aspect is not fully understood. While general adipose tissue inflammation has been suggested, other factors like abnormal adipogenesis and increased VEGF-C may also play roles. Our study revealed altered expression of calcitonin gene-related peptide (CGRP) and nerve growth factor (NGF) neuropeptides in lipedema skin, which are known to be involved in nociceptive pain pathways. Additionally, we observed a decrease in neuron body density in the abdominal skin of patients with lipedema, akin to findings in diabetic peripheral neuropathy.

Neurogenic inflammation, driven by neuropeptides like NGF, can result in chronic nerve sensitization, contributing to neurogenic inflammation. Our findings suggest that changes in CGRP or NGF expression in lipedema skin might stem from underlying tissue inflammation. The sequence of these changes, relative to vascular, immunological, and inflammatory markers in lipedema, needs further investigation.

Understanding the inflammatory processes and cellular mechanisms underlying lipedema provides critical insights into its pathogenesis. Targeting these processes in a multidisciplinary approach offers hope for improved management and quality of life for individuals living with this condition. Continued research in this field is essential for the development of innovative and effective therapeutic strategies for lipedema.

Suggested Reading

Okhovat JP, Alavi A. Lipedema: A review of the literature. *Int J Low Extrem Wounds.* (2015) 14(3):262–7. https://doi.org/10.1177/1534734614554284.

Priglinger E, Wurzer C, Steffenhagen C, Maier J, Hofer V, Peterbauer A, et al. The adipose tissue-derived stromal vascular fraction cells from lipedema patients: Are they different? *Cytotherapy* (2017) 19(7):849–60. https://doi.org/10.1016/j.jcyt.2017.03.073.

Al-Ghadban S, Diaz ZT, Singer HJ, Mert KB, Bunnell BA. Increase in leptin and PPAR-gamma gene expression in lipedema adipocytes differentiated in vitro from adipose-derived stem cells. *Cells* (2020) 9(2). https://doi.org/10.3390/cells9020430.

Ishaq M, Bandara N, Morgan S, Nowell C, Mehdi AM, Lyu R, et al. Key signaling networks are dysregulated in patients with the adipose tissue disorder, lipedema. *Int J Obes (Lond).* (2022) 46(3):502–14. https://doi.org/10.1038/s41366-021-01002-1.

Felmerer G, Stylianaki A, Hollmen M, Strobel P, Stepniewski A, Wang A, et al. Increased levels of VEGF-c and macrophage infiltration in lipedema patients without changes in lymphatic vascular morphology. *Sci Rep* (2020) 10(1):10947. https://doi.org/10.1038/s41598-020-67987-3.

Aron-Wisnewsky J, Tordjman J, Poitou C, Darakhshan F, Hugol D, Basdevant A, et al. Human adipose tissue macrophages: m1 and m2 cell surface markers in subcutaneous and omental depots and after weight loss. *J Clin Endocrinol Metab* (2009) 94(11):4619–23. https://doi.org/10.1210/jc.2009-0925.

Yuan Y, Arcucci V, Levy SM, Achen MG. Modulation of immunity by lymphatic dysfunction in lymphedema. *Front Immunol* (2019) 10:76. https://doi.org/10.3389/fimmu.2019.00076.

Avraham T, Zampell JC, Yan A, Elhadad S, Weitman ES, Rockson SG, et al. Th2 differentiation is necessary for soft tissue fibrosis and lymphatic dysfunction resulting from lymphedema. *FASEB J* (2013) 27(3):1114–26. https://doi.org/10.1096/fj.12-222695.

Wolf S, Deuel JW, Hollmen M, Felmerer G, Kim BS, Vasella M, et al. A distinct cytokine profile and stromal vascular fraction metabolic status without significant changes in the lipid composition characterizes lipedema. *Int J Mol Sci* (2021) 22(7). doi: https://doi.org/10.3390/ijms22073313.

Ellis B HP, Hahne F, Le Meur N, Gopalakrishnan N, Spidlen J, Jiang M, et al. flowCore: flowCore: Basic structures for flow cytometry data. (2020).

Van Gassen S, Callebaut B, Van Helden MJ, Lambrecht BN, Demeester P, Dhaene T, et al. FlowSOM: Using self-organizing maps for visualization and interpretation of cytometry data. *Cytometry A.* (2015) 87(7):636–45. https://doi.org/10.1002/cyto.a.22625.

James M. Uwot: The uniform manifold approximation and projection (UMAP) method for dimensionality reduction. (2018).

Gu Z, Eils R, Schlesner M. Complex heatmaps reveal patterns and correlations in multidimensional genomic data. *Bioinformatics* (2016) 32(18):2847–9. https://doi.org/10.1093/bioinformatics/btw313.

Chen S, Zhou Y, Chen Y, Gu J. Fastp: an ultra-fast all-in-one FASTQ preprocessor. *Bioinformatics* (2018) 34(17):i884–i90. https://doi.org/10.1093/bioinformatics/bty560.

Bray NL, Pimentel H, Melsted P, Pachter L. Near-optimal probabilistic RNA-seq quantification. *Nat Biotechnol* (2016) 34(5):525–7. https://doi.org/10.1038/nbt.3519.

Love MI, Huber W, Anders S. Moderated estimation of fold change and dispersion for RNA-seq data with DESeq2. *Genome Biol* (2014) 15(12):550. https://doi.org/10.1186/s13059-014-0550-8.

Dominici M, Le Blanc K, Mueller I, Slaper-Cortenbach I, Marini F, Krause D, et al. Minimal criteria for defining multipotent mesenchymal stromal cells. The international society for cellular therapy position statement. *Cytotherapy* (2006) 8(4):315–7. https://doi.org/10.1080/14653240600855905.

Eggerschwiler B, Canepa DD, Pape HC, Casanova EA, Cinelli P. Automated digital image quantification of histological staining for the analysis of the trilineage differentiation potential of mesenchymal stem cells. *Stem Cell Res Ther* (2019) 10(1):69. https://doi.org/10.1186/s13287-019-1170-8.

Barczyk K, Ehrchen J, Tenbrock K, Ahlmann M, Kneidl J, Viemann D, et al. Glucocorticoids promote survival of anti-inflammatory macrophages via stimulation of adenosine receptor A3. *Blood* (2010) 116(3):446–55. https://doi.org/10.1182/blood-2009-10-247106.

Huang SC, Smith AM, Everts B, Colonna M, Pearce EL, Schilling JD, et al. Metabolic reprogramming mediated by the mTORC2-IRF4 signaling axis is essential for macrophage alternative activation. *Immunity* (2016) 45(4):817–30. https://doi.org/10.1016/j.immuni.2016.09.016.

Park-Min KH, Antoniv TT, Ivashkiv LB. Regulation of macrophage phenotype by long-term exposure to IL-10. *Immunobiology* (2005) 210(2–4):77–86. https://doi.org/10.1016/j.imbio.2005.05.002.

Snodgrass RG, Brune B. Regulation and functions of 15-lipoxygenases in human macrophages. *Front Pharmacol* (2019) 10:719. https://doi.org/10.3389/fphar.2019.00719.

Koning N, van Eijk M, Pouwels W, Brouwer MS, Voehringer D, Huitinga I, et al. Expression of the inhibitory CD200 receptor is associated with alternative macrophage activation. *J Innate Immun* (2010) 2(2):195–200. https://doi.org/10.1159/000252803.

Li W, Wang Y, Zhu L, Du S, Mao J, Wang Y, et al. The P300/XBP1s/Herpud1 axis promotes macrophage M2 polarization and the development of choroidal neovascularization. *J Cell Mol Med* (2021) 25(14):6709–20. https://doi.org/10.1111/jcmm.16673.

Moeller JB, Nielsen MJ, Reichhardt MP, Schlosser A, Sorensen GL, Nielsen O, et al. CD163-L1 is an endocytic macrophage protein strongly regulated by mediators in the inflammatory response. *J Immunol* (2012) 188(5):2399–409. https://doi.org/10.4049/jimmunol.1103150.

van Tits LJ, Stienstra R, van Lent PL, Netea MG, Joosten LA, Stalenhoef AF. Oxidized LDL enhances pro-inflammatory responses of alternatively activated M2 macrophages: a crucial role for kruppel-like factor 2. *Atherosclerosis* (2011) 214(2):345–9. https://doi.org/10.1016/j.atherosclerosis.2010.11.018.

Zajac E, Schweighofer B, Kupriyanova TA, Juncker-Jensen A, Minder P, Quigley JP, et al. Angiogenic capacity of M1- and M2-polarized macrophages is determined by the levels of TIMP-1 complexed with their secreted proMMP-9. *Blood* (2013) 122(25):4054–67. https://doi.org/10.1182/blood-2013-05-501494.

Murray PJ. Macrophage polarization. *Annu Rev Physiol* (2017) 79:541–66. https://doi.org/10.1146/annurev-physiol-022516-034339.

Sun Y, Zhao J, Sun X, Ma G. Identification of TNFAIP8 as an immune-related biomarker associated with tumorigenesis and prognosis in cutaneous melanoma patients. *Front Genet* (2021) 12:783672. https://doi.org/10.3389/fgene.2021.783672.

Griffin C, Eter L, Lanzetta N, Abrishami S, Varghese M, McKernan K, et al. TLR4, TRIF, and MyD88 are essential for myelopoiesis and CD11c(+) adipose tissue macrophage production in obese mice. *J Biol Chem* (2018) 293(23):8775–86. https://doi.org/10.1074/jbc.RA117.001526.

Chistiakov DA, Myasoedova VA, Revin VV, Orekhov AN, Bobryshev YV. The impact of interferon-regulatory factors to macrophage differentiation and polarization into M1 and M2. *Immunobiology* (2018) 223(1):101–11. https://doi.org/10.1016/j.imbio.2017.10.005.

Kaneda MM, Messer KS, Ralainirina N, Li H, Leem CJ, Gorjestani S, et al. PI3Kgamma is a molecular switch that controls immune suppression. *Nature* (2016) 539(7629):437–42. https://doi.org/10.1038/nature19834.

Ribatti D. Bone marrow vascular niche and the control of tumor growth in hematological malignancies. *Leukemia* (2010) 24(7):1247–8. https://doi.org/10.1038/leu.2010.103.

Moestrup SK, Moller HJ. CD163: a regulated hemoglobin scavenger receptor with a role in the anti-inflammatory response. *Ann Med* (2004) 36(5):347–54. https://doi.org/10.1080/07853890410033171.

Goswami S, Anandhan S, Raychaudhuri D, Sharma P. Myeloid cell-targeted therapies for solid tumours. *Nat Rev Immunol* (2022). https://doi.org/10.1038/s41577-022-00737-w.

Miyazaki T, Ishikawa E, Matsuda M, Sugii N, Kohzuki H, Akutsu H, et al. Infiltration of CD163-positive macrophages in glioma tissues after treatment with anti-PD-L1 antibody and role of PI3Kgamma inhibitor as a combination therapy with anti-PD-L1 antibody in in vivo model using temozolomide-resistant murine glioma-initiating cells. *Brain Tumor Pathol* (2020) 37(2):41–9. https://doi.org/10.1007/s10014-020-00357-z.

Keuper M, Sachs S, Walheim E, Berti L, Raedle B, Tews D, et al. Activated macrophages control human adipocyte mitochondrial bioenergetics via secreted factors. *Mol Metab* (2017) 6(10):1226–39. https://doi.org/10.1016/j.molmet.2017.07.008.

Cinkajzlova A, Mraz M, Haluzik M. Lymphocytes and macrophages in adipose tissue in obesity: markers or makers of subclinical inflammation? *Protoplasma* (2017) 254(3):1219–32. https://doi.org/10.1007/s00709-017-1082-3.

Russo L, Lumeng CN. Properties and functions of adipose tissue macrophages in obesity. *Immunology* (2018) 155(4):407–17. https://doi.org/10.1111/imm.13002.

Kovacikova M, Sengenes C, Kovacova Z, Siklova-Vitkova M, Klimcakova E, Polak J, et al. Dietary intervention-induced weight loss decreases macrophage content in adipose tissue of obese women. *Int J Obes (Lond).* (2011) 35(1):91–8. https://doi.org/10.1038/ijo.2010.112.

Suga H, Araki J, Aoi N, Kato H, Higashino T, Yoshimura K. Adipose tissue remodeling in lipedema: adipocyte death and concurrent regeneration. *J Cutan Pathol* (2009) 36(12):1293–8. https://doi.org/10.1111/j.1600-0560.2009.01256.x.

Al-Ghadban S, Cromer W, Allen M, Ussery C, Badowski M, Harris D, et al. Dilated blood and lymphatic microvessels, angiogenesis, increased macrophages, and adipocyte hypertrophy in lipedema thigh skin and fat tissue. *J Obes* (2019) 2019:8747461. https://doi.org/10.1155/2019/8747461.

Felmerer G, Stylianaki A, Hagerling R, Wang A, Strobel P, Hollmen M, et al. Adipose tissue hypertrophy, an aberrant biochemical profile and distinct gene expression in lipedema. *J Surg Res* (2020) 253:294–303. https://doi.org/10.1016/j.jss.2020.03.055.

Mauer J, Chaurasia B, Goldau J, Vogt MC, Ruud J, Nguyen KD, et al. Signaling by IL-6 promotes alternative activation of macrophages to limit endotoxemia and obesity-associated resistance to insulin. *Nat Immunol* (2014) 15(5):423–30. https://doi.org/10.1038/ni.2865.

Kristiansen M, Graversen JH, Jacobsen C, Sonne O, Hoffman HJ, Law SK, et al. Identification of the haemoglobin scavenger receptor. *Nature* (2001) 409(6817):198–201. https://doi.org/10.1038/35051594.

Etzerodt A, Moestrup SK. CD163 and inflammation: biological, diagnostic, and therapeutic aspects. *Antioxid Redox Signal* (2013) 18(17):2352–63. https://doi.org/10.1089/ars.2012.4834.

Skytthe MK, Graversen JH, Moestrup SK. Targeting of CD163(+) macrophages in inflammatory and malignant diseases. *Int J Mol Sci* (2020) 21(15). https://doi.org/10.3390/ijms21155497.

Jung KY, Cho SW, Kim YA, Kim D, Oh BC, Park DJ, et al. Cancers with higher density of tumor-associated macrophages were associated with poor survival rates. *J Pathol Transl Med* (2015) 49(4):318–24. https://doi.org/10.4132/jptm.2015.06.01.

Nawaz A, Aminuddin A, Kado T, Takikawa A, Yamamoto S, Tsuneyama K, et al. CD206(+) M2-like macrophages regulate systemic glucose metabolism by inhibiting proliferation of adipocyte progenitors. *Nat Commun* (2017) 8(1):286. https://doi.org/10.1038/s41467-017-00231-1.

Ma H, Li YN, Song L, Liu R, Li X, Shang Q, et al. Macrophages inhibit adipogenic differentiation of adipose tissue derived mesenchymal stem/stromal cells by producing pro-inflammatory cytokines. *Cell Biosci* (2020) 10:88. https://doi.org/10.1186/s13578-020-00450-y.

Yi Y, Hu W, Lv W, Zhao C, Xiong M, Wu M, et al. FTY720 improves the survival of autologous fat grafting by modulating macrophages toward M2 polarization Via STAT3 pathway. *Cell Transplant.* (2021) 30:9636897211052975. https://doi.org/10.1177/09636897211052975.

Keuper M, Jastroch M, Yi CX, Fischer-Posovszky P, Wabitsch M, Tschop MH, et al. Spare mitochondrial respiratory capacity permits human adipocytes to maintain ATP homeostasis under hypoglycemic conditions. *FASEB J* (2014) 28(2):761–70. https://doi.org/10.1096/fj.13-238725.

Evans CA, Liu T, Lescarbeau A, Nair SJ, Grenier L, Pradeilles JA, et al. Discovery of a selective phosphoinositide-3-Kinase (PI3K)-gamma inhibitor (IPI-549) as an immuno-oncology clinical candidate. *ACS Med Chem Lett* (2016) 7(9):862–7. https://doi.org/10.1021/acsmedchemlett.6b00238.

Pemberton N, Mogemark M, Arlbrandt S, Bold P, Cox RJ, Gardelli C, et al. Discovery of highly isoform selective orally bioavailable phosphoinositide 3-kinase (PI3K)-gamma inhibitors. *J Med Chem* (2018) 61(12):5435–41. https://doi.org/10.1021/acs.jmedchem.8b00447.

Moller HJ. Soluble CD163. *Scand J Clin Lab Invest.* (2012) 72(1):1–13. https://doi.org/10.3109/00365513.2011.626868.

Mejia-Vilet JM, Zhang XL, Cruz C, Cano-Verduzco ML, Shapiro JP, Nagaraja HN, et al. Urinary soluble CD163: a novel noninvasive biomarker of activity for lupus nephritis. *J Am Soc Nephrol.* (2020) 31(6):1335–47. https://doi.org/10.1681/ASN.2019121285.

Stilund M, Reuschlein AK, Christensen T, Moller HJ, Rasmussen PV, Petersen T. Soluble CD163 as a marker of macrophage activity in newly diagnosed patients with multiple sclerosis. *PloS One* (2014) 9(6):e98588. https://doi.org/10.1371/journal.pone.0098588.

Abu El-Asrar AM, Ahmad A, Allegaert E, Siddiquei MM, Gikandi PW, De Hertogh G, et al. Interleukin-11 overexpression and M2 macrophage density are associated with angiogenic activity in proliferative diabetic retinopathy. *Ocul Immunol Inflamm* (2020) 28(4):575–88. https://doi.org/10.1080/09273948.2019.1616772.

Al-Ghadban S., Cromer W., Allen M., Ussery C., Badowski M., Harris D., Herbst K.L. Dilated Blood and Lymphatic Microvessels, Angiogenesis, Increased Macrophages, and Adipocyte Hypertrophy in Lipedema Thigh Skin and Fat Tissue. *J. Obes.* 2019;2019:8747461. https://doi.org/10.1155/2019/8747461.

Felmerer G., Stylianaki A., Hägerling R., Wang A., Ströbel P., Hollmén M., Lindenblatt N., Gousopoulos E. Adipose Tissue Hypertrophy, An Aberrant Biochemical Profile and Distinct Gene Expression in Lipedema. *J. Surg. Res.* 2020;253:294–303. https://doi.org/10.1016/j.jss.2020.03.055.

Suga H., Araki J., Aoi N., Kato H., Higashino T., Yoshimura K. Adipose tissue remodeling in lipedema: Adipocyte death and concurrent regeneration. *J. Cutan. Pathol.* 2009;36:1293–1298. https://doi.org/10.1111/j.1600-0560.2009.01256.x.

Herbst K.L., Kahn L.A., Iker E., Ehrlich C., Wright T., McHutchison L., Schwartz J., Sleigh M., MC Donahue P., Lisson K.H., et al. Standard of care for lipedema in the United States. *Phlebology.* 2021;36:779–796. https://doi.org/10.1177/02683555211015887.

Allen M., Schwartz M., Herbst K.L. Interstitial Fluid in Lipedema and Control Skin. *Womens Health Rep.* 2020;1:480–487. https://doi.org/10.1089/whr.2020.0086.

Crescenzi R., Marton A., Donahue P.M., Mahany H.B., Lants S.K., Wang P., Beckman J.A., Donahue M.J., Titze J. Tissue Sodium Content is Elevated in the Skin and Subcutaneous Adipose Tissue in Women with Lipedema. *Obesity.* 2018;26:310–317. https://doi.org/10.1002/oby.22090.

Rautiainen S., Laaksonen T., Koivuniemi R. Angiogenic Effects and Crosstalk of Adipose-Derived Mesenchymal Stem/Stromal Cells and Their Extracellular Vesicles with Endothelial Cells. *Int. J. Mol. Sci.* 2021;22:10890. https://doi.org/10.3390/ijms221910890.

Cao Y. Angiogenesis and vascular functions in modulation of obesity, adipose metabolism, and insulin sensitivity. *Cell Metab.* 2013;18:478–489. https://doi.org/10.1016/j.cmet.2013.08.008.

Herold J., Kalucka J. Angiogenesis in Adipose Tissue: The Interplay Between Adipose and Endothelial Cells. *Front. Physiol.* 2020;11:624903. https://doi.org/10.3389/fphys.2020.624903.

Starke R.D., Ferraro F., Paschalaki K.E., Dryden N.H., McKinnon T.A.J., Sutton R.E., Payne E.M., Haskard D.O., Hughes A.D., Cutler D.F., et al. Endothelial von Willebrand factor regulates angiogenesis. *Blood.* 2011;117:1071–1080. https://doi.org/10.1182/blood-2010-01-264507.

Ozel I., Duerig I., Domnich M., Lang S., Pylaeva E., Jablonska J. The Good, the Bad, and the Ugly: Neutrophils, Angiogenesis, and Cancer. *Cancers.* 2022;14:536. https://doi.org/10.3390/cancers14030536.

Crewe C., An Y.A., Scherer P.E. The ominous triad of adipose tissue dysfunction: Inflammation, fibrosis, and impaired angiogenesis. *J. Clin. Investig.* 2017;127:74–82. https://doi.org/10.1172/JCI88883.

Liao J.K. Linking endothelial dysfunction with endothelial cell activation. *J. Clin. Investig.* 2013;123:540–541. https://doi.org/10.1172/JCI66843.

Lip G.Y., Blann A. von Willebrand factor: A marker of endothelial dysfunction in vascular disorders? *Cardiovasc. Res.* 1997;34:255–265. https://doi.org/10.1016/S0008-6363(97)00039-4.

Randi A.M., Laffan M.A. Von Willebrand factor and angiogenesis: Basic and applied issues. *J. Thromb. Haemost.* 2017;15:13–20. https://doi.org/10.1111/jth.13551.

Ruiz-Ojeda F.J., Méndez-Gutiérrez A., Aguilera C.M., Plaza-Díaz J. Extracellular Matrix Remodeling of Adipose Tissue in Obesity and Metabolic Diseases. *Int. J. Mol. Sci.* 2019;20:4888. https://doi.org/10.3390/ijms20194888.

Zhang C. The role of inflammatory cytokines in endothelial dysfunction. *Basic Res. Cardiol.* 2008;103:398–406. https://doi.org/10.1007/s00395-008-0733-0.

Kwaifa I.K., Bahari H., Yong Y.K., Noor S.M. Endothelial Dysfunction in Obesity-Induced Inflammation: Molecular Mechanisms and Clinical Implications. *Biomolecules.* 2020;10:291. https://doi.org/10.3390/biom10020291.

Theofilis P., Sagris M., Oikonomou E., Antonopoulos A.S., Siasos G., Tsioufis C., Tousoulis D. Inflammatory Mechanisms Contributing to Endothelial Dysfunction. *Biomedicines.* 2021;9:781. https://doi.org/10.3390/biomedicines9070781.

Szmitko P.E., Wang C.H., Weisel R.D., de Almeida J.R., Anderson T.J., Verma S. New markers of inflammation and endothelial cell activation: Part I. *Circulation.* 2003;108:1917–1923. https://doi.org/10.1161/01.CIR.0000089190.95415.9F.

Al-Mansoori L., Al-Jaber H., Prince M.S., Elrayess M.A. Role of Inflammatory Cytokines, Growth Factors and Adipokines in Adipogenesis and Insulin Resistance. *Inflammation.* 2022;45:31–44. https://doi.org/10.1007/s10753-021-01559-z.

Gensior M.H.L., Cornely M. Pain in lipoedema, fat in lipoedema and its consequences: Results of a patient survey based on a pain questionnaire. *Handchir. Mikrochir. Plast. Chir.* 2019;51:249–254.

Aksoy H., Karadag A.S., Wollina U. Cause and management of lipedema-associated pain. *Dermatol. Ther.* 2020;34:e14364. https://doi.org/10.1111/dth.14364.

Malik R.A. Pathology of human diabetic neuropathy. *Handb. Clin. Neurol.* 2014;126:249–259.

Shillo P., Yiangou Y., Donatien P., Greig M., Selvarajah D., Wilkinson I.D., Anand P., Tesfaye S. Nerve and Vascular Biomarkers in Skin Biopsies Differentiate Painful From Painless Peripheral Neuropathy in Type 2 Diabetes. *Front. Pain Res.* 2021;2:731658. https://doi.org/10.3389/fpain.2021.731658.

Siems W., Grune T., Voss P., Brenke R. Anti-fibrosclerotic effects of shock wave therapy in lipedema and cellulite. *BioFactors.* 2005;24:275–282. https://doi.org/10.1002/biof.5520240132.

Amann-Vesti B.R., Franzeck U.K., Bollinger A. Microlymphatic aneurysms in patients with lipedema. *Lymphology.* 2001;34:170–175.

Zechner U., Kohlschmidt N., Kempf O., Gebauer K., Haug K., Engels H., Haaf T., Bartsch O. Familial Sotos syndrome caused by a novel missense mutation, C2175S, in NSD1 and associated with normal intelligence, insulin dependent diabetes, bronchial asthma, and lipedema. *Eur. J. Med. Genet.* 2009;52:306–310. https://doi.org/10.1016/j.ejmg.2009.06.001.

Angst F., Benz T., Lehmann S., Sandor P., Wagner S. Common and Contrasting Characteristics of the Chronic Soft-Tissue Pain Conditions Fibromyalgia and Lipedema. *J. Pain Res.* 2021;14:2931–2941. https://doi.org/10.2147/JPR.S315736.

Genetic of Lipedema

Lipedema is a complex condition with a multifactorial etiology, and its genetic basis is not yet fully understood. However, there is evidence to suggest that genetic factors may play a role in its development.

Several studies have investigated the genetics of lipedema and identified potential genetic associations. For example, a study published in 2016 found that variations in the FOXC2 gene, which is involved in the regulation of lymphatic vessel development, were associated with an increased risk of lipedema. Another study published in 2019 identified a genetic variant in the LAMA5 gene, which is involved in the development of adipose tissue and extracellular matrix, that was associated with an increased risk of lipedema. Additionally, several other genes have been implicated in the development of adipose tissue dysfunction and metabolic disorders, which are known risk factors for lipedema. These include genes involved in adipogenesis, lipid metabolism, and insulin signaling.

While genetic factors may contribute to the development of lipedema, it is important to note that the condition is also influenced by environmental and lifestyle factors. Obesity, hormonal imbalances, and trauma to the affected areas are all known risk factors for lipedema, and these factors can interact with genetic predispositions to increase the risk of developing the condition. The historical perspective of genetic studies in lipedema reveals a progressively evolving understanding of the condition's hereditary nature and its underlying genetic mechanisms. Initially, lipedema was primarily characterized by its clinical manifestations, with little attention paid to the potential genetic factors contributing to its development. Early observations noted the familial occurrence of lipedema, suggesting a hereditary component, but these observations lacked the molecular insights to elucidate specific genetic underpinnings.

As the field of genetics advanced, particularly with the advent of molecular biology techniques in the late twentieth century, researchers began to explore the genetic aspects of lipedema with greater specificity. Initial studies focused on mapping the inheritance patterns within affected families, which provided preliminary evidence supporting the idea that lipedema could be transmitted in a genetic manner, possibly

G. Laur, *Lipoedema*, https://doi.org/10.1007/978-981-96-8939-2_7

through an autosomal-dominant mode with variable penetrance. However, these studies were limited by the technology available at the time and often resulted in inconclusive findings.

The turn of the century marked a significant advancement in genetic research technologies, including the completion of the Human Genome Project and the development of high-throughput sequencing technologies. These breakthroughs enabled more detailed and comprehensive genetic analyses, leading to the identification of potential genetic markers associated with lipedema. Studies began to investigate specific genes related to adipose tissue regulation, lymphatic development, and inflammatory processes, although definitive genetic markers or mutations have yet to be universally recognized.

The current era of genetic research in lipedema is characterized by a focus on genome-wide association studies (GWAS) and whole-exome sequencing to uncover the complex genetic landscape of the condition. These studies aim not only to identify specific genes that may confer susceptibility to lipedema but also to understand the interaction between genetic predisposition and environmental or hormonal factors in the disease's pathogenesis.

The molecular pathways implicated in lipedema highlight the complex pathophysiological underpinnings of this condition, involving an intricate interplay of adipogenesis, lymphangiogenesis, inflammation, and fibrosis. At the core of lipedema's molecular landscape is the dysregulation of adipocyte proliferation and differentiation, mediated by signaling pathways such as the peroxisome proliferator-activated receptor (PPAR) pathway, which plays a crucial role in lipid metabolism and adipocyte life cycle. Abnormal activation or suppression of this pathway could contribute to the excessive and pathological fat accumulation observed in lipedema. Additionally, the disruption of lymphangiogenic signaling, particularly through the vascular endothelial growth factor (VEGF) pathways, including VEGF-C and its receptor VEGFR-3, underscores the compromised lymphatic architecture and function characteristic of lipedema, leading to impaired lymph drainage and subsequent tissue swelling.

Inflammatory processes are also central to lipedema's molecular pathology, with elevated levels of pro-inflammatory cytokines such as tumor necrosis factor-alpha (TNF-α), interleukin-6 (IL-6), and interleukin-1 beta (IL-1β), contributing to a chronic inflammatory state. This inflammation can further exacerbate adipose tissue fibrosis and lymphatic dysfunction, creating a feedback loop that perpetuates the disease process. Furthermore, the involvement of fibrotic pathways, mediated by transforming growth factor-beta (TGF-β) signaling, contributes to the excessive deposition of extracellular matrix components, leading to the hardening of adipose tissues and additional barriers to effective lymphatic drainage.

The evidence indicates that lipedema, a condition characterized by abnormal fat accumulation primarily in the legs, has a genetic basis, suggesting it can be inherited. However, determining the precise pattern of inheritance remains challenging.

In a study involving patients with lipedema, 73% reported having a family member with the condition, most commonly affecting mothers, grandmothers, aunts, sisters, and cousins, in descending order of frequency.

Research conducted in 2010 on six families, spanning more than three generations, identified an autosomal-dominant pattern of inheritance for lipedema. This pattern, along with studies showing a mother-to-daughter transmission, supports the theory that lipedema is genetically inherited, potentially involving the X-chromosome given its prevalence in families with female members.

The condition's onset around puberty and its predominance in females suggest hormones, especially estrogen, play a significant role in its development. Although the genetic basis of lipedema involves genes related to syndromic fat accumulation (like POU1F1A, NSD1, ELN, FZD9, MLXIPL, and ALDH18A1), the role of the AKR1C1 gene has been recently highlighted, opening new paths for understanding isolated lipedema.

Liposuction, a primary surgical option, suggests that understanding the genetic roots of lipedema could predict treatment outcomes. However, there is a lack of guidelines for molecular diagnosis, though genetic testing could exclude similar conditions. Advances in next-generation sequencing (NGS) technology enhance diagnostic and management capabilities by analyzing multiple genes simultaneously.

Specific gene variants, such as in PLIN1, LIPE, and PPARG, have been identified, which usually cause other fat distribution syndromes, raising questions about lipedema's diagnosis and its overlap with conditions like familial partial lipodystrophy.

This research underscores lipedema's genetic determination, possibly through X-linked dominant, autosomal dominant with sex limitation, or oligogenic inheritance. Most genes carrying deleterious variants are involved in steroidogenesis, lipid homeostasis, and the insulin signaling pathway, suggesting a complex interaction between these biological pathways and lipedema's manifestation.

Furthermore, the study explores genes associated with conditions that could model the molecular pathways involved in non-syndromic lipedema, such as mutations that cause distinct syndromes with features overlapping with lipedema.

Lipedema can be classified into three categories: non-syndromic, syndromic, and/or comorbid. The specific gene linked to primary isolated lipedema remains unidentified; nonetheless, it is plausible that it exists within a syndromic framework.

Lipedema can manifest in several forms, such as a germline missense variant in POU1F1A, a pathogenic mutual translocation occurring in the 10q25.2 and 15q11.2 bands, and Sotos syndrome 1, which arises from germline mutations in NSD1. These mutations could contribute to the formation of lipedema tissue mediated by estrogen. The presence of lipedema in certain cases of Williams-Beuren syndrome, a complex neurodevelopmental and metabolic condition, can be attributed to the deletion of a specific sequence of 27 genes located in the chromosomal region 7q11.2333.

Pseudoxanthoma elasticum (PXE) is a syndrome characterized by the presence of lipedema, which can impact many bodily systems such as the skin, eyes, cardiovascular system, and gastrointestinal system. Skin lesions of patients with lipedema have been shown to have abnormal elastic fibers that resemble those found in PXE. PXE fibroblasts have an elevated rate of cholesterol production, perhaps playing a significant role in the pathogenesis of lipedema-associated adipose tissue.

Cutis laxa type III is a complex connective tissue disorder that manifests as creased and rigid skin, accompanied with retinopathy and atypical adipose tissue accumulation in the gluteal region and upper thigh areas. Cutis laxa type III can have either an autosomal recessive or dominant inheritance pattern. It is caused by mutations in the ALDH18A139 gene, which encodes an enzyme responsible for reducing glutamate to delta1-pyrroline-5-carboxylate. This reduction process is crucial for the synthesis of proline, ornithine, and arginine.

In summary, lipedema is a hereditary condition that can be impacted by a range of factors, encompassing genetic predisposition, hormonal influences, and the presence of comorbidities. The comprehension of these hereditary elements and their potential contribution to the development of lipedema will facilitate the advancement of efficacious treatments and therapies for this particular ailment.

This study examines the correlation between lipedema and hypermobility, revealing that around 50% of women diagnosed with lipedema also have joint hypermobility. This finding implies a potential coexistence of hypermobile Ehlers-Danlos syndrome (hEDS), a prevalent condition. Ehlers-Danlos syndrome type III is caused by germline truncating mutations in TNXB and a single germline variant in COL3A1. Nevertheless, there have been no identified mutations in the aforementioned genes in relation to lipedema.

A unique germline truncating mutation in PALB2 has been discovered, resulting in a rare case of autosomal-dominant familial multiple subcutaneous lipomatosis (FML) and an increased susceptibility to malignancies. The presence of a KRAS somatic mutation c.436G > A (p.Ala146Thr) and an NF1 de novo germline truncating mutation has been identified in two individuals diagnosed with encephalocraniocutaneous lipomatosis, a congenital hamartomatous disorder characterized by unilateral skin lesions, lipomas, and ipsilateral ophthalmological and cerebral malformations.

In the afflicted tissue of patients with facial infiltrating lipomatosis, somatic activating mutations of PIK3CA, which have been previously documented in cancer and overgrowth syndromes, have been identified. Germline mutations in LIPE are responsible for the syndrome of multiple symmetric lipomatosis, partial lipodystrophy, and insulin resistance. These mutations significantly hinder the breakdown of fat from adipose tissue depots, potentially leading to fat accumulation in lipedema.

A de novo heterozygous missense mutation (p.Tyr446Cys) in the TBL1XR150 gene is responsible for the development of Pierpont syndrome, a condition characterized by plantar lipomatosis, limb deformities, atypical facies, and developmental delay. Hereditary retinoblastoma is a result of genetic variations in the RB1 gene. The susceptibility to lipomatosis in hereditary retinoblastoma is not linked to specific RB1 variants, but is likely influenced by other variables.

Multiple symmetric lipomatosis, also known as Madelung disease, is an uncommon condition affecting the differentiation of adipocytes. It is characterized by the presence of benign and widespread lipomatosis in the subcutaneous depots of the cephalic, cervical, and upper thoracic regions. This disorder is associated with biallelic mutations in the MFN2 gene, which encodes a mitochondrial protein that is already linked to Charcot-Marie-Tooth syndrome.

There are shared phenotypes between familial partial lipodystrophies and lipedema, characterized by the normal occurrence of fat loss in the buttocks and extremities, as well as fat increase in the face, neck, and abdomen. These illnesses are associated with metabolic problems such as insulin resistance, diabetes mellitus, hypertriglyceridemia, hepatic steatosis, hypertension, and coronary artery disease. However, it is important to note that none of these complications are directly related to the phenotype of lipedema. Nevertheless, genes that play a crucial role in partial lipodystrophy may also have a significant impact on altering the characteristics of lipedema.

Garg et al. conducted linkage analysis and whole-exome sequencing to find the disease-causing mutation in an African-American pedigree with a unique autosomal-dominant atypical FPLD. The patients that were impacted had significant adipose tissue reduction in the limbs, an excessive accumulation of fat in the face and neck, and metabolic problems. The researchers detected a genetic mutation (c.202C > T, p.Leu68Phe) in the adrenoceptor γ 2A (ADRA2A) in all individuals who were afflicted, while no such alteration was observed in the unaffected individuals. ADRA2A controls the release of norepinephrine, and its activation decreases the breakdown of fats in adipocytes.

GWAS and functional analysis have validated the relationship of many genes with subcutaneous adipose depots. These genes exhibit genetic regulation of the distribution of body fat, which is separate from the regulation of overall adiposity. The physiological significance of ATXN1 and UBE2E2 in adipogenesis has been established, and functional investigations of ATXN1 and UBE2E have demonstrated that the absence of Atxn1 or Ube2e2 in primary mouse adipose progenitor cells impedes the differentiation process of adipocytes.

The VEGFR3 signaling pathway plays a crucial role in the formation and upkeep of the lymphatic vascular system. The association between VEGFR3 and the development of lymphedema in humans has been established. Mice harboring heterozygous inactivating missense mutations in the VEGFR-3 gene exhibit subcutaneous adipose tissue hypertrophy and hypoplastic dermal lymphatics. VEGFR3 exerts inhibitory effects on fetal lymphangiogenesis and produces regression of pre-existing lymphatic vessels in the skin of transgenic mice, while the blood vasculature remains unaffected. The K14-VEGFR3–Ig mice, which have been genetically modified, have a higher accumulation of fat beneath the skin.

Mice lacking the Sirt6 gene that specifically targets fat have heightened susceptibility to obesity generated by a high-fat diet. This leads to the hypertrophy of adipocytes, which is attributed to impaired lipolytic activity resulting from the reduced expression of the lipolytic enzyme known as adipose tissue triglyceride lipase (ATGL). The fat-specific knockout of Sirt6 also demonstrated heightened inflammation in adipose tissue, thereby playing a role in the development of insulin resistance in mice fed a high-fat diet.

The promotion of healthy growth of subcutaneous adipose tissue by FGF21 leads to an improvement in systemic insulin sensitivity. Mice lacking FGF21 have reduced subcutaneous adipose tissue and heightened insulin resistance in response to a high-fat diet. There exists a favorable correlation between serum FGF21 levels and the area of subcutaneous adipose tissue in persons who are insulin-sensitive and obese.

Mice lacking the IL18 receptor 1 exhibit heightened vulnerability to obesity induced by dietary factors. Panx1 is responsible for encoding a glycoprotein called pannexin 1, which has a crucial function in controlling the development of adipocytes and the buildup of fat. The absence of the Panx1 gene in knockout mice results in a notable increase in total fat mass and a decrease in lean mass when subjected to a standard diet.

The gene PROX1 has been found to be associated with the presence of leaky lymphatic valves. In mice, a deficiency in the Prox1 gene leads to the accumulation of fat in the subcutaneous and intra-abdominal regions. ZPF423 is a gene that produces a transcription factor with many zinc fingers. This factor is found in preadipocytes and mature adipocytes in living organisms. It plays a crucial role in the final development of white adipose tissue beneath the skin. The decrease in lipid content within adipocytes in the absence of Zfp423 can be attributed to the reduced expression of PPARγ and other genes that are specific to adipocytes.

Suggested Reading

Bauer A.T., von Lukowicz D., Lossagk K., Aitzetmueller M., Moog P., Cerny M., Erne H., Schmauss D., Duscher D., Machens H.G. New Insights on Lipedema: The Enigmatic Disease of the Peripheral Fat. *Plast. Reconstr. Surg.* 2019;144:1475–1484. doi: https://doi.org/10.1097/PRS.0000000000006280.

Paolacci S., Precone V., Acquaviva F., Chiurazzi P., Fulcheri E., Pinelli M., Buffelli F., Michelini S., Herbst K.L., Unfer V., et al. GeneOb Project. Genetics of lipedema: New perspectives on genetic research and molecular diagnoses. *Eur. Rev. Med. Pharmacol. Sci.* 2019;23:5581–5594..

Precone V., Barati S., Paolacci S., Salgarello M., Visconti G., Gentileschi S., Guerri G., Gagliardi L., Aquilanti B., Matera G., et al. Genetic syndromes with localized subcutaneous fat tissue accumulation. *Acta Biomed.* 2019;90:90–92.

Van Pelt R.E., Gozansky W.S., Hickner R.C., Schwartz R.S., Kohrt W.M. Acute modulation of adipose tissue lipolysis by intravenous estrogens. *Obesity.* 2006;14:2163–2172. doi: https://doi.org/10.1038/oby.2006.253.

Gavin K.M., Cooper E.E., Hickner R.C. Estrogen receptor protein content is different in abdominal than gluteal subcutaneous adipose tissue of overweight-to-obese premenopausal women. *Metabolism.* 2013;62:1180–1188. doi: https://doi.org/10.1016/j.metabol.2013.02.010.

Orphanet. [(accessed on 22 December 2021)]. Available online: https://www.orpha.net/consor/cgi-bin/index.php

Warren A.G., Janz B.A., Borud L.J., Slavin S.A. Evaluation and management of the fat leg syndrome. *Plast. Reconstr. Surg.* 2007;119:9–15. doi: https://doi.org/10.1097/01.prs.0000244909.82805.dc.

Forner-Cordero I., Szolnoky G., Forner-Cordero A., Keméný L. Lipedema: An overview of its clinical manifestations, diagnosis and treatment of the disproportional fatty deposition syndrome-systematic review. *Clin. Obes.* 2012;2:86–95. doi: https://doi.org/10.1111/j.1758-8111.2012.00045.x.

Halk A.B., Damstra R.J. First Dutch guidelines on lipedema using the international classification of functioning, disability and health. *Phlebology.* 2017;32:152–159. doi: https://doi.org/10.1177/0268355516639421.

Hansson E., Svensson H., Brorson H. Review of Dercum's disease and proposal of diagnostic criteria, diagnostic methods, classification and management. *Orphanet J. Rare Dis.* 2012;7:23. doi: https://doi.org/10.1186/1750-1172-7-23.

Loh P-R, Tucker G, Bulik-Sullivan BK, Vilhjalmsson BJ, Finucane HK, Salem RM, et al. Efficient Bayesian mixed-model analysis increases association power in large cohorts. Nat Genet. 2015;47:284–90. https://doi.org/10.1038/ng.3190.

Loh P-R, Kichaev G, Gazal S, Schoech AP, Price AL. Mixed model association for biobank-scale data sets. bioRxiv. 2017. https://doi.org/10.1101/194944.

Klarin D, Zhu QM, Emdin CA, Chaffin M, Horner S, McMillan BJ, et al. Genetic analysis in UK Biobank links insulin resistance and transendothelial migration pathways to coronary artery disease. Nat Genet. 2017;49:1392–7. https://doi.org/10.1038/ng.3914.

Klarin D, Emdin CA, Natarajan P, Conrad MF, Kathiresan S. Genetic Analysis of Venous Thromboembolism in UK Biobank Identifies the ZFPM2 Locus and Implicates Obesity as a Causal Risk Factor CLINICAL PERSPECTIVE. Circ Cardiovasc Genet. 2017;10. https://doi.org/10.1161/CIRCGENETICS.116.001643.

R Core Team. R: A language and environment for statistical computing. R Foundation for Statistical Computing, Vienna, Austria. 2021. https://www.R-project.org/.

Zheng J, Erzurumluoglu AM, Elsworth BL, Kemp JP, Howe L, Haycock PC, et al. LD Hub: a centralized database and web interface to perform LD score regression that maximizes the potential of summary level GWAS data for SNP heritability and genetic correlation analysis. Bioinformatics. 2017;33:272. https://doi.org/10.1093/bioinformatics/btw613.

Bulik-Sullivan B, Finucane HK, Anttila V, Gusev A, Day FR, Loh PR, et al. An atlas of genetic correlations across human diseases and traits. Nat Genet. 2015;47:1236–41. https://doi.org/10.1038/ng.3406.

Bulik-Sullivan BK, Loh P-R, Finucane HK, Ripke S, Yang J, Consortium SWG of the PG. et al. LD Score regression distinguishes confounding from polygenicity in genome-wide association studies. Nat Genet. 2015;47:291–5. https://doi.org/10.1038/ng.3211.

Watanabe K, Taskesen E, van Bochoven A, Posthuma D. Functional mapping and annotation of genetic associations with FUMA. Nat Commun. 2017;8:1826. https://doi.org/10.1038/s41467-017-01261-5.

Consortium TGte. The Genotype-Tissue Expression (GTEx) pilot analysis: Multitissue gene regulation in humans. Sci 2015;348:648–60. https://doi.org/10.1126/science.1262110.

Veno-Lymphatic Relationship in Lipedema

Lipedema is a condition characterized by the abnormal accumulation of fat primarily in the lower extremities, often accompanied by pain and swelling. While the exact cause of lipedema is not fully understood, there is evidence to suggest that venous and lymphatic dysfunction may play a role in its development.

Veins are blood vessels with thinner walls that consist of intimal, medial, and adventitial layers. The intimal layer, which is located on the basement membrane, has antithrombogenic properties. It produces prostaglandin I2, glycosaminoglycan cofactors of antithrombin, thrombomodulin, and tissue-type plasminogen activator (t-PA). The middle layer comprises three layers of smooth muscle intertwined with collagen and elastin, which receive innervation from adrenergic nerves. Veins possess a less robust muscle layer and a lower amount of elastic tissue in comparison to arteries. The adventitia, which is the outermost layer, is thicker in veins compared to arteries due to a higher concentration of collagen. This results in veins being more rigid than arteries. The calf "muscle pump" relies on the venous system's high capacitance, which is mostly attributed to the elliptical shape of the lower leg veins.

The superficial (Fig. 1), deep (Fig. 2), and most perforating veins are equipped with bicuspid valves that are composed of folds of endothelium supported by a thin layer of connective tissue. These valves partition the hydrostatic column of blood into sections and guarantee the movement from the outermost layer to the innermost layer and from the tail end to the head end. Valve closure is a passive occurrence that is triggered by the reversal of the initial forward pressure difference across the valve. Reflux that lasts for less than 0.5 seconds is considered normal and anticipated; however, retrograde flow that continues for more than 0.5 seconds is typically classified as pathological reflux.

The veins of the lower extremities are categorized based on their positioning relative to the muscle fascia and can be found in either the superficial or deep compartment.

The lower extremities possess a venous system that consists of deep veins, located beneath the muscular fascia, responsible for draining the muscles of the lower extremities; superficial veins, situated above the deep fascia, responsible for

G. Laur, *Lipoedema*, https://doi.org/10.1007/978-981-96-8939-2_8

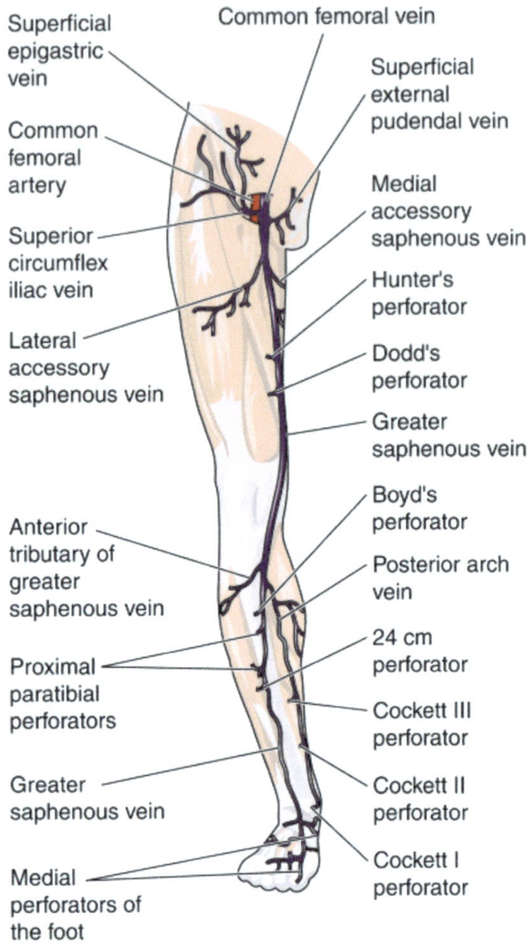

Fig. 1 Anatomy of the superficial venous system on the leg

draining the cutaneous microcirculation; and perforating veins, which traverse the muscular fascia and establish connections between the superficial and deep veins. Communicating veins establish connections between veins that are part of the same system, specifically between deep veins and deep veins and between superficial veins and superficial veins.

The superficial venous system comprises the reticular veins, as well as the great (larger) and small (lesser) saphenous veins and their tributaries. Reticular veins are responsible for draining the skin and subcutaneous tissue of the lower extremities. They connect with either saphenous tributaries or deep veins through perforators. Approximately 60% of patients with widespread thigh telangiectasias have been shown to have direct contact between inadequate reticular veins and the deep venous system via perforating veins.

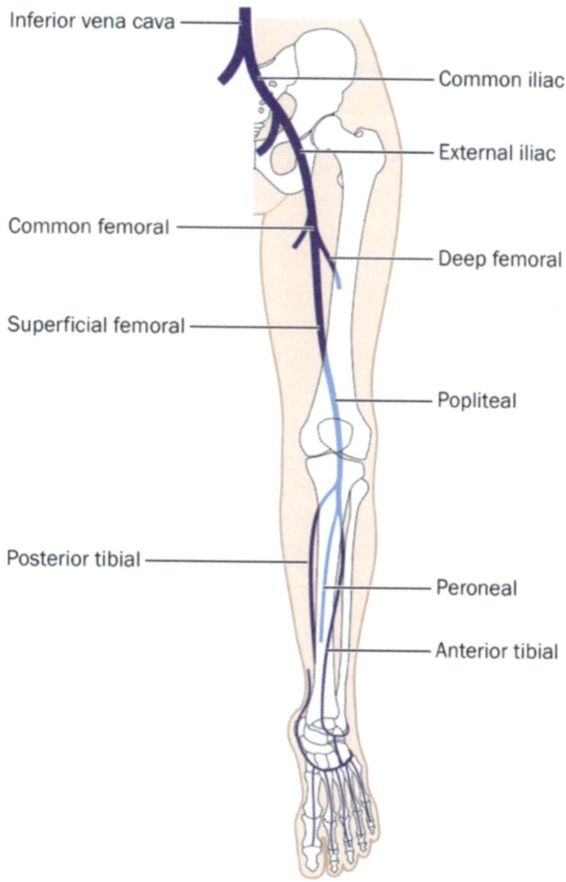

Fig. 2 Anatomy of the deep venous system on the leg

The great saphenous vein originates from the inner side of the dorsal pedal venous arch and moves upward in front of the inner ankle bone, crossing the tibia at the point where the lower and middle parts of the calf meet and then passing behind and toward the inner side of the knee. The vein thereafter rises toward the center of the thigh, penetrating the deep fascia, and converges with the common femoral vein approximately 3–4 cm (equivalent to 2 fingerbreadths) below and to the side of the pubic tubercle. The saphenous nerve is positioned in front of the great saphenous vein in the calf and can be damaged by procedures that reach into the calf area.

The presence of accessory branches and tributaries of the great saphenous vein may have a significant role in the development of chronic venous illness. Typically, the calf has two primary saphenous tributaries: an anterior branch and the posterior arch (Leonardo's) vein. These tributaries collect blood from a network of veins in the medial ankle. It is noteworthy that the posterior tibial perforators connect to this vein instead of the main trunk of the great saphenous vein. Treatments focused on the great saphenous vein in the calf region will not resolve these perforators.

The anterior and posterior accessory saphenous veins run alongside the major saphenous vein in the thigh, outside the saphenous fascia. The perineum and lower abdominal wall are typically drained by the superficial external pudendal, superficial circumflex iliac, and superficial epigastric veins, which often connect with the great saphenous vein around the saphenofemoral junction. The saphenofemoral junction contains a valve in 94–100% of people, and 81% of persons have at least one valve in the external iliac—common femoral segment located above the junction.

The tiny saphenous vein, previously referred to as the short or lesser saphenous vein, begins at the dorsal pedal arch and rises diagonally toward the back and side before ending at several points in the popliteal vein. The structure usually consists of seven to ten valves that are tightly positioned and is linked to the sural nerve. Approximately 60% of small saphenous veins connect to the popliteal vein within a distance of 8 cm from the knee joint. Another 20% of these veins merge with the great saphenous vein through anterior or posterior tributaries. The remaining 20% of small saphenous veins join either the femoral, deep femoral, or internal iliac veins.

There are alternative drainage channels that go from the surface to the deep layers, and they can sometimes play a significant role in the development of chronic venous illness. The lateral superficial veins are residual structures of the embryonic vena marginalis lateralis and can be a significant characteristic of the Klippel-Trenaunay syndrome. Additional routes consist of the sciatic drainage system, which transports blood from the back of the thigh to the internal iliac system, the lateral subdermic system that drains toward the deep femoral and inferior gluteal veins, drainage via the obturator veins, and alternate venous paths via the round ligament.

The principal deep veins of the lower extremity generally parallel the path of the corresponding arteries, except for the femoral vein. The deep venous system of the calf comprises the tibial and peroneal veins, together with the soleal and gastrocnemius veins. In 38% of limbs, the femoral vein has a direct connection to the popliteal vein, while in 48% of limbs, it interacts with the popliteal vein through a tributary. In current terminology, the term "superficial femoral vein" has been discarded to prevent any misunderstanding with the superficial venous system.

The structure of the iliac veins is less clearly defined compared to the infrainguinal veins. In most cases, a solitary internal iliac trunk typically empties into the external iliac vein, resulting in the formation of the common iliac vein. This occurrence can be observed in approximately 27% of the limbs. The internal iliac vein collects blood from both the outer and inside parts of the body, which have several interconnected pathways without valves. Pelvic venous insufficiency and incompetent tributaries of the internal iliac vein are often the cause of varicosities in the vulva, vagina, and posteromedial thigh, as well as symptoms of pelvic congestion syndrome.

The inferior vena cava is formed during the process of development and selective regression of the paired fetal posterior cardinal, subcardinal, and supracardinal veins. Anomalies in the formation of the subcardinal and supracardinal veins can result in the interruption of the inferior vena cava, leading to either a continuation

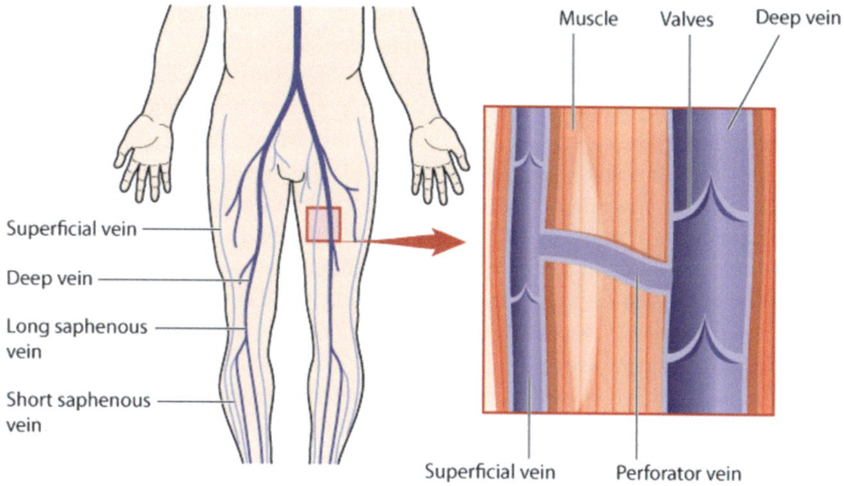

Fig. 3 Vein perforator

with the azygous or hemiazygos vein, or the presence of a duplicated or left-sided inferior vena cava, respectively.

The quantity of deep venous valves progressively rises from the head toward the tail. Valves are infrequently found in the iliac veins, in contrast to the infrainguinal veins. Anatomical dissections have revealed that valves are present in just 1.2% of common iliac veins, 27% of external iliac veins, and 10.1% of internal iliac veins. Typically, there is an average of five deep venous valves located between the inguinal ligament and popliteal fossa. However, the actual number might range from two to nine.

Perforating veins (Fig. 3) can be categorized into four clinically significant types, which include those located in the foot, medial and lateral calf, and thigh. Foot perforators are distinctive because they typically guide blood flow toward the superficial veins, whereas all other perforators typically send blood flow toward the deep system. The medial calf and thigh are primarily supplied by major perforators, which are equipped with one to three valves that facilitate the passage of blood from the superficial veins to the deep veins.

The calf is composed of four sets of perforators. These include the paratibial perforators, which connect the great saphenous and posterior tibial veins; the posterior tibial perforators, which connect the posterior accessory great saphenous (posterior arch) and posterior tibial veins; and the lateral and anterior leg perforators. The paratibial and posterior tibial perforators, which are located in the medial calf, are of utmost clinical significance.

The Hunterian perforators, which are located in the femoral canal, provide a connection between the great saphenous vein approximately 15 cm above the knee and the distal superficial femoral vein or the proximal popliteal vein. The presence of a competent proximal great saphenous vein can lead to the development of varicose veins in the medial thigh due to this perforator.

The CEAP categorization system, devised by the American Venous Forum, serves as a diagnostic and comparative tool for venous illnesses.

The classification has four elements: clinical illness class (C), etiology (E), anatomic distribution of reflux and blockage (A), and underlying pathophysiology (P). The approach identifies seven distinct clinical illness groups, namely, asymptomatic limbs (class 0), limbs with telangiectasias (class 1), limbs with varicose veins (class 2), limbs with edema (class 3), limbs with skin abnormalities but no ulceration (class 4), limbs with healed ulcers (class 5), and limbs with active ulcers (class 6).

The root cause might be categorized as congenital, primary, or secondary. Primary venous diseases may not have a clearly identified cause of venous dysfunction, whereas secondary venous disorders are the outcome of a previous event, typically an episode of acute deep venous thrombosis (DVT). The anatomical distribution of reflux and blockage is categorized into 18 venous segments, each of which is further characterized based on the underlying pathology.

The pooling of blood in the veins of the lower extremities when standing is constrained by the physical characteristics of the venous wall, the role of the venous valves, and the activity of the calf muscle pump. The deep veins in the lower extremities facilitate around 90% of the venous return, thanks to the foot, calf, and thigh muscle pumps. The calf muscle pump exhibits the highest capacitance, creates the biggest pressures, and holds the utmost significance.

Reflux, also known as pathologic retrograde flow, happens when the valves in the veins are either missing or unable to function properly due to degenerative processes (primary venous disease) or a previous incident of deep vein thrombosis (secondary venous disease). In these conditions, when the calf muscles relax, retrograde flow prevents the normal decrease in pressure, leading to a quick filling of veins from the backward flow of blood, as well as a gradual input of blood into the capillaries. Incompetent perforators can convey high venous pressure from the deep veins to the superficial veins.

The main cause of severe clinical symptoms in chronic venous insufficiency is ambulatory venous hypertension, which refers to the inability to sufficiently reduce venous pressure during physical activity. The degree of chronic venous illness is directly linked to the level of venous hypertension, which is assessed by measuring the pressure in a dorsal foot vein with a 21-gauge needle after performing ten tiptoe maneuvers. Ulceration typically does not occur when the venous pressure is below 30 mm Hg during normal activities. However, when the pressure exceeds 90 mm Hg, the incidence of ulceration is 100%. Ambulatory venous pressure is influenced by various factors, such as venous reflux, blockage, and calf muscle pump dysfunction, which collectively contribute to its determination.

Primary venous illness is an intricate and diverse condition marked by varicose veins, which are enlarged, easily felt twisted veins that are more than 4 mm in diameter and do not cause the skin above them to change color. Reticular veins are enlarged but not easily felt, appearing as blue veins in the skin that are less than 4 mm in width. They can be differentiated from smaller red to purple telangiectasias. Telangiectasias and reticular veins often do not affect the major saphenous trunks, although varicose veins often result in their incompetence.

Varicose veins exhibit a wide range of histologic characteristics that differ across different sections of the vein. The characteristic changes observed are uneven thickening of the innermost layer of the blood vessel, fibrosis between the innermost and outermost layers, shrinkage and disruption of elastic fibers, thickening of individual collagen fibers, and disarray in the layers of smooth muscle. The irregularities are unevenly spread across the great saphenous vein and its branches, with certain regions showing excessive growth while others display underdevelopment or normal characteristics. The varices, which are saccular dilations, are regularly positioned immediately downstream of the valve cusps.

Reflux is the main aberration in the blood flow of primary venous illness. However, there is little evidence to support the idea that varicose veins arise from sequential valve failure or a primary valve problem. Research conducted on surgical specimens indicates that varices can develop at any point along the path of the great saphenous vein, rather than exclusively beginning at the saphenofemoral junction. Ultrasound investigations indicate that primary valvular incompetence is a condition that affects multiple centers and develops at the same time in noncontinuous segments of veins. Evidence suggests that varicose alterations occur before the onset of obvious valve failure, indicating that valve dysfunction is a consequence of the former. Hypotheses have primarily concentrated on intrinsic structural and biochemical abnormalities of the vein wall. For instance, "weak wall" hypotheses propose that varicose veins arise due to underlying connective tissue deficiencies and modified venous tone.

Histologic investigations have indicated that varicose veins exhibit diminished contractility and compliance and that the ability to contract effectively may be further hindered by the fragmentation of the muscle layers. Smooth muscle cells undergo a transformation from a state of contraction to a state of secretion. This transformation is accompanied by alterations in the extracellular matrix of both affected and unaffected sections of veins. Varicose saphenous veins have elevated levels of collagen and decreased levels of elastin. Reduced venous elasticity has been observed in both limbs with visible varicose veins and in limbs without varicose veins but with a high likelihood of developing them. Forearm veins of patients with varicosities have also exhibited comparable connective tissue abnormalities.

Secondary venous disease is characterized by a higher probability of exhibiting both reflux and blockage, rather than either abnormality occurring in isolation.

The symptoms (Fig. 4) are mostly associated with a decrease in the time it takes for the veins to refill, rather than with ongoing issues in the outflow of blood from the veins. As a result, valvular incompetence is frequently considered to be the more significant of these concerns. The structures of reflux and venous blockage are also significant factors in determining the severity of post-thrombotic symptoms.

The process by which valve incompetence occurs after venous recanalization is still a significant question. In 50% of cases, individuals with chronic venous insufficiency show the fusion of the leaflet to the valve sinus due to the presence of a thrombus. In the other cases, there is endothelial degradation along with thickening of the basement membrane. Nevertheless, the loss of valves does not seem to be a widespread outcome of acute deep vein thrombosis (DVT).

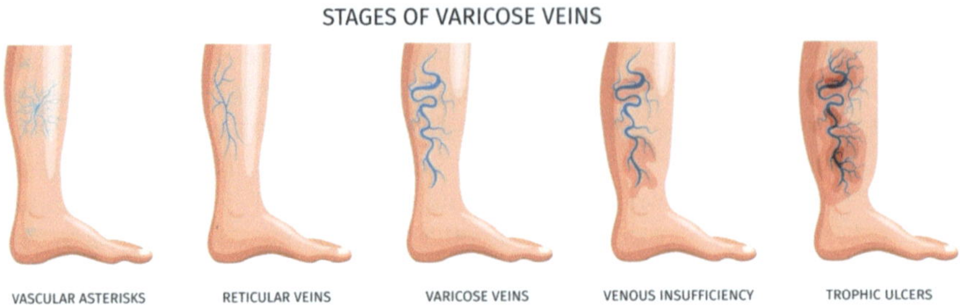

Fig. 4 Diagram of the evolution of chronic venous insufficiency

From a physiological perspective, the interactions between the venous and lymphatic systems are critical for maintaining fluid homeostasis and immune function within the body. The venous system, responsible for returning deoxygenated blood to the heart, works in tandem with the lymphatic system, which manages the clearance of interstitial fluid, proteins, and cellular debris from the tissues back into the circulatory system. This partnership ensures the efficient removal of excess fluid and waste products, thereby preventing tissue swelling and promoting tissue health. The lymphatic system also plays a role in fat and lipid transport, particularly in the gut, where it absorbs and processes dietary fats. In the context of lipedema, the pathological changes in adipose tissue distribution and function can significantly impact the veno-lymphatic interactions. Excessive adipose tissue can lead to mechanical compression of lymphatic vessels and impaired lymph flow, a condition known as lymphostasis. Simultaneously, the added burden on the venous system can exacerbate venous insufficiency, further complicating the fluid dynamics and contributing to the progressive swelling and pain characteristic of lipedema. Additionally, the inflammatory milieu associated with adipose tissue in lipedema can affect the structural integrity and function of lymphatic vessels, further impairing lymphatic drainage and exacerbating the condition. Thus, understanding the nuanced interplay between these two systems from a physiological standpoint is crucial for elucidating the pathogenesis of lipedema and developing targeted therapeutic strategies.

The mechanisms underpinning veno-lymphatic dysfunction in lipedema are multifaceted, involving both structural and functional aberrations within the venous and lymphatic systems. Structurally, the excessive accumulation of adipose tissue characteristic of lipedema can physically obstruct lymphatic vessels and impede venous return, leading to reduced lymphatic drainage and venous flow. This mechanical compression not only exacerbates fluid accumulation but also predisposes individuals to venous insufficiency, further complicating the clinical presentation of lipedema. Functionally, adipose tissue in lipedema is often associated with a pro-inflammatory state, where increased levels of adipokines and inflammatory cytokines can damage the endothelial lining of lymphatic vessels and impair their contractile function. This endothelial dysfunction reduces the efficiency of lymphatic pumping mechanisms, diminishing the transport capacity of the lymphatic system and contributing to lymph stasis. Furthermore, the altered microenvironment can promote fibrosis around lymphatic vessels, stiffening the tissue matrix and further restricting lymph flow. These combined structural and functional disruptions in the veno-lymphatic system contribute to the progressive nature of lipedema, leading to chronic edema, pain, and mobility issues, underscoring the complexity of veno-lymphatic dysfunction in the pathogenesis of lipedema.

Inflammatory pathways play a role in the pathogenesis of various diseases, significantly impacting veno-lymphatic health through a cascade of cellular and molecular events. In the context of conditions like lipedema, the chronic, low-grade inflammation within adipose tissue can lead to a detrimental cycle affecting the integrity and function of the venous and lymphatic systems. Adipocytes in diseased states secrete a plethora of inflammatory mediators, including cytokines such as tumor necrosis factor-alpha (TNF-α), interleukin-6 (IL-6), and adipokines, which can directly damage the endothelial cells lining the venous and lymphatic vessels. This endothelial dysfunction not only increases vascular permeability, leading to enhanced fluid extravasation into the interstitial space, but also impairs the contractility of lymphatic vessels, crucial for the propulsion of lymph. Furthermore, these inflammatory mediators can stimulate the proliferation of fibroblasts, leading to fibrosis around lymphatic vessels and impeding lymphatic drainage. The resultant lymph stasis further exacerbates the inflammatory response, creating a feedback loop that perpetuates veno-lymphatic dysfunction. Understanding these inflammatory pathways and their deleterious effects on veno-lymphatic health is crucial for identifying therapeutic targets to mitigate the progression of diseases characterized by inflammation-induced veno-lymphatic impairment.

Distinguishing lipedema from lymphedema and venous insufficiency is pivotal for accurate diagnosis and effective management, as these conditions share overlapping symptoms but have distinct pathophysiologies and therapeutic implications. Lipedema is characterized by the bilateral and symmetrical accumulation of adipose tissue, primarily in the lower extremities, sparing the feet, and is often associated with pain and tenderness. Unlike lipedema, lymphedema involves asymmetric swelling due to impaired lymphatic drainage, affecting one or both limbs and often extending to the dorsum of the feet. Lymphedema may also present with skin changes such as thickening and hyperpigmentation, which are less common in lipedema. Venous insufficiency, on the other hand, results from dysfunctional venous valves leading to chronic venous hypertension, edema, and skin changes like varicosities, stasis dermatitis, and ulcers, primarily affecting the lower legs and ankles. While venous insufficiency can cause fluid accumulation, it lacks the distinctive fatty tissue distribution and pain associated with lipedema. Diagnostic differentiation involves clinical evaluation, patient history, and specific investigations such as lymphoscintigraphy for lymphedema and duplex ultrasonography for venous insufficiency. Understanding these differences is crucial for tailoring treatment strategies, as interventions vary significantly across these conditions, emphasizing the importance of precise diagnostic approaches in the management of veno-lymphatic disorders.

The impact of veno-lymphatic dysfunction on the progression and severity of lipedema is profound, influencing both the rate at which the condition advances and the intensity of symptoms experienced by patients. Veno-lymphatic dysfunction, characterized by impaired venous return and lymphatic drainage, exacerbates the pathological accumulation of adipose tissue and fluid in the affected limbs, leading to increased swelling, pain, and fibrosis. This dysfunction not only contributes to the characteristic features of lipedema, such as bilateral and symmetrical fatty deposition in the lower extremities, but also predisposes individuals to secondary lymphedema, further complicating the clinical picture. The severity of lipedema is closely linked to the degree of veno-lymphatic impairment, with more advanced dysfunction associated with greater adipose tissue proliferation, fibrotic changes, and mobility restrictions.

Additionally, the chronic inflammatory state induced by adipose tissue expansion can further deteriorate veno-lymphatic health, creating a vicious cycle that accelerates disease progression. Early intervention to address veno-lymphatic dysfunction is crucial for slowing the progression of lipedema and mitigating its severity, underscoring the need for comprehensive diagnostic and therapeutic strategies that specifically target the veno-lymphatic components of the disease.

The management and treatment of lipedema with veno-lymphatic involvement require a multifaceted approach, addressing both the adipose tissue distribution and the underlying veno-lymphatic dysfunction to alleviate symptoms and halt progression. Conservative management strategies, such as compression therapy and manual lymphatic drainage (MLD), are foundational, aiming to improve lymphatic flow and reduce fluid accumulation. Compression garments exert controlled pressure on affected limbs, facilitating venous return and lymphatic drainage, whereas MLD, a specialized form of massage, encourages the movement of lymph fluids out of the swollen areas. Exercise and lifestyle modifications, including low-impact aerobics activities, strength training, and dietary adjustments, further support venous and lymphatic function, promoting overall health and potentially reducing lipedema progression. Surgical interventions, such as liposuction, can remove excess adipose tissue, thereby relieving mechanical pressure on the lymphatic system, while lymphaticovenous anastomosis (LVA) aims to restore lymphatic drainage by directly connecting lymphatic vessels to the venous system. Emerging therapies and pharmacological approaches focus on targeting the molecular and inflammatory pathways involved in lipedema and veno-lymphatic dysfunction. These include trials of drugs that enhance lymphangiogenesis, reduce inflammation, or modulate fat metabolism, offering hope for more targeted and effective treatments. Together, these strategies underscore the importance of a personalized, comprehensive treatment plan, integrating both established and innovative therapies to manage lipedema with veno-lymphatic involvement effectively.

In conclusion, the exploration of veno-lymphatic dysfunction in the context of lipedema has unveiled its significant impact on disease progression and severity. The key points underscore the intricate relationship between the venous and lymphatic systems in maintaining fluid homeostasis and highlight how their dysfunction contributes to the pathophysiology of lipedema, exacerbating adipose tissue accumulation, pain, and mobility impairments. The importance of a multidisciplinary approach in managing lipedema cannot be overstated, as it necessitates the collaboration of healthcare professionals across various specialties—including vascular medicine, physical therapy, nutrition, and plastic surgery—to offer comprehensive care tailored to the individual needs of patients. This integrative strategy not only addresses the multifactorial aspects of lipedema but also ensures that both physical and psychological impacts of the condition are duly considered. Looking ahead, future directions in the management of lipedema with veno-lymphatic involvement should focus on advancing our understanding through research, particularly in the areas of pathogenesis, diagnostic markers, and novel treatment modalities. There is a growing need for high-quality clinical trials to evaluate emerging therapies, including pharmacological interventions targeting the underlying mechanisms of veno-lymphatic dysfunction. Moreover, the development of standardized guidelines for diagnosis, staging, and treatment will be crucial in improving patient outcomes. As we continue to unravel the complexities of lipedema and its association with veno-lymphatic health, fostering a collaborative, patient-centered approach remains paramount in mitigating the burden of this challenging condition.

Suggested Reading

Gould DJ, El-Sabawi B, Goel P, et al. . Uncovering lymphatic transport abnormalities in patients with primary lipedema. J Reconstr Microsurg. 2020;36:136–141.

Rasmussen JC, Aldrich MB, Fife CE, et al. . Lymphatic function and anatomy in early stages of lipedema. Obesity. 2022;30:1391–1400.

Sandhofer M, Hanke CW, Habbema L, et al. . Prevention of progression of lipedema with liposuction using tumescent local anesthesia: results of an international consensus conference. Dermatol Surg. 2020;46:220–228.

Aksoy H, Karadag AS, Wollina U. Cause and management of lipedema-associated pain. Dermatol Ther. 2021;34:e14364.

van de Pas CB, Boonen RSM, Stevens S, et al. . Does tumescent liposuction damage the lymph vessels in lipoedema patients? Phlebology. 2020a;35:231.

Villa G, Campisi CC, Ryan M, et al. Procedural recommendations for lymphoscintigraphy in the diagnosis of peripheral lymphedema: the genoa protocol. Nucl Med Mol Imaging. 2019;53:47.

Bilancini S, Lucchi M, Tucci S, et al.. Functional lymphatic alterations in patients suffering from lipedema. Angiology. 1995;46:333–339.

Wright TF, Herbst KL. A case series of lymphatic injuries after suction lipectomy in women with lipedema. Am J Case Rep. 2022;23:e935016–e935011.

van de Pas CB, Boonen RSM, Stevens S, et al.. Does tumescent liposuction damage the lymph vessels in lipoedema patients? Phlebology. 2020b;35:231.

Jiang X, Nicolls MR, Tian W, et al. . Lymphatic dysfunction, leukotrienes, and lymphedema. Annu Rev Physiol. 2018;80:49–70.

Norden PR, Kume T. The role of lymphatic vascular function in metabolic disorders. Front Physiol. 2020;11:404.

Carter C J, Anderson F A, Wheeler H B. In: Hull RD, Raskob GE, Pineo GF, editor. Venous Thromboembolism: An Evidence-Based Atlas. Armonk, NY: Futura Publishing Company; 1996. Epidemiology and pathophysiology of venous thromboembolism. pp. 3–20.

Nawroth P P, Handley D A, Esmon C T, Stern D M. Interleukin 1 induces endothelial cell procoagulant while suppressing cell-surface anticoagulant activity. Proc Natl Acad Sci USA. 1986;83:3460–3464.

Stewart G J. Neutrophils and deep venous thrombosis. Haemostasis. 1993;23(suppl 1):127–140.

Moneta G L, Nehler M R. In: Gloviczki P, Yao JST, editor. Handbook of Venous Disorders: Guidelines of the American Venous Forum. 1st ed. London: Chapman and Hall Medical; 1996. The lower extremity venous system: anatomy and physiology of normal venous function and chronic venous insufficiency. pp. 3–26.

Browse N, Burnand K, Thomas M. Diseases of the Veins: Pathology, Diagnosis, and Treatment. London: Edward Arnold; 1988.

van Bemmelen P S, Beach K, Bedford G, Strandness D E. The mechanism of venous valve closure. Arch Surg. 1990;125:617–619.

van Bemmelen P S, Bedford G, Beach K, Strandness D E. Quantitative segmental evaluation of venous valvular reflux with duplex ultrasound scanning. J Vasc Surg. 1989;10:425–431.

Caggiati A, Bergan J J, Gloviczki P, Jantet G, Wendell-Smith C P, Partsch H. Nomenclature of the veins of the lower limbs: an international interdisciplinary consensus statement. J Vasc Surg. 2002;36:416–422.

Somjen G M. Anatomy of the superficial venous system. Dermatol Surg. 1995;21:35–45.

Thomson H. The surgical anatomy of the superficial and perforating veins of the lower limb. Ann R Coll Surg Engl. 1979;61:198–205.

Mozes G, Gloviczki P, Menawat S S, Fisher D R, Carmichael S W, Kadar A. Surgical anatomy for endoscopic subfascial division of perforating veins. J Vasc Surg. 1996;24:800–808.

Leu H J, Vogt M, Pfrunder H. Morphological alterations of non-varicose and varicose veins. (A morphological contribution to the discussion on pathogenesis of varicose veins) Basic Res Cardiol. 1979;74:435–444.

Mozes G, Carmichael S W, Gloviczki P. In: Gloviczki P, Yao JST, editor. Handbook of Venous Disorders: Guidelines of the American Venous Forum. 2nd ed. London: Arnold; 2001. Development and anatomy of the venous system. pp. 11–24.

Cotton L T. Varicose veins: gross anatomy and development. Br J Surg. 1961;48:589–597.

LePage P A, Villavicencio J L, Gomez E R, Sheridan M N, Rich N M. The valvular anatomy of the iliac venous system and its clinical implications. J Vasc Surg. 1991;14:678–683.

Mathews R, Smith P A, Fishman E K, Marshall F F. Anomalies of the inferior vena cava and renal veins: embryologic and surgical considerations. Urology. 1999;53:873–880.

Negus D. In: Dodd H, Cockett FB, editor. The Pathology and Surgery of the Veins of the Lower Limb. 2nd ed. Edinburgh: Churchill Livingstone; 1976. The surgical anatomy of the veins of the lower limb. pp. 18–49.

Burnand K G. In: Gloviczki P, Yao JST, editor. Handbook of Venous Disorders: Guidelines of the American Venous Forum. 2nd ed. London: Arnold; 2001. The physiology and hemodynamics of chronic venous insufficiency of the lower limb. pp. 49–57.

Porter J, Moneta G. Reporting standards in venous disease: an update. J Vasc Surg. 1995;21:635–645.

Goldman M P, Fronek A. Anatomy and pathophysiology of varicose veins. J Dermatol Surg Oncol. 1989;15:138–145.

Ludbrook J. The musculovenous pumps of the human lower limb. Am Heart J. 1966;71:635–641.

Back T L, Padberg F T, Jr, Araki C T, Thompson P N, Hobson R W. Limited range of motion is a significant factor in venous ulceration. J Vasc Surg. 1995;22:519–523.

Nicolaides A N, Hussein M K, Szendro G, Christopoulos D, Vasdekis S, Clarke H. The relationship of venous ulceration with ambulatory venous pressure measurements. J Vasc Surg. 1993;17:414–419.

Nicolaides A N. Investigation of chronic venous insufficiency: a consensus statement (France, March 5–9, 1997) Circulation. 2000;102:E126–E163.

Hosoi Y, Zukowski A, Kakkos S K, Nicolaides A N. Ambulatory venous pressure measurements: new parameters derived from a mathematic hemodynamic model. J Vasc Surg. 2002;36:137–142.

Labropoulos N, Giannoukas A D, Nicolaides A N, Veller M, Leon M, Volteas N. The role of venous reflux and calf muscle pump function in nonthrombotic chronic venous insufficiency: correlation with severity of signs and symptoms. Arch Surg. 1996;131:403–406.

Cordts P R, Hartono C, LaMorte W W, Menzoian J O. Physiologic similarities between extremities with varicose veins and with chronic venous insufficiency utilizing air plethysmography. Am J Surg. 1992;164:260–264.
van Bemmelen P S, Mattos M A, Hodgson K J, et al. Does air plethysmography correlate with duplex scanning in patients with chronic venous insufficiency? J Vasc Surg. 1993;18:796–807.
Araki C T, Back T L, Padberg F T, et al. The significance of calf muscle pump function in venous ulceration. J Vasc Surg. 1994;20:872–877.
Bouissou H, Julian M, Pieraggi M T, Louge L. Vein morphology. Phlebology. 1988;3(suppl 1):1–11.
Lowell R C, Gloviczki P, Miller V M. In vitro evaluation of endothelial and smooth muscle function of primary varicose veins. J Vasc Surg. 1992;16:679–686.
Porto L C, Azizi M A, Pelajo-Machado M, Matos da S P, Lenzi H L. Elastic fibers in saphenous varicose veins. Angiology. 2002;53:131–140.
Jones G T, Solomon C, Moaveni A, van Rij A M, Thomson I A, Galvin I. Venous morphology predicts class of chronic venous insufficiency. Eur J Vasc Endovasc Surg. 1999;18:349–354.
Ascher E, Jacob T, Hingorani A, Tsemekhin B, Gunduz Y. Expression of molecular mediators of apoptosis and their role in the pathogenesis of lower-extremity varicose veins. J Vasc Surg. 2001;33:1080–1086.
Labropoulos N, Giannoukas A D, Delis K, et al. Where does venous reflux start? J Vasc Surg. 1997;26:736–742.
Gandhi R H, Irizarry E, Nackman G B, Halpern V J, Mulcare R J, Tilson M D. Analysis of the connective tissue matrix and proteolytic activity of primary varicose veins. J Vasc Surg. 1993;18:814–820.
Rose S S, Ahmed A. Some thoughts on the aetiology of varicose veins. J Cardiovasc Surg (Torino) 1986;27:534–543.
Vanhoutte P M, Corcaud S, de Montrion C. Venous disease: from pathophysiology to quality of life. Angiology. 1997;48:559–567.
Clarke G H, Vasdekis S N, Hobbs J T, Nicolaides A N. Venous wall function in the pathogenesis of varicose veins. Surgery. 1992a;111:402–408.
Travers J P, Brookes C E, Evans J, et al. Assessment of wall structure and composition of varicose veins with reference to collagen, elastin and smooth muscle content. Eur J Vasc Endovasc Surg. 1996;11:230–237.
Michiels C, Arnould T, Thibaut-Vercruyssen R, Bouaziz N, Janssens D, Remacle J. Perfused human saphenous veins for the study of the origin of varicose veins: role of the endothelium and of hypoxia. Int Angiol. 1997;16:134–141.
Clarke G H, Vasdekis S N, Hobbs J T, Nicolaides A N. Venous wall function in the pathogenesis of varicose veins. Surgery. 1992b;111:402–408.
Alexander C J. The theoretical basis of varicose vein formation. Med J Aust. 1972;1:258–261.
Haardt B. A comparison of the histochemical enzyme pattern in normal and varicose veins. Phlebology. 1987;2:135–158.
Barber D A, Wang X, Gloviczki P, Miller V M. Characterization of endothelin receptors in human varicose veins. J Vasc Surg. 1997;26:61–69.
Johnson B F, Manzo R A, Bergelin R O, Strandness D E. Relationship between changes in the deep venous system and the development of the postthrombotic syndrome after an acute episode of lower limb deep vein thrombosis: a one- to six-year follow-up. J Vasc Surg. 1995;21:307–313.
Johnson B F, Manzo R A, Bergelin R O, Strandness D E. The site of residual abnormalities in the leg veins in long-term follow-up after deep venous thrombosis and their relationship to the development of the post-thrombotic syndrome. Int Angiol. 1996;15:14–19.
Killewich L A, Martin R, Cramer M, Beach K W, Strandness D E. An objective assessment of the physiological changes in the postthrombotic syndrome. Arch Surg. 1985;120:424–426.
Hanrahan L M, Araki C T, Rodriguez A A, Kechejian G J, LaMorte W W, Menzoian J O. Distribution of valvular incompetence in patients with venous stasis ulceration. J Vasc Surg. 1991;13:805–811.

Classification of Lipedema

The classification systems for lipedema (Fig. 1) have evolved significantly as understanding of the disease has advanced, with a growing emphasis on evidence-based approaches. Initially, lipedema was classified solely based on clinical presentation and morphology of the affected limbs. However, recent classification systems have integrated pathophysiological insights, genetic data, and imaging findings to create a more nuanced categorization. For instance, the differentiation between types of lipedema based on fat distribution patterns—such as predominantly hips, buttocks, or legs—has been refined with the understanding that adipose tissue in lipedema has distinct metabolic and histopathological features compared to normal adipose tissue. Advanced imaging techniques like lymphoscintigraphy and MRI have also been incorporated to identify early lymphatic dysfunction, even when clinical signs of lymphedema are not yet present. Genetic studies have begun to uncover potential hereditary patterns and markers, suggesting a polygenic influence which may inform future subclassifications. These evolving classification systems are crucial for tailoring treatment strategies to individual patients, enabling targeted therapies that address the specific manifestations and stages of lipedema, and for facilitating robust clinical research that can yield further insights into this complex and often misdiagnosed condition.

Lipedema is classified based on the extent and severity of the condition. Here are the main classifications of lipedema (Fig. 2):

1. Stage 1 lipedema: This stage is characterized by the presence of small nodules or bumps under the skin, typically in the buttocks or thighs. The skin may appear normal or slightly discolored, but there is no pitting edema (i.e., no visible indentation when pressure is applied to the skin).

Stage 1 lipedema represents the initial phase in the clinical progression of this chronic condition, marked by subtle yet distinct changes in the subcutaneous adipose tissue. Clinically, patients with stage 1 lipedema may observe the emergence of small nodules or bumps under the skin, akin to a grainy texture, which are

G. Laur, *Lipoedema*, https://doi.org/10.1007/978-981-96-8939-2_9

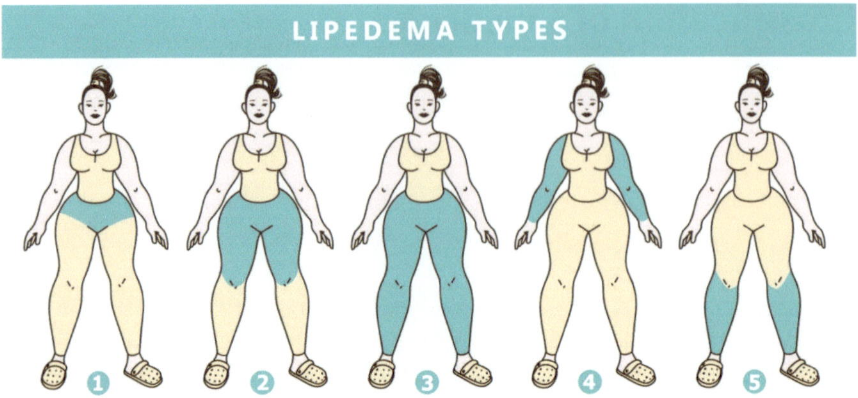

Fig. 1 Classification of the different types of lipedema

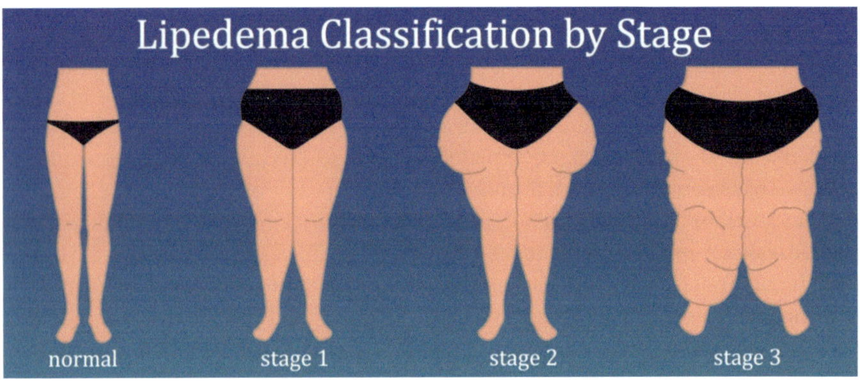

Fig. 2 Classification of the different stages of lipedema

particularly palpable in areas with high fat deposition such as the buttocks or thighs. The skin overlying the affected areas typically retains its normal appearance or may display a slight discoloration or temperature change compared to unaffected regions.

At this initial stage, the adipose tissue undergoes hypertrophy and hyperplasia, leading to an increased number of fat cells and a slight increase in their size. This proliferation does not yet significantly alter the overlying skin's appearance, nor does it produce the severe edematous changes seen in later stages. Histologically, there may be evidence of early lymphatic involvement, though not pronounced enough to cause visible pitting edema.

The diagnosis at this stage is often challenging due to the subtlety of symptoms and the lack of overt, distinguishing features that may be more apparent in advanced lipedema. A high index of suspicion is required, particularly in patients with a family history of the condition or when the fat distribution does not conform to typical patterns of obesity. Diagnosis is largely clinical but can be supported by imaging modalities such as ultrasound or MRI, which may reveal the characteristic nodular fat pattern.

The absence of pitting edema is a key diagnostic criterion differentiating stage 1 lipedema from lymphedema or common obesity. In lymphedema, the edema is typically evident and may leave an indentation when pressure is applied, a feature not present in early lipedema.

Management strategies at this stage are predominantly conservative, focusing on mitigating progression. Patients may benefit from a combination of a well-balanced diet, regular exercise, and physical therapies such as manual lymphatic drainage (MLD) to optimize lymphatic function. Compression garments may also be introduced early to support the tissue and prevent deterioration of lymphatic flow.

The prognosis for stage 1 lipedema, if identified and managed appropriately, can be favorable with interventions aimed at maintaining normal body weight and preventing the progression to more advanced stages. However, a lack of awareness and understanding can lead to misdiagnosis and delayed treatment, underscoring the importance of education and research.

Current research efforts are directed toward understanding the molecular and genetic basis of lipedema to refine diagnostic criteria and develop targeted interventions. Clinical trials are exploring various pharmacological and non-pharmacological treatments to establish evidence-based guidelines for early-stage lipedema management.

In summary, stage 1 lipedema, characterized by the presence of small nodules and the absence of pitting edema, lays the foundation for understanding the condition's trajectory. Accurate classification and early intervention are crucial to alter the course of the disease, prevent complications, and improve patient outcomes. As research advances, it holds the promise of unveiling novel insights that could lead to more definitive treatments and, ultimately, a cure for lipedema.

2. Stage 2 lipedema: This stage is characterized by the presence of more pronounced nodules and increased swelling in the affected areas. The skin may appear discolored and have a peau d'orange (orange peel) appearance, and there may be mild pitting edema.

Stage 2 lipedema signifies a progression from the initial phase of the condition, with patients typically exhibiting more pronounced and palpable subcutaneous nodules. The adipose tissue in affected areas—commonly the thighs, hips, and buttocks—undergoes further hypertrophy and begins to form larger fatty lobules that give the skin a characteristic peau d'orange or orange peel texture. This stage is often accompanied by an increase in swelling, contributing to a heavier and more uncomfortable sensation in the limbs.

Clinically, the skin overlying the affected adipose tissue may appear discolored, taking on a bruised or inflamed look, which reflects the underlying vascular changes and potential microvascular damage. Mild pitting edema becomes more evident in stage 2 lipedema; when pressure is applied to the skin, a temporary indentation may be visible, indicating an exacerbation of fluid accumulation within the interstitial spaces. However, this pitting is typically less pronounced than that observed in lymphedema.

The structural changes in the adipose tissue and skin are often more discernible in imaging studies at this stage. Ultrasound may reveal an increased echogenicity of the subcutaneous tissue, while MRI can show the enlarged fatty lobules in greater detail. These imaging findings, along with the clinical presentation, aid in the differentiation of stage 2 lipedema from other edematous or adipose conditions.

Management of stage 2 lipedema focuses on controlling symptoms and preventing further progression. This includes meticulous skin care to prevent infections, compression therapy to reduce swelling and improve lymphatic drainage, and potential use of advanced pneumatic compression devices. Nutritional counseling and physical therapy remain integral components of the treatment plan, emphasizing the importance of a multidisciplinary approach to care.

The transition from stage 1 to stage 2 lipedema highlights the condition's progressive nature and underscores the need for ongoing monitoring and adaptability in management strategies. As the condition advances, the importance of a supportive healthcare framework and patient education becomes paramount to address the multifaceted challenges posed by lipedema.

3. Stage 3 lipedema: This stage is characterized by the presence of large, confluent nodules and significant swelling in the affected areas. The skin may be thickened and fibrotic and have a spongy consistency. There may be significant pitting edema, and the affected areas may be painful or tender to the touch.

Stage 3 lipedema is the more advanced and severe phase of the condition, signifying considerable progression from the earlier stages. It is characterized by large, confluent nodules that form extensive areas of adipose tissue overgrowth, leading to significant swelling and deformation of the affected regions. At this stage, the skin texture undergoes notable changes; it may thicken and become fibrotic, acquiring a spongy consistency that can be readily discerned both visually and by palpation.

The nodular and uneven texture of the skin may resemble the surface of an orange, known as "peau d'orange." This feature is a consequence of the hypertrophy and hyperplasia of adipocytes coupled with the expansion of the fibrous septa that compartmentalize the fat lobules. This extensive tissue remodeling is often accompanied by increased fluid accumulation, resulting in significant pitting edema where a pressed finger leaves a visible indentation in the skin, a sign of the tissue's compromised fluid handling capacity.

In stage 3 lipedema, the functional impact becomes more pronounced. The enlarged limbs may become increasingly painful or tender, with the affected individual frequently experiencing discomfort or pain upon touch or pressure, limiting mobility and daily activities. The excessive and abnormal fat accumulation can also lead to joint pain, gait disturbances, and secondary health issues such as venous insufficiency.

From a clinical perspective, stage 3 lipedema requires a comprehensive management approach that may include manual lymphatic drainage, advanced compression therapy, and, in some cases, surgical intervention, such as liposuction, to remove the dysfunctional adipose tissue. It is critical for patients to receive multidisciplinary care, including physiotherapy, pain management, and psychological support to address the broad spectrum of challenges posed by this stage of lipedema.

The profound changes in tissue structure and function seen in stage 3 lipedema highlight the urgent need for increased awareness, early detection, and proactive treatment strategies to prevent or slow the progression to this debilitating stage. Research efforts continue to focus on unraveling the pathophysiological mechanisms at play and exploring novel therapeutic targets that could offer relief and improve quality of life for those living with this challenging condition.

In addition to the clinical stages, lipedema can also be classified based on the distribution of the affected areas:

1. Type 1 lipedema: This type involves the lower extremities, typically from the waist down to the ankles.

Lipedema type 1 is characterized by an abnormal accumulation of adipose tissue predominantly affecting the pelvis, buttocks, and hips. This type often presents with a symmetric enlargement of the areas around the hips, leading to a distinct "pear-shaped" body profile. The adipose tissue distribution in this type tends to start from the waist and extends to the buttocks and hips, sparing the legs below the groin area. Individuals with type 1 lipedema may notice that the fat accumulation in these areas is unusually soft and can be painful or tender to touch, differing markedly from the firmer, more evenly distributed fat seen in general obesity. Unlike typical fat, the lipedema fat in type 1 is often resistant to diet and exercise, making weight loss from these areas particularly challenging. The onset of type 1 lipedema is frequently linked to hormonal changes, such as puberty, pregnancy, or menopause, suggesting a hormonal sensitivity of the adipose tissue. While the upper body may remain unaffected or slim, the disproportion caused by the accumulation in the pelvis, buttocks, and hips can lead to psychosocial distress and physical discomfort, including mobility issues and joint pain due to the altered biomechanics of the lower body. Early diagnosis and management are crucial to alleviate symptoms and prevent progression to more advanced stages of the condition.

2. Type 2 lipedema: This type involves the upper extremities, typically from the shoulders down to the wrists.

Lipedema type 2 typically manifests as an excess accumulation of fatty tissue on the limbs, which may include both the legs and arms, though the legs are more commonly affected. This subtype is characterized by a disproportionate accumulation of adipose tissue extending from the hips down to the ankles, creating a column-like shape of the legs, often referred to as "riding breeches" fat distribution. The involvement of arms, while less common, follows a similar pattern of adipose tissue accumulation without affecting the hands. The adipose tissue in lipedema type 2 is usually tender, bruises easily, and can be accompanied by a feeling of heaviness or discomfort in the limbs.

Clinically, type 2 lipedema can be differentiated from other types of fat distribution disorders by its symmetrical presentation and the absence of pitting edema, which is characteristic of lymphedema. The skin in the affected areas often retains its elasticity but may become increasingly indented or exhibit a cellulite-like appearance as the condition progresses. Unlike common obesity, lipedema fat is generally unresponsive to caloric restriction and exercise, which may lead to frustration and psychological distress in affected individuals.

Early intervention is vital to managing symptoms, improving limb function, and preventing secondary health complications such as joint pain or the development of lipolymphedema. Management strategies often involve a combination of conservative treatments such as manual lymphatic drainage, compression therapy, and, possibly, surgical options like liposuction to remove non-lymphatic excess fat tissue.

3. Type 3 lipedema: This type involves both the upper and lower extremities.

Lipedema type 3 is a progressive condition that encompasses both the upper and lower extremities, marking a more advanced and widespread distribution of lipedematous adipose tissue. In this type, patients experience significant fat accumulation starting from the hips and extending to the ankles, often with involvement of the arms as well. The adiposity in the limbs can lead to a column-like appearance, with the fat typically being non-pitting, soft, and easily bruised. Unlike typical obesity, this abnormal deposition of fat is often resistant to lifestyle modifications, such as diet and exercise, and does not result from caloric excess alone.

The pathophysiology of type 3 lipedema is complex and not fully understood, but it is believed to involve a combination of lymphatic dysfunction, hormonal imbalances, and genetic factors. The condition can significantly impair mobility due to the added bulk and weight of the limbs, and the excess fat can cause joint pain, particularly in the knees, hips, and ankles. As the disease progresses, patients may also develop secondary health issues, including venous insufficiency, orthopedic complications like flat feet, and psychosocial problems due to altered body image and reduced quality of life.

Patients with type 3 lipedema often require a multidisciplinary approach for management, including physiotherapy, compression therapy, psychological support, and, in some cases, surgical interventions such as liposuction or lipectomy to remove excess adipose tissue. Early diagnosis and intervention are crucial to halt the progression, manage symptoms, and improve the patient's overall well-being.

4. Type 4 lipedema: This type involves the trunk, including the abdomen, chest, and back.

Lipedema type 4, although less commonly discussed than the types affecting the limbs, is characterized by the accumulation of adipose tissue in the trunk, including the abdomen, chest, and back. Unlike more typical forms of weight gain that are responsive to caloric restriction and increased physical activity, the fat distribution in type 4 lipedema is disproportionate and often does not respond to lifestyle changes. Patients with this type may present with a relatively normal BMI for their limbs but exhibit significant adiposity in the trunk region, which can be tender to touch and may exhibit the same bruising tendencies seen in other types of lipedema.

This type of lipedema can lead to a significant impact on the individual's body image and physical comfort, as the excessive fat accumulation can alter the body's contour and lead to psychosocial distress. The trunk adiposity in type 4 lipedema may also interfere with the mechanics of respiration and mobility due to the added weight in the central part of the body. The pathophysiology behind type 4 lipedema suggests a hormonal or genetic predisposition, which might affect the adipocyte regulation differently than in typical obesity. Due to the potential for misdiagnosis as common obesity, careful clinical evaluation is required, potentially supplemented by imaging or histological studies, to differentiate type 4 lipedema from other conditions with central obesity. Management strategies may include lymphatic drainage therapy, compression garments, and, in some cases, liposuction to remove the resistant adipose tissue. Understanding and recognizing this subtype of lipedema are essential for providing comprehensive care and appropriate management to those affected.

Staging lipedema involves a set of criteria that assesses the extent and nature of fat deposition, the presence of pain, and the degree of mobility impairment. These criteria are critical for determining the appropriate clinical interventions and for prognostic assessment. The generally accepted stages of lipedema are based on the physical characteristics and progression of the disease. Stage 1 is characterized by a normal skin surface with an underlying layer of small nodules or fat lobules. In stage 2, the skin becomes uneven with larger fatty nodules, and there may be indentations when the skin is pressed. Stage 3 is identified by larger folds of skin and fat, which can extend to the ankles and cause significant contour deformities, leading to mobility issues. Some classifications also consider a stage 4, which involves the onset of lymphedema, or lipolymphedema, in addition to lipedema. Pain, a hallmark of lipedema at all stages, is assessed through patient history and clinical examination. Mobility is evaluated based on the patient's ability to perform daily activities and is often correlated with the stage of fat accumulation. The staging of lipedema not only guides treatment approaches but also serves as a tool for monitoring disease progression and response to treatment. Accurate staging requires a comprehensive clinical evaluation and may be supported by diagnostic imaging to elucidate the structure of the adipose tissue and the status of the lymphatic system.

Lipedema progresses through distinct stages, each characterized by specific clinical features that reflect the severity and extent of adipose tissue involvement. In the early stage, or stage 1, individuals may notice a disproportionate accumulation of fat in the lower extremities, often with a smooth skin surface overlying a layer of enlarged fat cells. This stage is typically marked by a symmetrical increase in fat below the waist, sparing the feet, creating a "bracelet" effect around the ankles. Pain and bruising may occur with minor trauma. In the middle stage, or stage 2, the skin surface becomes nodular or uneven due to further fat accumulation and the development of fibrosis within the adipose tissue. Patients may experience increased pain, sensitivity, and spontaneous bruising, alongside the cosmetic changes. The late stage, or stage 3, involves significant fat deposits leading to large skin folds and lobules, which can extend over the knees and ankles, severely affecting mobility. The skin may become harder and more fibrotic, and lymphatic dysfunction may become evident, leading to additional swelling and increased risk of infections. Each stage of lipedema brings about a progressive impact on physical appearance, mobility, and quality of life, underscoring the importance of early diagnosis and management to halt or slow the progression of the disease.

The progression of lipedema through its stages carries significant clinical implications, impacting both management strategies and patient quality of life. In the early stage, lipedema is characterized by an accumulation of fat in the lower limbs, often without noticeable skin changes. Patients may report a feeling of heaviness or discomfort in the affected areas, but mobility is generally not impaired, and pain, if present, is mild. This stage presents an optimal window for intervention, as lifestyle modifications and conservative treatments can potentially slow disease progression.

As lipedema advances to the middle stage, the fat accumulation becomes more pronounced, and nodularity of the subcutaneous tissue can be observed, leading to an uneven skin texture. Pain and sensitivity in the affected areas may increase, and patients might start to experience mobility issues due to the added mass and discomfort. The increased fat deposition can also begin to interfere with lymphatic drainage, setting the stage for compounded lymphatic dysfunction.

In the late stage of lipedema, large fat masses and significant skin folds can develop, severely impacting the patient's mobility and daily functioning. The risk of developing secondary lymphedema (lipolymphedema) increases, with patients experiencing exacerbated swelling and an elevated risk of infections. Pain can become a major issue, severely affecting the patient's quality of life. At this stage, treatment options become more limited and may include surgical interventions such as liposuction to remove lipedemic fat.

The clinical implications of each stage of lipedema underline the importance of early detection and intervention. Effective management strategies tailored to the stage of disease can help mitigate the progression of symptoms, reduce the risk of complications, and improve overall patient outcomes.

Lipedema is characterized by a spectrum of phenotypic variations, with considerable variability in fat distribution and texture among affected individuals. This variability is evident in the different types of lipedema, which range from fat accumulation primarily in the lower extremities to involvement of the arms or trunk. The texture of adipose tissue in lipedema can also vary, from soft and doughy to fibrotic and nodular, often progressing in texture as the disease advances. These phenotypic differences are influenced by a multitude of factors, including genetic predispositions, which may dictate the pattern of fat deposition and the propensity for progression of the disease. Ethnic backgrounds can also play a role, as certain body shapes and fat distribution patterns are more prevalent in different populations, which may affect the presentation of lipedema. Lifestyle factors, including diet, physical activity, and hormonal influences such as puberty, pregnancy, and menopause, can further modify the expression of lipedema. For instance, a high-calorie diet and sedentary lifestyle may exacerbate the accumulation of lipedema fat, while regular exercise and a balanced diet might mitigate the progression, albeit without reducing the lipedema fat significantly. The interaction between these factors contributes to the clinical heterogeneity of lipedema, making it a complex condition that requires individualized approaches to diagnosis and management. Understanding the nuances of these phenotypic variations is crucial for clinicians to provide tailored treatments and to advance research into the underlying pathophysiological mechanisms.

The severity and functional impact of lipedema on patients are multifaceted, encompassing both physical manifestations and psychosocial repercussions. Assessment of severity in lipedema is typically based on the extent of adipose tissue accumulation and the degree of associated symptoms such as pain, tenderness, and swelling. Physical implications may include mobility restrictions due to limb size and joint stress, circulatory disturbances, and increased susceptibility to bruising. Functionally, this can translate into difficulties with daily activities, exercise intolerance, and lymphatic complications such as recurrent infections.

However, the assessment of lipedema severity must also take into account the psychosocial impact on the patient. Lipedema can lead to significant body image disturbances and emotional distress due to its visible nature and societal perceptions of body size. This distress is often exacerbated by misdiagnosis or dismissal by healthcare professionals, leading to a sense of isolation and frustration. Patients may experience anxiety, depression, and a diminished quality of life, which are integral components of the disease's severity.

Quality of life considerations are increasingly recognized as crucial in the classification and staging of lipedema. Comprehensive management strategies are therefore not limited to addressing the physical symptoms but must also include psychological support, patient education, and community engagement to improve overall well-being. Tools such as the Lipedema Quality of Life questionnaire can aid in quantifying the impact and guiding treatment approaches that are sensitive to the full scope of the disorder's impact on the individual.

Distinguishing lipedema from other conditions such as lymphedema and obesity is crucial for accurate diagnosis and appropriate management. Lipedema is typically characterized by the symmetrical buildup of painful, fatty tissue in the legs and arms, sparing the feet and hands, which distinguishes it from lymphedema where swelling can affect the distal extremities and is not necessarily symmetrical or painful. Unlike obesity, which is characterized by generalized adipose tissue accumulation that can be influenced by dietary and lifestyle changes, lipedema fat is resistant to diet and exercise and has a distinct nodular texture.

Imaging and diagnostic tests play a role in differentiating these conditions. Lymphoscintigraphy can assess lymphatic function and help identify lymphedema, while MRI and ultrasound imaging can visualize the quality and distribution of adipose tissue characteristic of lipedema. Dual-energy X-ray absorptiometry (DEXA) scans can provide detailed assessments of body composition, further aiding differentiation. In addition, a careful clinical examination including a thorough patient history is fundamental, as it reveals the typical lipedema symptoms, such as pain and bruising, and the often familial pattern of fat distribution. Together, clinical assessment combined with targeted imaging and diagnostic tests can effectively distinguish lipedema from lymphedema and obesity, leading to more accurate diagnoses and tailored treatment strategies.

In conclusion, the accurate classification of lipedema is not merely a taxonomic concern but a critical step toward ensuring effective patient care and advancing research. The refinement of lipedema classification systems to encompass the nuances of its presentation—varying distributions of adipose tissue, stages of progression, and associated symptoms—enables healthcare professionals to devise personalized management strategies that address the specific needs of each patient. Such stratification also facilitates the development of targeted therapies and interventions that can mitigate the physical and psychosocial burdens of the disease.

Moreover, accurate classification underpins research efforts by providing a structured framework for studying the condition. It allows for the standardization of patient groups in clinical trials, the comparison of data across studies, and the comprehensive analysis of therapeutic outcomes. This is particularly important for identifying the underlying pathophysiological mechanisms of lipedema and for exploring the genetic, hormonal, and environmental factors contributing to its development.

As our understanding of lipedema deepens, classification systems will likely continue to evolve, incorporating emerging insights from clinical practice and scientific inquiry. The ultimate goal is to transform the landscape of lipedema care from one of obscurity and misunderstanding to one of clarity and precision. Through meticulous classification, we pave the way for breakthroughs in treatment and the potential for improved quality of life for those living with lipedema.

Suggested Reading

La Torre Y.S.-D., Wadeea R., Rosas V., Herbst K.L. Lipedema: Friend and Foe. *Horm. Mol. Biol. Clin. Investig.* 2018;33:1. doi: https://doi.org/10.1515/hmbci-2017-0076.

Buso G., Depairon M., Tomson D., Raffoul W., Vettor R., Mazzolai L. Lipedema: A Call to Action! *Obesity.* 2019;27:1567. doi: https://doi.org/10.1002/oby.22597.

Shavit E., Wollina U., Alavi A. Lipoedema Is Not Lymphoedema: A Review of Current Literature. *Int. Wound J.* 2018;15:921–928. doi: https://doi.org/10.1111/iwj.12949.

Herbst K.L. Rare Adipose Disorders (RADs) Masquerading as Obesity. *Acta Pharmacol. Sin.* 2012;33:155–172. doi: https://doi.org/10.1038/aps.2011.153.

Buck D.W., Herbst K.L. Lipedema: A Relatively Common Disease with Extremely Common Misconceptions. *Plast. Reconstr. Surg. Glob. Open.* 2016;4:e1043. doi: https://doi.org/10.1097/GOX.0000000000001043.

Herbst K.L., Kahn L.A., Iker E., Ehrlich C., Wright T., McHutchison L., Schwartz J., Sleigh M., Donahue P.M.C., Lisson K.H., et al. Standard of Care for Lipedema in the United States. *Phlebology.* 2021;36:779–796. doi: https://doi.org/10.1177/02683555211015887.

Suga H., Araki J., Aoi N., Kato H., Higashino T., Yoshimura K. Adipose Tissue Remodeling in Lipedema: Adipocyte Death and Concurrent Regeneration. *J. Cutan. Pathol.* 2009;36:1293–1298. doi: https://doi.org/10.1111/j.1600-0560.2009.01256.x.

Crescenzi R., Marton A., Donahue P.M.C., Mahany H.B., Lants S.K., Wang P., Beckman J.A., Donahue M.J., Titze J. Tissue Sodium Content Is Elevated in the Skin and Subcutaneous Adipose Tissue in Women with Lipedema. *Obesity.* 2018;26:310–317. doi: https://doi.org/10.1002/oby.22090.

Forner-Cordero I., Szolnoky G., Forner-Cordero A., Kemény L. Lipedema: An Overview of Its Clinical Manifestations, Diagnosis and Treatment of the Disproportional Fatty Deposition Syndrome – Systematic Review. *Clin. Obes.* 2012;2:86–95. doi: https://doi.org/10.1111/j.1758-8111.2012.00045.x.

Child A.H., Gordon K.D., Sharpe P., Brice G., Ostergaard P., Jeffery S., Mortimer P.S. Lipedema: An Inherited Condition. *Am. J. Med. Genet. Part A.* 2010;152:970–976. doi: https://doi.org/10.1002/ajmg.a.33313.

Reich-Schupke S., Schmeller W., Brauer W.J., Cornely M.E., Faerber G., Ludwig M., Lulay G., Miller A., Rapprich S., Richter D.F., et al. S1 Guidelines: Lipedema. *JDDG J. Dtsch. Dermatol. Ges.* 2017;15:758–767. doi: https://doi.org/10.1111/ddg.13036.

Bauer A.T., Von Lukowicz D., Lossagk K., Hopfner U., Kirsch M., Moog P., Bauer H., Machens H.G., Schmauss D. Adipose Stem Cells from Lipedema and Control Adipose Tissue Respond Differently to Adipogenic Stimulation In Vitro. *Plast. Reconstr. Surg.* 2019;144:623–632. doi: https://doi.org/10.1097/PRS.0000000000005918.

Lee M.J., Wu Y., Fried S.K. Adipose Tissue Heterogeneity: Implication of Depot Differences in Adipose Tissue for Obesity Complications. *Mol. Asp. Med.* 2013;34:1–11. doi: https://doi.org/10.1016/j.mam.2012.10.001.

Jeffery E., Wing A., Holtrup B., Sebo Z., Kaplan J.L., Saavedra-Peña R., Church C.D., Colman L., Berry R., Rodeheffer M.S. The Adipose Tissue Microenvironment Regulates Depot-Specific Adipogenesis in Obesity. *Cell Metab.* 2016;24:142–150. doi: https://doi.org/10.1016/j.cmet.2016.05.012.

Ioannidou A., Fisher R.M., Hagberg C.E. The Multifaceted Roles of the Adipose Tissue Vasculature. *Obes. Rev.* 2022;23:e13403. doi: https://doi.org/10.1111/obr.13403.

Lipoedema

Risk Factors

Lipedema is a debilitating disease caused by abnormal and excessive accumulation of subcutaneous fat, primarily affecting the lower and upper limbs. It is primarily affecting women and is influenced by sex hormones. The global prevalence of lipedema is estimated to be 1–9/100,000. However, it can be misdiagnosed and confused with other diseases like obesity and lymphedema. Lipedema is generally limited to the limbs and may be normal, while obesity has generalized fat accumulation with a high body mass index (BMI). Lymphedema is bilateral and associated with pain and bruising, while lipedema can be unilateral and characterized by a positive Stemmer sign. Dieting cannot effectively improve lipedema, but it can reduce obesity associated with it. Lipedema can be an independent disease or part of a syndrome, with diagnosis based on medical history, physical examination, blood tests, and imaging techniques.

The exact cause of lipedema is unknown, but there are several risk factors that have been identified. Here are some of the most commonly recognized risk factors:

1. Gender: Lipedema is almost exclusively found in women, with only rare cases reported in men.
2. Genetics: Lipedema appears to have a genetic component, with a family history of the condition being commonly reported. Lipedema is a medical disorder characterized by the abnormal buildup of fat beneath the skin, mainly in the lower and/or upper limbs, resulting in symmetrical expansion. This illness, frequently misunderstood, can present itself as either primary lipedema or as a component of a syndrome, exhibiting similarities with other disorders. The paper you mentioned examines the genetic basis of lipedema, emphasizing its intricate nature and the use of next-generation sequencing (NGS) for diagnosing and treating the condition. Lipedema demonstrates a hereditary pattern, indicating a genetic origin.

The user did not provide any text. The inheritance pattern may manifest as X-linked dominant, autosomal-dominant with sex limitation, or oligogenic (involving many genes).The elucidation of the role of certain genes, such as AKR1C1, in isolated lipedema is becoming evident. The use of next-generation sequencing

G. Laur, *Lipoedema*, https://doi.org/10.1007/978-981-96-8939-2_10

(NGS) in this work signifies a noteworthy progression in comprehending the genetic aspects of lipedema. This technique has the potential to enhance diagnosis accuracy, facilitate distinction from comparable illnesses, and enable more customized treatment options, such as predicting the efficacy of procedures such as liposuction. As research progresses, these findings could be crucial in improving the care and quality of life for persons suffering from lipedema.

3. Hormones: It is believed that lipedema pathophysiology begins during times of hormonal changes like puberty, pregnancy, or menopause. While our understanding of lipedema has advanced, its root causes are still unclear. Estrogen, which is crucial in controlling fat and sugar metabolism in fat cells and the distribution of fat in women, is suspected to contribute to lipedema's pathophysiology. The mismanagement of fat buildup in the body due to estrogen is likely caused by two processes: (1) a change in the distribution of estrogen receptors in fat cells (ERα/ERß ratio) affecting metabolic signaling and (2) a heightened release of steroidogenic enzymes from fat cells, leading to more paracrine estrogen release. These changes might enhance the activation of peroxisome proliferator-activated receptor γ (PPARγ), increase the entry of free fatty acids into fat cells, raise glucose absorption, and promote angiogenesis, while reducing fat breakdown, the creation of mitochondria, and mitochondrial efficiency. Collectively, these metabolic shifts could cause increased fat cell formation and fat accumulation in fat cells, leading to a larger mass of fat deposits.
4. Obesity: Lipedema and obesity are distinct conditions, but they frequently coexist, with up to 85% of patients with lipedema also being obese. The presence of obesity in individuals with lipedema increases their risk of developing lymphedema. Diagnosing lipedema, distinguishing it from lymphedema or obesity, or recognizing the co-occurrence of these conditions can be challenging. Body mass index (BMI) is a measure that shows the relationship between an individual's weight and height, offering healthcare professionals a tool to assess a patient's general health. BMI categorizes individuals as underweight, normal weight, overweight, or obese. However, BMI does not provide a complete assessment of a patient's health or their full body composition, though it is widely used in diagnosing various diseases.

Lipedema is metabolically different from obesity; both involve excessive fat accumulation, but they differ in fat distribution. Obesity typically results in central body fat, especially in the abdomen, and is linked to conditions like diabetes, high blood pressure, high cholesterol, and cardiovascular disease. In contrast, lipedema is characterized by peripheral fat accumulation in the extremities, usually not affecting the abdomen or waist. Yet, as both conditions can increase a patient's BMI, misdiagnosis is common and problematic. This demonstrates why BMI is not a reliable biological method for diagnosing either obesity or lipedema.

5. Sedentary lifestyle: Lack of exercise and physical activity can contribute to the development and worsening of lipedema. People with lipedema often suffer from quadriceps weakness, which impairs their ability to effectively strengthen

these muscles for walking or running. This weakness might impede the ability to raise their legs, causing quick exhaustion and frequently leading to a sedentary way of life. Maintaining a consistent regimen of physical exercise is essential for those with lipedema in order to mitigate the risk of mobility impairments.

Lipedema can result in edema and fluid retention as adipose tissue expands, potentially resulting in lipoatrophy or adipose tissue degeneration. This ailment may result in ambulatory challenges due to discomfort experienced when extending the legs. Edema may also manifest in the axillary region, inguinal area, and inner femoral region, resulting in discomfort when raising the legs due to the presence of prominent adipose tissue in these regions. It is recommended to regularly evaluate symptoms and seek medical advice if any changes occur.

Ankles may experience pain when excessive weight is placed on the fatty tissue that supports the foot, resulting in continuous pressure. Special footwear with inner soles or ankle straps may be necessary for alleviation. The pain can worsen when wearing high heels since they exert additional strain on the feet and ankles. Achilles tendon weakness is a frequent problem in individuals with lipedema, which can be relieved by wearing shoes with lower heels or ankle straps. Applying cushioning around the Achilles tendon can alleviate discomfort and stress. Lipedema does not inherently impair muscle strength, even while fatty tissue is present. Primarily impacting females between the ages of 20 and 50, this condition may also manifest in children.

Lipedema can cause decreased blood circulation in the ankles, resulting in edema and alterations in skin color. Adopting nonrestrictive footwear and applying sunscreen when exposed to the sun for extended periods are preventative methods. Compression garments can additionally aid in diminishing the accumulation of fluid and alleviating discomfort. Gastrocnemius muscle weakness can lead to a sluggish and fatigued walking pattern, as well as hindered running ability, due to inadequate strength in the calves and foot. This condition is predominantly prevalent among women, with a mere 15% reporting no occurrence of calf muscle weakness.

A considerable number of individuals with lipedema experience substantial adipose tissue buildup in the abdominal region, which adversely impacts their respiratory function and ability to ambulate effectively. Maintaining a consistent exercise routine is essential for preventing severe belly edema.

Excessive accumulation of adipose tissue can cause reduced flexibility in the abdomen region and ankles, resulting in challenges when assuming an upright sitting or standing position and necessitating the use of specialized footwear or supportive equipment. The swelling in the flexor hallucis longus, which leads to the outward turning of the feet, can be effectively controlled by choosing suitable footwear.

Lipedema can also impair flexibility in the thighs, rendering it difficult to extend the knees while in an upright position or during locomotion and resulting in discomfort.

Properly fitting shoes and supportive devices are crucial for facilitating mobility and minimizing discomfort. Foot pain caused by excessive adipose tissue can be effectively alleviated by utilizing appropriate arch support in footwear.

6. Poor diet: Consuming a diet high in processed foods, sugar, and unhealthy fats can contribute to inflammation and fluid retention, worsening lipedema symptoms.
7. Injuries and surgeries: Trauma, surgery, or other forms of tissue damage can trigger the onset of lipedema or worsen existing symptoms.

It is important to note that while these risk factors have been identified, they do not necessarily guarantee the development of lipedema. The condition can still occur in individuals without any identifiable risk factors, and not all individuals with risk factors will develop lipedema.

Understanding risk factors is crucial in various fields such as health, finance, environmental science, and safety. These factors are characteristics, conditions, or behaviors that increase the probability of an event or condition occurring. Recognizing and understanding these factors is essential for several reasons, including prevention and early intervention, targeted screening and monitoring, resource allocation, policy and regulation development, risk reduction strategies, personalized healthcare approaches, educational and behavioral interventions, research and development, legal and insurance implications, and global health and epidemic preparedness.

In healthcare, identifying risk factors allows for early intervention and prevention strategies, such as targeting smoking cessation programs for lung cancer. In public health and safety, understanding risk factors helps in efficient resource allocation, such as allocating more resources for emergency preparedness and response.

Suggested Reading

Allen EV, Hines EA, Hines EA. Lipedema of the legs: a syndrome characterized by fat legs and orthostatic edema. *Proc Staff Meet Mayo Clin.* 1940;15:184–187.

Wold L, Hines EA, Jr, Allen EV. Lipedema of the legs: a syndrome characterized by fat legs and edema. *Ann Intern Med.* 1951;34(5):1243–1250. doi: https://doi.org/10.7326/0003-4819-34-5-1243.

Whonamedit? *Allen-Hines syndrome.* 2021. [citado 2021 out 28]. https://www.whonamedit.com/synd.cfm/2015.html.

Kruppa P, Georgiou I, Biermann N, Prantl L, Klein-Weigel P, Ghods M. Lipedema-Pathogenesis, Diagnosis, and Treatment Options. *Dtsch Arztebl Int.* 2020;117(22–23):396–403.

Amato ACM. Is lipedema a unique entity? *EC Clin Med Cases Reports.* 2020;2:1–7.

Dudek JE, Białaszek W, Gabriel M. Quality of life, its factors, and sociodemographic characteristics of Polish women with lipedema. *BMC Womens Health.* 2021;21(1):27. doi: https://doi.org/10.1186/s12905-021-01174-y.

Fife CE, Maus EA, Carter MJ. Lipedema: a frequently misdiagnosed and misunderstood fatty deposition syndrome. *Adv Skin Wound Care.* 2010;23(2):81–92. doi: https://doi.org/10.1097/01.ASW.0000363503.92360.91.

Beninson J, Edelglass JW. Lipedema: the non-lymphatic masquerader. *Angiology.* 1984;35(8):506–510. doi: https://doi.org/10.1177/000331978403500806.
Amato ACM, Amato FCM, Benitti DA, Santos RV. Translation, cultural adaptation, and validation of a lipedema symptoms questionnaire. *J Vasc Bras.* 2020a;19:e20200049. doi: https://doi.org/10.1590/1677-5449.200049.
Amato ACM, Saucedo DZ, Santos KS, Benitti DA. Ultrasound criteria for lipedema diagnosis. *Phlebol J Venous Dis.* 2021;36(8):026835552110023.
Cellina M, Gibelli D, Soresina M, et al. Non-contrast MR Lymphography of lipedema of the lower extremities. *Magn Reson Imaging.* 2020;71:115–124. doi: https://doi.org/10.1016/j.mri.2020.06.010.
Monnin-Delhom ED, Gallix BP, Achard C, Bruel JM, Janbon C. High resolution unenhanced computed tomography in patients with swollen legs. *Lymphology.* 2002;35(3):121–128.
Amato ACM, Amato FCM, Benitti DA, Amato LGL. Criação de questionário e modelo de rastreamento de lipedema. *J Vasc Bras.* 2020b;19:e20200114. doi: https://doi.org/10.1590/1677-5449.200114.
Mandrekar JN. Receiver operating characteristic curve in diagnostic test assessment. *J Thorac Oncol.* 2010;5(9):1315–1316. doi: https://doi.org/10.1097/JTO.0b013e3181ec173d.
Choy M, Switzer P, De Martel C, Parsonnet J. Estimating disease prevalence using census data. *Epidemiol Infect.* 2008;136(9):1253–1260. doi: https://doi.org/10.1017/S0950268807009752.
Herpertz U. Krankheitsspektrum des lipodems an einer lymphologischen fachklinik – erscheinungsformen, mischbilder und behandlungsmoglichkeiten. *Vasomed.* 1997;9:301–307.
Amato ACM, Markus DV, dos Santos RV. Lipedema associado a obesidade, linfedema e insuficiência venosa: relato de um caso. *Diagnóstico e Trat.* 2020c;25:4–8.
Schwahn-Schreiber C, Marshall M. Prävalenz des Lipödems bei berufstätigen Frauen in Deutschland. *Phlebologie.* 2011;40(03):127–134. doi: https://doi.org/10.1055/s-0037-1621766.
Instituto Brasileiro de Geografia e Estatística – IBGE *Projeção da população brasileira.* 2021. [citado 2021 out 28]. https://www.ibge.gov.br/apps/populacao/projecao/index.html .
Heen MSJ, Lieberman JD, Miethe TD. A comparison of different online sampling approaches for generating national samples. *Cent Crime Justice Policy.* 2014;1:1–8.
Instituto Brasileiro de Geografia e Estatística – IBGE *Tabela 5919: população, por níveis de instrução.* 2021. [citado 2021 out 28]. SIDRA. https://sidra.ibge.gov.br/tabela/5919.
Nunnaly J, Bernstein I. *No psychometric theory.* 3rd. New York: McGraw-Hill; 1994.
Asmussen PD, Földi M, Strößenreuther R, et al. *Földi's textbook of lymphology for physicians and lymphedema therapists.* München: Elsevier Urban & Fischer; 2012.
Forner-Cordero I, Szolnoky G, Forner-Cordero A, Kemény L. Lipedema: an overview of its clinical manifestations, diagnosis and treatment of the disproportional fatty deposition syndrome – systematic review. *Clin Obes.* 2012;2(3–4):86–95. doi: https://doi.org/10.1111/j.1758-8111.2012.00045.x.
Schmeller W, Hueppe M, Meier-Vollrath I. Tumescent liposuction in lipoedema yields good long-term results. *Br J Dermatol.* 2012;166(1):161–168. doi: https://doi.org/10.1111/j.1365-2133.2011.10566.x.
Harwood CA, Bull RH, Evans J, Mortimer PS. Lymphatic and venous function in lipoedema. *Br J Dermatol.* 1996;134(1):1–6. doi: https://doi.org/10.1111/j.1365-2133.1996.tb07831.x.
Ruopp MD, Perkins NJ, Whitcomb BW, Schisterman EF. Youden index and optimal cut-point estimated from observations affected by a lower limit of detection. *Biom J.* 2008;50(3):419–430. doi: https://doi.org/10.1002/bimj.200710415.
Moraes IN. Cânones da beleza. *Rev Cult e Saude.* 2003;1:25–30.
Child AH, Gordon KD, Sharpe P, et al. Lipedema: an inherited condition. *Am J Med Genet A.* 2010;152A(4):970–976. doi: https://doi.org/10.1002/ajmg.a.33313.
Dudek JE, Białaszek W, Ostaszewski P. Quality of life in women with lipoedema: a contextual behavioral approach. *Qual Life Res.* 2016;25(2):401–408. doi: https://doi.org/10.1007/s11136-015-1080-x.

Romeijn JRM, de Rooij MJM, Janssen L, Martens H. Exploration of Patient Characteristics and Quality of Life in Patients with Lipoedema Using a Survey. *Dermatol Ther (Heidelb)* 2018;8(2):303–311. doi: https://doi.org/10.1007/s13555-018-0241-6.

Amato ACM, Silva AEC, Bernal IM, et al. Combined nutcracker and Ehlers-Danlos syndromes: a case report. *EJVES Vasc Forum.* 2020d;47:12–17. doi: https://doi.org/10.1016/j.ejvsvf.2020.02.005.

Buck DW, 2nd, Herbst KL. Lipedema: a relatively common disease with extremely common misconceptions. *Plast Reconstr Surg Glob Open.* 2016;4(9):e1043. doi: https://doi.org/10.1097/GOX.0000000000001043.

Wollina U, Heinig B. Treatment of lipedema by low-volume micro-cannular liposuction in tumescent anesthesia: results in 111 patients. *Dermatol Ther.* 2019;32(2):e12820. doi: https://doi.org/10.1111/dth.12820.

Herbst KL, Kahn LA, Iker E, et al. Standard of care for lipedema in the United States. *Phlebology.* 2021;36(10):779–796. doi: https://doi.org/10.1177/02683555211015887.

La Torre YSD, Wadeea R, Rosas V, Herbst KL. Lipedema: friend and foe. *Horm Mol Biol Clin Investig.* 2018;33(1):20170076. doi: https://doi.org/10.1515/hmbci-2017-0076.

Reich-Schupke S, Altmeyer P, Stücker M. Thick legs: not always lipedema Stefanie. *J Dtsch Dermatol Ges.* 2013;11(3):225–234.

Dayan E, Kim JN, Smith ML, et al. *Lipedema – The Disease They Call FAT: An Overview for Clinicians.* Lipedema Simplified Publications; 2017

Clinical Manifestation

The clinical manifestations of lipedema are diverse and necessitate a discerning approach for accurate recognition and diagnosis. Lipedema is a chronic condition characterized by an abnormal and symmetrical accumulation of adipose tissue in the extremities, primarily affecting the legs and, in some cases, the arms. This accumulation is often resistant to diet and exercise and typically spares the feet, creating a "bracelet" effect above the ankles. The clinical features of lipedema include a disproportionate lower body size, a column-like shape of the legs, and a soft texture of the subcutaneous tissue, which may become more fibrotic over time. Patients frequently report tenderness, easy bruising, and pain within the affected areas, which are not typical of general obesity. The presence of these symptoms, particularly in conjunction with a family history of similar characteristics, is suggestive of lipedema.

Recognizing these clinical features is crucial, as lipedema is often misunderstood as simple obesity or lymphedema. Early and accurate recognition of lipedema is important for several reasons: It facilitates earlier intervention, which may help to manage symptoms and prevent progression. It informs appropriate patient counseling and support, which is essential given the condition's impact on physical and psychological well-being. It helps to delineate lipedema from other conditions, ensuring that patients receive the most effective, targeted treatment. Ultimately, awareness of lipedema's clinical manifestations enables healthcare professionals to offer better care and support to those living with this condition.

The early signs and symptoms of lipedema are distinctive and can be markedly different from normal adiposity, warranting a thorough understanding for timely recognition and intervention. Lipedema typically presents initially as a symmetrical enlargement of the legs, often beginning at the hips and buttocks and extending down to the ankles, with the feet remaining unaffected—a characteristic known as the "ankle bracelet" sign. This disproportionate fat distribution is often unresponsive to dieting and exercise, which is a stark contrast to normal adiposity where weight loss is more uniform. Common symptoms in the early stages include a tendency to bruise easily; a dull, aching discomfort in the legs; and a heaviness that

G. Laur, *Lipoedema*, https://doi.org/10.1007/978-981-96-8939-2_11

may not correlate with the actual weight of the limbs. Unlike normal adipose tissue, lipedema fat can be tender to the touch, and patients may report pain when pressure is applied, even if it is gentle. The skin over the affected areas may retain a normal texture in the initial stages, which helps differentiate it from later stages of lipedema where nodularity and fibrosis become more apparent. These early clinical presentations are key to differentiating lipedema from typical fat accumulation, setting the stage for accurate diagnosis and management of the condition before progression to more advanced and challenging stages.

The physical characteristics of lipedema are distinct and play a central role in the diagnosis of this chronic condition. Lipedema is primarily characterized by symmetrical fat distribution that affects the lower body, most notably the legs, and can also affect the arms. This adiposity typically starts at the hips and extends to the ankles, sparing the feet, thus creating a "bracelet" effect above the ankles. The upper body remains relatively unaffected, which can result in a dramatic disproportion between the two halves of the body. The typical areas of involvement are the legs (including the thighs, inner knees, calves) and the arms, particularly the upper arms. Uncommonly, lipedema may also involve the trunk or the upper body, although this is less frequent.

The texture and feel of lipedema fat are distinctive; in the early stages, the adipose tissue often feels soft, like a gelatinous substance, and is unusually tender to the touch. As the condition progresses, the texture can become more nodular or lumpy, resembling the texture of an orange peel or mattress foam, indicative of fibrotic changes within the tissue. These palpable qualities, along with the pain and bruising often associated with lipedema fat, set it apart from the more even distribution and firmness of normal adiposity or the pitting edema seen in conditions such as lymphedema. Understanding the physical characteristics of lipedema is crucial for healthcare providers as it aids in the differential diagnosis from other forms of adipose tissue accumulation and guides appropriate management strategies.

Pain and sensitivity are hallmark features of lipedema, profoundly affecting patient experience and quality of life. The types of pain associated with lipedema are multifaceted; patients often report a chronic, dull ache or heaviness in the affected limbs, accompanied by episodes of sharp, shooting pains. Additionally, there is a characteristic tenderness and sensitivity to pressure and touch, even light contact, which is not observed in normal adiposity or other forms of edema. This heightened pain response is thought to be due to increased pressure in the fatty tissue leading to hypoxia and inflammation, as well as possibly an abnormality in the pain processing pathways.

The impact of this pain and sensitivity on daily activities can be substantial. The discomfort may limit mobility and endurance, leading to difficulties with standing for long periods, climbing stairs, and engaging in physical activities that are otherwise necessary for maintaining health. The persistent pain can also interfere with sleep and lead to chronic fatigue, which further diminishes the ability to perform daily tasks. Moreover, the psychosocial impact, including body image dissatisfaction and social stigma, can exacerbate stress and contribute to a cycle of pain and emotional distress. Thus, pain and sensitivity are not merely symptoms of lipedema but are central to the patient's clinical presentation and require targeted strategies within the management plan to improve overall function and well-being.

The progression of lipedema is typically categorized into stages, each characterized by distinct changes in symptoms and physical appearance, and is influenced by various factors. The disease generally initiates with stage 1, where patients present with a smooth skin surface overlying enlarged subcutaneous fat tissue with a normal skin texture. Transitioning into stage 2, the skin begins to exhibit a nodular or "mattress" appearance due to the enlargement of the fat lobules and the development of fibrotic tissue. By stage 3, the hypertrophic fat lobules become more pronounced, leading to significant contour deformities and skin folds, which may impede mobility. In some cases, lipedema may progress to include lymphedema, characterized as stage 4 or lipolymphedema, where lymphatic dysfunction exacerbates the swelling and skin changes.

The symptoms of lipedema, such as tenderness, heaviness, and pain, typically intensify as the condition advances. Factors influencing the progression of lipedema include hormonal changes, genetic predisposition, lifestyle, and weight management. Hormonal events such as puberty, pregnancy, and menopause are often associated with the onset or exacerbation of lipedema, suggesting a strong hormonal component to its progression. Moreover, individuals with a family history of lipedema are more likely to experience a more rapid or severe course of the disease. Lifestyle factors, including diet and physical activity, though not directly causative, can influence the severity of symptoms and overall disease burden. Understanding the stages and progression of lipedema is imperative for clinicians to provide timely interventions, to prevent complications, and to mitigate the impact on patients' quality of life.

In patients with lipedema, dermatological changes are both characteristic and diagnostic. As the disease progresses, alterations in skin texture manifest, initially presenting as a soft, dough-like consistency and eventually progressing to a more nodular, rubbery texture reminiscent of cellulite.

This change in texture is a result of increased fibrosis within the subcutaneous tissue. Concurrently, the overlying skin may demonstrate changes in coloration, ranging from pallor due to underlying circulatory compromise to erythema associated with inflammation. The skin of patients with lipedema displays a marked susceptibility to bruising, a phenomenon attributed to increased fragility of blood vessels within the fatty deposits.

Wound healing can be notably impaired in these individuals, often due to the compromised local vascular supply and secondary lymphatic dysfunction, leading to prolonged healing times and increased risk of infection. Secondary dermatological conditions that may arise include stasis dermatitis, which results from venous insufficiency often coexisting with lipedema, and lymphorrhea, the leakage of lymph fluid through the skin, which can occur when lipedema progresses to lipolymphedema. Moreover, the chronic inflammatory state of lipedema tissue may predispose patients to develop cellulitis, further complicating the clinical picture. Recognizing these skin and dermatological changes is essential for the comprehensive care of patients with lipedema, guiding both the diagnostic process and the subsequent management strategies, which must incorporate skin care to maintain integrity and prevent secondary complications.

Ultrasound studies have revealed distinct characteristics of lipedema tissue, including thinner skin, increased thickness, and heightened hypoechogenicity of subcutaneous fat, particularly pronounced in the medial calf and distal extremities. The severity of lipedema is often assessed by the thickness of the subcutaneous fat layer, with classifications ranging from mild (12 to 15 mm) to severe (>30 mm).

Interestingly, these measurements overlap with those observed in cases of obesity, highlighting the need for a comprehensive assessment of other symptoms for an accurate diagnosis. Common clinical features of lipedema include an onset during puberty, an inability to reduce fat above the waist through diet alone, disproportionate fat distribution primarily affecting the lower extremities, tenderness upon pressure, easy bruising, varicose veins, vein telangiectasia, and the presence of fat pads (bulging protuberances) above or below the knee, known as pretibial fat pads.

Surprisingly, lipedema can affect individuals across a wide BMI range, including those with normal BMI, pre-obesity, overweight, and various obesity classes. Lipedema is further categorized into stages, with stage 1 showing pea-sized fat nodules within the hypodermis but normal skin appearance. In stage 2, the skin exhibits dimpling, indentations, and mattress-like patterns due to connective tissue thickening over increased fat. Stage 3 involves lobular extrusions of skin, fat, and fascia tissue, resulting in compromised blood and lymph flow, potentially impacting joint integrity, mobility, and balance. Stage 4 is associated with lipolymphedema, a combination of lipedema and lymphedema, characterized by severe swelling and fat deposition.

Types of lipedema are anatomically classified, with type 1 affecting the region from the umbilicus to the hips, type 2 extending from the pelvis to the knees, type 3 involving the region from the pelvis to the ankles with an ankle cuff, type 4 covering the shoulders to the wrists, and type 5 being a rare occurrence that encompasses fat distribution from below the knees to the ankles while sparing the dorsum of the feet. Various combinations of these types are also observed, with arm involvement varying from the elbows to the wrists or extending from the shoulders to the wrists.

These dermatological manifestations highlight the complexity and variability of lipedema, necessitating a multidimensional approach to diagnosis and management.

The lymphatic system is a complex network of vessels and nodes that helps to maintain fluid balance in the body and defend against infection. In lipedema, the abnormal accumulation of fat can compress the lymphatic vessels, leading to impaired lymphatic drainage and fluid accumulation in the tissues. This can lead to the development of lymphedema, a condition characterized by swelling and inflammation of the affected limbs.

Mobility and functional impairments are significant concerns in the clinical management of lipedema, given their profound impact on patients' quality of life. The characteristic adipose tissue deposition around the lower extremities can lead to a reduction in mobility, often altering gait patterns. Patients may adopt a wider stance to accommodate the increased girth of the limbs, which can lead to an abnormal gait and secondary musculoskeletal issues due to altered biomechanics. Joint pain, particularly in the knees, hips, and ankles, is commonly reported, likely due to the increased load and stress on the joints from the excess weight of the adipose tissue.

These musculoskeletal issues are often compounded by the inherent pain and tenderness of the lipedematous tissue, which may further restrict movement. The cumulative effect of these factors results in considerable limitations in daily living activities. Tasks such as climbing stairs, running, and even prolonged standing become increasingly challenging, leading to a sedentary lifestyle that can exacerbate the condition. In advanced stages, the mobility impairment may lead to disability and the need for assistive devices. Addressing these functional impairments through targeted physical therapy, pain management, and weight control is crucial to improving the overall functionality and well-being of individuals with lipedema. Research on the orthopedic manifestations of lipedema has shed light on the significant burden this condition places on the musculoskeletal system. A study involving 138 participants with lipedema revealed that 30% of them had a high arch, a condition known as pes cavus, which can affect balance and stability. Additionally, 15% of participants had flat feet, which can lead to various foot and ankle issues.

Furthermore, knee abnormalities were prevalent in this study cohort, with less than 4% of participants exhibiting varus knee (bowlegged) alignment, while 39% had valgus knee (knock-knee) alignment. Valgus knee alignment can result in increased stress on the medial compartment of the knee joint, potentially contributing to joint pain and degeneration.

Knee pain was a prevalent and distressing symptom among individuals with lipedema, affecting 63% of the study participants. On average, the severity of knee pain was rated at 6 out of 10, indicating a significant level of discomfort. Osteoarthritis, a degenerative joint condition, was identified in 13% of the participants. Notably, the severity of osteoarthritis was found to be more pronounced in older individuals with higher body mass indices (BMI) and advanced stages of lipedema.

The high prevalence of knee pain and orthopedic alterations underscores the critical importance of including orthopedic evaluation in the comprehensive assessment of patients with lipedema.

Clinicians should consider the musculoskeletal impact of lipedema and be vigilant in identifying orthopedic abnormalities, such as pes cavus, flat feet, and knee misalignments. Early detection and intervention can be crucial in preventing further musculoskeletal deterioration.

Moreover, the increased incidence and severity of osteoarthritis associated with lipedema highlight the need for proactive management strategies. It is essential to address pain and mobility issues promptly to enhance the patient's overall quality of life. Management should encompass a multidisciplinary approach, including physical therapy, orthopedic consultations, and, potentially, surgical interventions when indicated.

The clinical presentation of lipedema is marked by significant variability, influenced by individual, ethnic, and genetic factors. Individual variations in manifestation are considerable; some patients may present with early-onset lipedema that rapidly progresses, while others may experience a slow evolution of symptoms over decades. The distribution of adipose tissue can also vary, with some individuals predominantly affected in the lower extremities and others displaying involvement of the arms or even the upper torso. Ethnic background plays a role in the clinical expression of lipedema, affecting both the pattern of fat distribution and the progression of the disease. For example, certain ethnic groups may exhibit more pronounced lower body adiposity due to genetic predisposition, potentially masking or mimicking the appearance of lipedema.

Furthermore, genetic factors can influence not only the likelihood of developing lipedema but also the severity and specific characteristics of the disease. Familial aggregation studies suggest a hereditary component, with many patients reporting a family history of similar symptoms. Research into specific genetic markers and pathways is ongoing, with the aim of elucidating the pathophysiology and inheritance patterns of lipedema. This variability in clinical presentation underscores the need for a personalized approach to diagnosis and management, taking into account the unique aspects of each patient's condition. Understanding the individual and demographic factors that influence the presentation of lipedema is critical for healthcare providers to deliver culturally competent and genetically informed care.

The clinical manifestations of lipedema comprise a spectrum of symptoms, including disproportionate and symmetrical fat accumulation in the lower extremities, a tendency for easy bruising, and a characteristic pain and tenderness in the adipose tissue. These manifestations can lead to significant physical discomfort and mobility limitations, affecting patients' quality of life. The disease typically spares the feet, creating a "bracelet" effect at the ankles, and may also involve the arms. Over time, the affected areas may develop a nodular texture, and secondary lymphatic complications such as lipolymphedema can arise. The variability in presentation, influenced by genetic and ethnic factors, necessitates a discerning approach to diagnosis.

Early recognition of lipedema is crucial; it enables timely intervention, which can slow disease progression, alleviate symptoms, and mitigate associated psychosocial impacts.

A holistic management plan is essential, not only addressing the physical aspects of lipedema through modalities, such as compression therapy and manual lymphatic drainage, but also incorporating dietary guidance, psychological support, and physical rehabilitation. Such comprehensive care is pivotal in managing this chronic condition effectively, as it considers the multifaceted challenges faced by individuals with lipedema. Healthcare providers must maintain a high index of suspicion for lipedema in patients presenting with its characteristic features, despite a prevalence of obesity in the population, to distinguish it from other causes of limb enlargement and to offer specialized care that can significantly improve patient outcomes.

Suggested Reading

Zaleska MT, Olszewski WL, Krzesniak NE. Lower Limb Lipedema-Superficial Lymph Flow, Skin Water Concentration, Skin and Subcutaneous Tissue Elasticity. Lymphat Res Biol. 2023 Feb;21(1):60–69. doi: https://doi.org/10.1089/lrb.2022.0010. Epub 2022 Jun 8. PMID: 35675661.

Herbst KL. Subcutaneous Adipose Tissue Diseases: Dercum Disease, Lipedema, Familial Multiple Lipomatosis, and Madelung Disease. 2019 Dec 14. In: Feingold KR, Anawalt B, Blackman MR, Boyce A, Chrousos G, Corpas E, de Herder WW, Dhatariya K, Dungan K, Hofland J, Kalra S, Kaltsas G, Kapoor N, Koch C, Kopp P, Korbonits M, Kovacs CS, Kuohung W, Laferrère B, Levy M, McGee EA, McLachlan R, New M, Purnell J, Sahay R, Shah AS, Singer F, Sperling MA, Stratakis CA, Trence DL, Wilson DP, editors. Endotext [Internet]. South Dartmouth (MA): MDText.com, Inc.; 2000–. PMID: 31895524.

Földi M, Földi E, Strößenreuther R, Kubik S. *Urban & Fischer.* München, Germany: 2012. Lipedema Földi's textbook of lymphology: for physicians and lymphedema therapists 3rd Edition; pp. 364–369.

Meier-Vollrath I, Schneider W, Schmeller W. Lipödem: Verbesserte Lebensqualität durch Therapiekombination. *Dtsch Arztebl.* 2005;102:A1061–A-1067.

Forner-Cordero I, Szolnoky G, Forner-Cordero A, Kemeny L. Lipedema: an overview of its clinical manifestations, diagnosis and treatment of the disproportional fatty deposition syndrome – systematic review. *Clin Obes.* 2012;2:86–95.

Peled AW, Kappos EA. Lipedema: diagnostic and management challenges. *Int J Womens Health.* 2016;8:389–395.

Deutsche Gesellschaft für Phlebologie D. S1-Leitlinie Lipödem. *AWMF.* 2015

Buck DW 2nd, Herbst KL. Lipedema: a relatively common disease with extremely common misconceptions. *Plast Reconstr Surg Glob Open.* 2016;4

Allen EV, Hines EA. Lipedema of the legs: a syndrome characterized by fat legs and orthostatic edema. *Proc Staff Mayo Clinic.* 1940:184–187.

Bauer AT, von Lukowicz D, Lossagk K, et al. New insights on lipedema: the enigmatic disease of the peripheral fat. *Plast Reconstr Surg.* 2019;144:1475–1484.

Fife CE, Maus EA, Carter MJ. Lipedema: a frequently misdiagnosed and misunderstood fatty deposition syndrome. *Adv Skin Wound Care.* 2010;23:81–92. quiz 3–4.

Langendoen SI, Habbema L, Nijsten TE, Neumann HA. Lipoedema: from clinical presentation to therapy A review of the literature. *Br J Dermatol.* 2009;161:980–986.

Clinical Examination

Lipedema is a chronic, progressive medical condition predominantly affecting women, marked by the pathological accumulation of adipose tissue, which symmetrically engulfs the lower extremities and occasionally the arms. Despite its distinct clinical presentation, lipedema is often misdiagnosed or overlooked, leading to a significant impact on quality of life due to pain, mobility restrictions, and psychosocial distress. The pathophysiology of lipedema is not fully understood but is believed to involve genetic, hormonal, and inflammatory factors that contribute to its development and progression. Clinically significant due to its differentiation from obesity and lymphedema, lipedema fat is resistant to both diet and exercise interventions. Furthermore, the condition is associated with a heightened risk of comorbidities, including venous insufficiency, joint disorders, and psychosocial issues. Lipedema's significance in the medical field is amplified by its potential to transition to lipolymphedema, a more complex condition resulting from secondary lymphatic dysfunction, which exacerbates the risk of infection and skin changes. The importance of lipedema lies not only in its physical manifestations but also in the need for increased awareness and research to improve diagnostic accuracy, develop effective treatment modalities, and ultimately enhance patient care and outcomes.

The clinical examination for lipedema is quintessential for establishing a definitive diagnosis and formulating an appropriate management strategy. The objectives of this examination are multifold: initially, it aims to identify the characteristic features of lipedema, such as symmetrical enlargement of the limbs, disproportionate fat accumulation, and tenderness to palpation. A precise assessment distinguishes lipedema from other adipose disorders like lymphedema and obesity, which can present with similar phenotypes but differ in pathophysiology and treatment approach. The examination includes evaluating the consistency of the adipose tissue, the presence of a positive Stemmer sign (which is indicative of lymphedema), and the absence of pitting edema, which is typically not associated with lipedema. Additionally, the clinical examination is instrumental in assessing the stage of lipedema, based on the extent of fat deposition and the presence of secondary

G. Laur, *Lipoedema*, https://doi.org/10.1007/978-981-96-8939-2_12

changes, such as fibrosis and nodularity. A comprehensive physical evaluation also screens for associated comorbidities, including venous insufficiency, joint pain, and mobility limitations. By establishing the severity and impact of lipedema on a patient's quality of life, the examination informs a tailored treatment plan that addresses both physical and psychosocial health components. Ultimately, the clinical examination serves not only to elucidate the diagnosis but also to monitor the progression of the disease and the effectiveness of interventions over time.

The collection of a detailed medical and family history is a critical step in the evaluation of patients suspected of having lipedema, as it assists clinicians in distinguishing this condition from other adipose and lymphatic disorders. A comprehensive history should document the onset of symptoms, particularly the age at which fat accumulation began and whether it correlates with hormonal changes such as puberty, pregnancy, or menopause, which are often reported triggers in lipedema. The pattern of symptom development, including bilaterality, distribution of fat, and presence of pain or bruising, provides insight into the characteristic features of the disorder. Family history is equally essential, as lipedema shows a genetic predisposition; therefore, the presence of similar symptoms in family members can be a significant diagnostic clue. Additionally, lifestyle factors including diet, exercise, and occupation are important to document, as they can influence the severity of lipedema symptoms and overall health. These factors may also provide a foundation for developing individualized management plans that address weight management and mobility, which are central to the treatment of lipedema. Accurate documentation of these components facilitates a comprehensive approach to care, guiding potential genetic counseling and informing decisions about further diagnostic assessments or referrals to specialists. Recognizing the importance of these elements underscores the need for a holistic approach to patient assessment, which is paramount in the management of lipedema.

The physical examination of lipedema is a nuanced process that necessitates a systematic approach, beginning with a detailed inspection of the affected areas. Clinicians visually assess for the hallmark lipedema characteristics: a disproportionate accumulation of adipose tissue, typically manifesting as symmetrical enlargement of the legs, often with a distinct demarcation just above the ankles where the feet remain unaffected. This visual inspection must evaluate the color, texture, and any visible vascular abnormalities or skin changes. Palpation follows, which is critical for assessing the texture of the adipose tissue; early lipedema is characterized by a soft, dough-like consistency, whereas advanced stages may present with increased fibrosis and nodularity. Palpation also discerns tenderness, a distinguishing feature of lipedema that may not be present in other conditions such as simple obesity. Tenderness is typically diffuse rather than localized to specific nodules. Additionally, the examination includes an assessment of the symmetry and distribution of swelling, as lipedema typically presents with a bilaterally symmetrical pattern, contrasting with the often asymmetric swelling seen in lymphedema. Together, these examination techniques form a comprehensive assessment that not only assists in the diagnosis of lipedema but also contributes to staging the disease, which is crucial for treatment planning and establishing a baseline for monitoring disease progression.

Assessing pain and sensitivity in lipedema is a complex yet crucial aspect of the clinical evaluation, as pain is a defining symptom of the condition. Methods for evaluating pain levels typically include the use of standardized pain assessment tools such as visual analog scales (VAS), numeric rating scales (NRS), or the McGill Pain Questionnaire, which enable patients to quantify their pain and describe its nature. These tools aid clinicians in identifying the chronic, often aching pain characteristic of lipedema, which is typically exacerbated by pressure or touch. Distinguishing lipedema pain from other causes is imperative; lipedema-associated pain is usually not responsive to common weight loss methods and may not correlate with the size of the affected limbs, unlike the mechanical pain due to excess weight in obesity. Patients may report a unique sensitivity, describing the pain as a bruise-like sensation even in the absence of visible bruising. Furthermore, it is essential to differentiate the pain of lipedema from neuropathic pain, which may have a burning or shooting quality, and from the heaviness associated with venous insufficiency. By accurately assessing and documenting the pain and sensitivity specific to lipedema, clinicians can tailor pain management strategies effectively and monitor the impact of therapeutic interventions over time.

Measurement and documentation are components in the physical examination of lipedema, providing objective data to track the progression of the disease and the efficacy of treatments.

Circumferential measurements of the limbs at consistent anatomical landmarks are essential for quantifying the extent of lipedema. Standardized techniques, such as using a flexible, non-stretchable measuring tape, ensure consistent and accurate measurement. The tape should be placed horizontally around the limb at specific points, such as the ankle, the point of maximal calf circumference, the knee, and the thigh at set intervals above the patella. These measurements should be taken with the patient in a standing position, ensuring that the tape is snug but not compressing the tissue. Baseline measurements are critical for future comparisons, documenting both the absolute values and any changes in limb size over time. Repeated measurements, ideally by the same practitioner to minimize inter-observer variability, are necessary for monitoring the natural history of lipedema or the response to interventions such as compression therapy, diet, or surgery. Accurate and repeated circumferential measurements are invaluable in creating a comprehensive picture of disease progression, guiding clinical decisions, and measuring treatment outcomes.

Mobility and functional assessment form an integral part of the clinical evaluation for patients with lipedema, as the condition frequently imposes significant limitations on daily activities. Evaluating gait and mobility involves observing the patient's walking pattern, stride length, and speed to detect any alterations that may arise from the excess adipose tissue, such as a widened gait or shortened stride. Clinicians assess joint range of motion to identify restrictions in movement that may be due to the mechanical effects of lipedema on the lower extremities. This assessment often includes measuring the active and passive range of motion of the hips, knees, and ankles using a goniometer, a device that ensures precise angular measurements. Additionally, the impact of lipedema on daily activities is assessed through patient-reported outcomes and functional performance tests. Patients may report difficulty with tasks such as climbing stairs, running, or prolonged standing. Standardized functional assessments like the Timed Up and Go (TUG) test can be employed to objectively measure the patient's functional mobility. Together, these assessments provide a comprehensive understanding of the functional implications of lipedema, aiding in the development of personalized treatment plans that aim to maintain or enhance mobility, reduce pain, and improve overall quality of life.

Skin and tissue assessment is a critical aspect of the comprehensive evaluation of lipedema, necessitating a meticulous and systematic approach. The examination commences with a detailed inspection of the skin for alterations in color, which may suggest circulatory changes, and for texture, which may reveal the presence of the characteristic "mattress" appearance or fibrotic nodules typical of advanced lipedema. Palpation assists in evaluating the temperature of the skin, where localized warmth can indicate inflammation or infection. The propensity for easy bruising in lipedema requires careful inspection for ecchymosis, which can serve as an index for the fragility of the blood vessels within the affected tissues. Moreover, the clinician must vigilantly search for any wounds or signs of infection, as the compromised circulation and lymphatic drainage can result in delayed healing and increased risk of cellulitis. Alongside these assessments, the examiner must evaluate for lymphatic and vascular changes, including the presence of varicosities, telangiectasias, or lymphangiectases, which may signal concurrent lymphatic or venous insufficiency. This skin and tissue assessment not only aids in the staging of lipedema but also in the identification of potential complications that may necessitate targeted interventions.

Accurate and repeated assessments are vital for monitoring the course of the disease and the response to treatment, thereby forming an essential component of the ongoing management of individuals with lipedema.

The staging of lipedema is a critical process in the clinical management of the condition, providing a framework for treatment planning and prognostication. Lipedema is commonly classified into four stages based on clinical criteria that include the appearance and texture of the skin, the presence of pain, and the degree of mobility impairment. Stage 1 is characterized by a smooth skin surface with an underlying layer of small, palpable nodules or fat lobules. In stage 2, the skin becomes uneven or mattress-like due to the growth of larger fat lobules, and there may be some skin discoloration. Stage 3 is marked by large, deforming fat lobules that can create overhanging skin folds, significantly affecting mobility. The most advanced stage, stage 4, is characterized by the presence of lipolymphedema, where lipedema progresses to include lymphedema, exacerbating swelling and skin changes.

Each stage of lipedema carries specific clinical implications. Early stages may be managed with conservative measures such as compression therapy, manual lymphatic drainage, and lifestyle modifications. As lipedema progresses, pain and mobility issues become more pronounced, often necessitating a multidisciplinary approach to treatment that can include physiotherapy, pain management, and psychological support. In the advanced stages, surgical interventions such as liposuction or excisional procedures may be considered to alleviate symptoms and improve function.

Staging is guiding treatment, as it allows clinicians to tailor interventions according to the severity and specific characteristics of the lipedema. It also provides a means for standardizing communication between healthcare providers, facilitating research, and enabling the comparison of treatment outcomes. Accurate staging is, therefore, essential not only for individualized patient care but also for the advancement of knowledge regarding the optimal management of lipedema.

The psychosocial and emotional evaluation of patients with lipedema is an indispensable facet of comprehensive care, addressing the profound impact this chronic condition can have on mental health. Lipedema is not merely a physical ailment; its conspicuous nature and resistance to conventional weight loss strategies often lead to misdiagnosis and social stigma, exacerbating psychological distress. Assessment tools such as questionnaires and structured interviews are employed to gauge the extent of the impact on mental well-being, identifying symptoms of depression, anxiety, and social isolation that patients may experience. Body image and self-esteem are particularly vulnerable in lipedema due to the visible and progressive nature of the disease, which can diverge markedly from societal norms of body shape and size.

Clinicians are tasked with the sensitive role of addressing these issues, recognizing that body image disturbances and diminished self-esteem can significantly hinder patients' quality of life and engagement with treatment. This underscores the importance of integrating psychological support into the treatment regimen, including counseling, support groups, and possibly cognitive-behavioral therapy, tailored to help patients develop coping strategies and resilience. Such support is not ancillary but central to the management of lipedema, as it can alleviate the emotional burden of the condition, enhance adherence to treatment protocols, and ultimately contribute to better overall outcomes.

The inclusion of psychological evaluation and support in the care of patients with lipedema acknowledges the complexity of the condition and affirms the necessity of treating the individual holistically, addressing both the physical and emotional dimensions of their health.

The integration of clinical findings with diagnostic imaging is an aspect of the comprehensive evaluation and management of lipedema. Advanced imaging modalities such as ultrasound and magnetic resonance imaging (MRI) play a vital role in substantiating the clinical diagnosis, assessing the extent of adipose tissue distribution, and identifying underlying tissue changes that may not be apparent on physical examination alone. High-resolution ultrasound serves as a first-line imaging tool, offering real-time visualization of the subcutaneous fat architecture and facilitating the detection of edema, fibrosis, and vascular anomalies. It can also be used to monitor the progression of the disease over time. MRI provides a more detailed view, allowing for the assessment of both the superficial and deep fat compartments and the differentiation between lipedema and other conditions such as lymphedema or lipomatosis.

Correlating imaging findings with physical examination is essential to ensure a holistic understanding of the condition. For instance, the identification of skin thickening and nodular fat lobules on imaging can confirm the stage of lipedema observed during palpation. Moreover, imaging can uncover the extent of involvement of the lymphatic system, which has direct implications for treatment planning. By integrating clinical examination with imaging studies, healthcare providers can achieve a more accurate diagnosis, tailor interventions more precisely, and better predict treatment outcomes. Consequently, diagnostic imaging not only complements the physical examination but also enhances the clinician's ability to deliver personalized care to patients with lipedema.

In concluding the physical examination of patients with lipedema, it is imperative to synthesize the findings to construct a comprehensive picture of the individual's condition. This involves summarizing the clinical observations regarding the distribution and texture of adipose tissue, the presence of tenderness or pain, mobility restrictions, and any skin or lymphatic changes noted during the examination. The integration of these findings with patient history and, if applicable, diagnostic imaging results allows for the accurate staging of lipedema and identification of any concurrent conditions that may impact management. Formulating a management plan then necessitates a multidisciplinary approach, incorporating interventions such as compression therapy, manual lymphatic drainage, dietary counseling, and psychological support, tailored to the patient's specific needs and the severity of their condition.

Organizing necessary referrals to specialists, such as dietitians, physiotherapists, or mental health professionals, is critical to ensure comprehensive care. Moreover, establishing a schedule for follow-up recommendations is essential for monitoring the progression of lipedema and adjusting the management plan as needed. Follow-up visits should focus on assessing changes in symptoms, evaluating the effectiveness of the treatment regimen, and addressing any emerging needs of the patient. Through a structured approach to the conclusion and next steps following the physical examination, healthcare providers can ensure that patients with lipedema receive coordinated, patient-centered care that optimizes their quality of life and health outcomes.

Suggested Reading

Wold LE, Hines EA, Allen EV. Lipedema of the legs: a syndrome characterized by fat legs and edema. *Ann Intern Med.* 1951;**34**(5):1243–1250.

Garfein ES, Borud LJ, Warren AG, Slavin SA. Learning from a lymphedema clinic: an algorithm for the management of localized swelling. *Plast Reconstr Surg.* 2008;**121**(2):521–528.

Allen EV, Hines EA. Jr, Lipedema of the legs: a syndrome characterized by fat legs and orthostatic edema. *Mayo Clin Proc.* 1940;**15**:184–187.

Rudkin GH, Miller TA. Lipedema: a clinical entity distinct from lymphedema. *Plast Reconstr Surg.* 1994;**94**(6):841–847.

Harwood CA, Bull RH, Evans J, Mortimer PS. Lymphatic and venous function in lipoedema. *Br J Dermatol.* 1996;**134**(1):1–6.
Beninson J, Edelglass JW. Lipedema – the non-lymphatic masquerader. *Angiology.* 1984;**35**(8):506–510.
Stemmer R. A clinical symptom for the early and differential diagnosis of lymphedema. *Vasa.* 1976;**5**(3):261–262.
Warren AG, Janz BA, Borud LJ, Slavin SA. Evaluation and management of the fat leg syndrome. *Plast Reconstr Surg.* 2007a;**119**(1):9e–15e.
Warren AG, Brorson H, Borud LJ, Slavin SA. Lymphedema: a comprehensive review. *Ann Plast Surg.* 2007b;**59**(4):464–472.
Bilancini S, Lucchi M, Tucci S, Eleuteri P. Functional lymphatic alterations in patients suffering from lipedema. *Angiology.* 1995;**46**(4):333–339.
Jagtman BA, Kuiper JP, Brakkee AJ. Measurements of skin elasticity in patients with lipedema of the Moncorps "rusticanus" type. *Phlebologie.* 1984;**37**(3):315–319.

References

La Torre Y.S.-D., Wadeea R., Rosas V., Herbst K.L. Lipedema: Friend and Foe. *Horm. Mol. Biol. Clin. Investig.* 2018;33:1. doi: https://doi.org/10.1515/hmbci-2017-0076.
Buso G., Depairon M., Tomson D., Raffoul W., Vettor R., Mazzolai L. Lipedema: A Call to Action! *Obesity.* 2019;27:1567. doi: https://doi.org/10.1002/oby.22597.
Shavit E., Wollina U., Alavi A. Lipoedema Is Not Lymphoedema: A Review of Current Literature. *Int. Wound J.* 2018;15:921–928. doi: https://doi.org/10.1111/iwj.12949.
Herbst K.L. Rare Adipose Disorders (RADs) Masquerading as Obesity. *Acta Pharmacol. Sin.* 2012;33:155–172. doi: https://doi.org/10.1038/aps.2011.153.
Buck D.W., Herbst K.L. Lipedema: A Relatively Common Disease with Extremely Common Misconceptions. *Plast. Reconstr. Surg. Glob. Open.* 2016;4:e1043. doi: https://doi.org/10.1097/GOX.0000000000001043.
Herbst K.L., Kahn L.A., Iker E., Ehrlich C., Wright T., McHutchison L., Schwartz J., Sleigh M., Donahue P.M.C., Lisson K.H., et al. Standard of Care for Lipedema in the United States. *Phlebology.* 2021;36:779–796. doi: https://doi.org/10.1177/02683555211015887.
Suga H., Araki J., Aoi N., Kato H., Higashino T., Yoshimura K. Adipose Tissue Remodeling in Lipedema: Adipocyte Death and Concurrent Regeneration. *J. Cutan. Pathol.* 2009;36:1293–1298. doi: https://doi.org/10.1111/j.1600-0560.2009.01256.x.
Crescenzi R., Marton A., Donahue P.M.C., Mahany H.B., Lants S.K., Wang P., Beckman J.A., Donahue M.J., Titze J. Tissue Sodium Content Is Elevated in the Skin and Subcutaneous Adipose Tissue in Women with Lipedema. *Obesity.* 2018;26:310–317. doi: https://doi.org/10.1002/oby.22090.
Forner-Cordero I., Szolnoky G., Forner-Cordero A., Kemény L. Lipedema: An Overview of Its Clinical Manifestations, Diagnosis and Treatment of the Disproportional Fatty Deposition Syndrome – Systematic Review. *Clin. Obes.* 2012;2:86–95. doi: https://doi.org/10.1111/j.1758-8111.2012.00045.x.
Child A.H., Gordon K.D., Sharpe P., Brice G., Ostergaard P., Jeffery S., Mortimer P.S. Lipedema: An Inherited Condition. *Am. J. Med. Genet. Part A.* 2010;152:970–976. doi: https://doi.org/10.1002/ajmg.a.33313.
Reich-Schupke S., Schmeller W., Brauer W.J., Cornely M.E., Faerber G., Ludwig M., Lulay G., Miller A., Rapprich S., Richter D.F., et al. S1 Guidelines: Lipedema. *JDDG J. Dtsch. Dermatol. Ges.* 2017;15:758–767. doi: https://doi.org/10.1111/ddg.13036.
Bauer A.T., Von Lukowicz D., Lossagk K., Hopfner U., Kirsch M., Moog P., Bauer H., Machens H.G., Schmauss D. Adipose Stem Cells from Lipedema and Control Adipose Tissue Respond

Differently to Adipogenic Stimulation In Vitro. *Plast. Reconstr. Surg.* 2019;144:623–632. doi: https://doi.org/10.1097/PRS.0000000000005918.
Lee M.J., Wu Y., Fried S.K. Adipose Tissue Heterogeneity: Implication of Depot Differences in Adipose Tissue for Obesity Complications. *Mol. Asp. Med.* 2013;34:1–11. doi: https://doi.org/10.1016/j.mam.2012.10.001.
Jeffery E., Wing A., Holtrup B., Sebo Z., Kaplan J.L., Saavedra-Peña R., Church C.D., Colman L., Berry R., Rodeheffer M.S. The Adipose Tissue Microenvironment Regulates Depot-Specific Adipogenesis in Obesity. *Cell Metab.* 2016;24:142–150. doi: https://doi.org/10.1016/j.cmet.2016.05.012.
Ioannidou A., Fisher R.M., Hagberg C.E. The Multifaceted Roles of the Adipose Tissue Vasculature. *Obes. Rev.* 2022;23:e13403. doi: https://doi.org/10.1111/obr.13403.
Van Dijk C.G.M., Nieuweboer F.E., Pei J.Y., Xu Y.J., Burgisser P., Van Mulligen E., El Azzouzi H., Duncker D.J., Verhaar M.C., Cheng C. The Complex Mural Cell: Pericyte Function in Health and Disease. *Int. J. Cardiol.* 2015;190:75–89. doi: https://doi.org/10.1016/j.ijcard.2015.03.258.
Krüger-Genge A., Blocki A., Franke R.P., Jung F. Vascular Endothelial Cell Biology: An Update. *Int. J. Mol. Sci.* 2019;20:4411. doi: https://doi.org/10.3390/ijms20184411.
Hasan S.S., Fischer A. The Endothelium: An Active Regulator of Lipid and Glucose Homeostasis. *Trends Cell Biol.* 2021;31:37–49. doi: https://doi.org/10.1016/j.tcb.2020.10.003.
Hammarstedt A., Gogg S., Hedjazifar S., Nerstedt A., Smith U. Impaired Adipogenesis and Dysfunctional Adipose Tissue in Human Hypertrophic Obesity. *Physiol. Rev.* 2018;98:1911–1941. doi: https://doi.org/10.1152/physrev.00034.2017.
Yucel N., Arany Z. Fat, Obesity, and the Endothelium. *Curr. Opin. Physiol.* 2019;12:44–50. doi: https://doi.org/10.1016/j.cophys.2019.09.003.

Causes

The precise etiology of lipedema remains incompletely elucidated, while several variables are thought to contribute to its pathogenesis. Many possible etiologies for lipedema have been suggested.

To start with, the hereditary nature of lipedema and its genetic propensity have been confirmed via an increasing amount of data, providing insight into how the ailment is passed on and its likely genetic basis. Observational research and clinical reports consistently indicate a heritable component in the development of lipedema, suggesting a family propensity. The presence of family patterns, especially in female lineages, is a strong indication of a genetic propensity for lipedema that may be inherited throughout generations. This assertion has been reinforced by research that has documented instances when many female relatives in consecutive generations exhibit distinct symptoms of lipedema, thereby emphasizing the influence of genetics in its formation. Studies on the genetic structure of lipedema have shown the potential presence of several genetic markers and mutations linked to the illness. Although the specific genetic locations and mutations have not been definitively determined, initial studies have investigated other possibilities, such as genes associated with the control of adipose tissue, the development of the lymphatic system, and inflammatory pathways. Research have initiated investigations into the involvement of genes associated with the extracellular matrix and adipogenesis in lipedema. These research propose that mutations in these regions may contribute to the aberrant accumulation of fat and fibrosis found in lipedema. Moreover, the possible contribution of genes that regulate the integrity of the lymphatic system implies a connection between hereditary variables and the impaired flow of lymphatic fluid that is typical of the illness. However, due to the intricate nature of the genetic foundation of lipedema, further research is required. Modern genetic research approaches, including as genome-wide association studies (GWAS) and whole-exome sequencing, may help uncover the complex genetic variables that contribute to lipedema. The objective of such study is to not only uncover precise genetic markers and mutations linked to the disorder, but also to comprehend the interaction between genetic predisposition and environmental triggers. In the end, clarifying the genetic

G. Laur, *Lipoedema*, https://doi.org/10.1007/978-981-96-8939-2_13

components and processes of inheritance in lipedema will lead to early diagnosis, personalized treatment methods, and maybe preventative initiatives. This will greatly improve the management and comprehension of this ailment.

In addition to this, the complex connection between hormonal impacts and lipedema highlights the important function of estrogens and other sex hormones in the development and advancement of this illness. Estrogens, specifically, have been linked to the formation and worsening of lipedema. Clinical observations and studies indicate that hormonal changes during puberty, pregnancy, and menopause might trigger or intensify lipedema symptoms. Puberty is believed to initiate the first signs of lipedema in persons who are genetically susceptible, as a result of increased amounts of estrogen. This suggests a direct connection between hormonal changes and the start of the disorder.

Pregnancy, characterized by significant hormonal changes, particularly the rise in estrogen and progesterone, is a crucial phase during which lipedema may either develop or pre-existing symptoms may become more severe. The hormones have an impact on fluid retention, the storage of fat, and perhaps the modification of the extracellular matrix. These actions may worsen the distinctive uneven distribution of fat and discomfort in lipedema. Menopause is a major hormonal shift that causes a decrease in estrogen levels. This decrease may lead to changes in how fat is distributed in the body and how metabolism works, which may worsen symptoms of lipedema. The connection between hormonal imbalances and the development of lipedema is made more complex by the fact that not just estrogen but also other hormones including progesterone, insulin, and thyroid hormones may have a role in contributing to it. Insulin resistance has been observed in a specific group of patients with lipedema, indicating a connection between metabolic and hormonal variables. Furthermore, the probable role of androgens and their imbalance may possibly impact the growth of adipocytes in lipedema; however, further research is needed to confirm this. The understanding of the hormonal factors highlights the possible effectiveness of hormonal modulation as a therapeutic option, such as using hormone replacement therapy or contraceptives to control symptoms. Nevertheless, the intricate nature of hormonal interactions in lipedema requires a subtle and detailed approach to therapy, highlighting the need of more study to clarify the exact pathways via which hormones impact lipedema pathology. This will facilitate the development of personalized care strategies that target not just the lymphatic and adipose components of lipedema, but also the hormonal oscillations that may contribute to its advancement.

On the other hand, the malfunction of the lymphatic system is a key factor in the development of lipedema, a disorder characterized by the abnormal buildup of fatty tissue mostly in the lower limbs. The lymphatic system plays a vital role in avoiding edema by maintaining fluid balance and immunological activities. It does this by carrying lymph, a fluid that contains lymphocytes, waste materials, and excess fluids, back to the venous circulation. Lipedema is characterized by a notable decline in lymphatic function, which is believed to play a role in the disease's progressive nature. Patients with lipedema have aberrant lymphatic drainage and function, as seen by clinical examinations and imaging techniques like lymphoscintigraphy.

These findings indicate a clear connection between the severity of the ailment and the damage of the lymphatic system. The results of this study provide evidence that lymphatic malfunction may cause a buildup of fluid in the interstitial space. This accumulation of fluid might potentially contribute to the development and worsening of fibrotic adipose tissue, which is a typical feature of lipedema. Various theories suggest numerous processes that connect lymphatic dysfunction to the buildup of fat in lipedema. One dominant hypothesis is that a compromised lymphatic drainage system results in persistent inflammation, which, in turn, produces an increase in the size and number of fat cells as the body tries to retain surplus fluid. Inadequate lymphatic clearance may lead to the buildup of proteins in the interstitial fluid. This can attract water and worsen tissue swelling and fibrosis. This creates a harmful loop that worsens both lymphatic dysfunction and the accumulation of adipose tissue. Another hypothesis is that the mechanical strain on lymphatic capillaries resulting from the increased fat content can limit lymphatic function, hence impeding the elimination of surplus interstitial fluid. Present treatment approaches focus on enhancing lymphatic drainage and diminishing the buildup of adipose tissue using techniques such as manual lymphatic drainage, compression therapy, and, sometimes, surgical procedures. Nevertheless, the intricate relationship between lymphatic dysfunction and the buildup of fat in lipedema highlights the need for a comprehensive therapeutic strategy that tackles both components of the condition.

Additional investigation into the fundamental processes of lymphatic dysfunction in patients with lipedema might help to slow down the advancement of lipedema and enhance patient results.

Lipedema is characterized by severe anomalies in adipocyte activity and fat accumulation, which indicate a dysregulation in adipose tissue. This dysregulation deviates from the typical functioning of healthy adipose tissue. Lipedema is a condition where fat cells undergo abnormal growth and enlargement, resulting in an excessive and irregular buildup of fat, especially in the lower limbs. This atypical accumulation of fat is not only unresponsive to traditional methods of weight reduction, such as dietary changes and physical activity, but also exhibits unique physical and biochemical characteristics when compared to regular adipose tissue. Lipedema fat often exhibits characteristics such as elevated fibrosis, decreased blood flow, and heightened sensitivity to pressure and pain. These features are caused by the excessive growth of connective tissue and an aberrant network of blood vessels around the fat cells. The aforementioned attributes add to the distressing symptoms seen by persons with lipedema and complicate the treatment of the disorder.

Moreover, there are metabolic disruptions that worsen the growth of lipedema due to variations between lipedema fat and regular adipose tissue. Research has shown that adipose tissue in lipedema may be metabolically active in a way that encourages inflammation and oxidative stress, leading to a long-lasting, low-level inflammatory condition. The presence of inflammation may negatively affect the way adipocytes process lipids and respond to insulin, resulting in an even greater accumulation of fat tissue and possibly worsening metabolic disorders including insulin resistance and dyslipidemia. The precise processes responsible for these metabolic abnormalities are still being actively investigated. Current ideas include that changes in the production of adipokines, the breakdown of fats (lipolysis), and the intake of fatty acids all play a role in the disrupted metabolism of adipose tissue seen in lipedema. The identification of adipose tissue dysregulation in lipedema highlights the need for specific treatment strategies that target the distinct pathophysiological characteristics of the illness. Existing methods that prioritize alleviating symptoms and decreasing swelling are essential, but they may not completely target the underlying abnormalities in adipocytes and metabolic imbalances. Therefore, it is crucial to do more study on the molecular and cellular pathways that cause dysregulation of adipose tissue in lipedema. This research will not only enhance our comprehension of the disorder but also facilitate the creation of innovative treatment approaches that may more efficiently impede or reverse the development of lipedema, hence enhancing patient outcomes and quality of life.

In the development of lipedema, inflammatory processes are crucial, and persons afflicted by this condition often have chronic inflammation as a prominent characteristic in their adipose tissue. This persistent inflammatory condition is defined by the invasion of immune cells, specifically macrophages, into the adipose tissue. This invasion leads to the generation and discharge of pro-inflammatory cytokines, including tumor necrosis factor-alpha (TNF-α), interleukin-6 (IL-6), and interleukin-1 beta (IL-1β). These cytokines have the dual effect of causing inflammation and worsening the fibrosis of adipose tissue. Additionally, they hinder the function of the lymphatic system and contribute to discomfort and sensitivity in regions affected by lipedema. Several investigations have demonstrated the presence of increased levels of inflammatory markers and cytokines in lipedema tissue, indicating the important involvement of inflammation in the development of this illness.

In the clinical course of lipedema, inflammation has a complex role, affecting both the buildup of fatty tissue and the deterioration of lymphatic function. Chronic inflammation may cause alterations in the extracellular matrix, which encourages the development of fibrosis. This, in turn, hinders the normal flow of lymphatic drainage, leading to the worsening of edema and the accumulation of fat. Moreover, the presence of inflammation may disturb the normal functioning of adipocytes, resulting in changes to lipid metabolism and an increase in the size of adipocytes. The process of inflammation, fibrosis, and enlargement of adipose tissue adds to the gradual progression of lipedema, leading to the worsening of symptoms as time goes on. Treatments that reduce inflammation, such as medications that target particular cytokines or pathways, lifestyle changes to decrease overall inflammation, and therapies that enhance lymphatic drainage, may provide relief and improve results for individuals with lipedema. However, further investigation is required to completely understand the processes that cause inflammation in lipedema and to discover efficient anti-inflammatory approaches that can be included into comprehensive treatment programs for this complex disorder.

Vascular variables are crucial in the pathophysiology of lipedema, and the condition's influence on the afflicted tissues is mostly due to abnormalities in the microvasculature. Lipedema is characterized by specific changes in the microcirculation of adipose tissue, such as decreased blood flow, heightened vascular permeability, and the possible development of microaneurysms. The presence of these vascular anomalies is a contributing factor to the distinctive symptoms of lipedema, including discomfort, tenderness, and the tendency for patients to bruise easily. The damaged microvascular network in lipedema tissues results in ineffective transport of oxygen and nutrients, which might worsen the oxygen-deprived environment and encourage the development of fibrous adipose tissue. Moreover, the heightened permeability of blood vessels allows plasma proteins to escape into the surrounding tissue, worsening swelling and adding to the gradual progression of the illness. Reduced blood flow and malfunction in blood vessels not only directly impact the well-being of fatty tissues but also indirectly reduce the efficiency of lymphatic drainage. The accumulation of lymphatic fluid, together with the intrinsic structural and functional defects of lipedema, hinders the removal of interstitial fluid. This creates a harmful loop where edema worsens and adipose tissue expands. This cycle emphasizes the significance of preserving vascular health in reducing the advancement of lipedema. Treating the vascular aspects of lipedema includes implementing treatment approaches focused on enhancing microvascular performance and decreasing vascular permeability. Interventions such as compression therapy, exercise, and pharmaceutical medications that specifically target vascular health have shown promising advantages in the management of lipedema symptoms and enhancing the quality of life for patients. Further study is needed to understand the intricate vascular involvement in lipedema, including the underlying processes of vascular alterations. This will enable the development of tailored therapies that may successfully address this crucial part of the disorder.

Ultimately, the cause of lipedema is complex and involves several elements such as genetics, hormones, inflammation, vascular issues, and dysregulation of adipose tissue. According to current understanding, lipedema is believed to be caused by a mixture of these factors, with each one contributing to the distinct characteristics of the condition, such as the abnormal buildup of fat, as well as the discomfort and soreness experienced in the lower limbs. Genetic propensity is very influential, as seen by family studies that demonstrate a hereditary tendency, especially via maternal lines. The presence of hormones, particularly the changes that occur during puberty, pregnancy, and menopause, has a key role in causing or worsening lipedema symptoms.

This indicates a close connection between sex hormones and the development and evolution of the disorder. The presence of long-lasting inflammation in lipedema tissue, characterized by increased levels of pro-inflammatory cytokines and the infiltration of immune cells, plays a role in the development of fibrosis and discomfort. Vascular variables, such as compromised microcirculation and heightened vascular permeability, worsen edema and impede effective transportation of nutrients and oxygen to tissues.

A comprehensive strategy is required to treat and control lipedema due to the intricate interaction of these variables. Gaining a comprehensive understanding of the root causes has substantial ramifications for the development of precise and focused treatments. Genetic research has the potential to pave the way for personalized medical strategies, while hormonal investigations may provide hormone-modulating therapies. Implementing anti-inflammatory methods and therapies targeting vascular health might effectively alleviate the symptoms associated with lipedema, hence enhancing the overall quality of life for patients. Moreover, it is essential to acknowledge lipedema as a unique medical illness, different from obesity and lymphedema, in order to properly manage it and establish efficient treatment procedures.

As knowledge of the illness advances, the capacity to provide patients with more thorough and efficient treatment will also increase, eventually enhancing outcomes and quality of life for those impacted by this sometimes incapacitating disorder.

Diagnosis

Lipedema is a chronic, progressive medical condition characterized by the symmetric accumulation of adipose tissue, primarily in the lower extremities, which can lead to pain, mobility issues, and psychological distress. Unlike typical fat distribution, lipedema fat is resistant to diet and exercise and often coexists with a tendency toward easy bruising and pain upon pressure. This condition predominantly affects women and is frequently misdiagnosed or underdiagnosed, partly because of a lack of awareness among healthcare providers and overlapping symptoms with other conditions such as lymphedema and obesity.

The importance of accurate diagnosis cannot be overstated, as it is the cornerstone for effective management and treatment of lipedema. An accurate diagnosis involves a comprehensive clinical evaluation, including a detailed medical history and physical examination, and may be supported by imaging studies such as lymphoscintigraphy to rule out lymphedema. Early and precise diagnosis is critical for several reasons. First, it enables the implementation of appropriate treatment strategies, such as manual lymphatic drainage, compression therapy, dietary management, and, in some cases, surgical interventions like liposuction, which can significantly improve symptoms and quality of life. Second, it helps in preventing the progression of the condition to more advanced stages, which are associated with increased pain, mobility restrictions, and psychosocial impact. Lastly, recognizing lipedema as a distinct medical entity empowers patients, reducing the stigma and frustration often associated with misdiagnosis and contributing to a more compassionate and informed approach to care.

The clinical presentation and history taking are fundamental steps in the diagnostic process of lipedema, emphasizing the identification of key symptoms and signs, gathering comprehensive patient history, and acknowledging the importance of family history. The hallmark symptoms of lipedema include bilateral and symmetrical fatty deposits on the legs and arms, pain, tenderness, and a tendency to bruise easily.

Unlike common obesity, these fat accumulations are typically resistant to diet and exercise. A thorough patient history should explore the onset, progression, and

G. Laur, *Lipoedema*, https://doi.org/10.1007/978-981-96-8939-2_14

impact of these symptoms on daily activities and quality of life. The *Journal of Lymphoedema* (2015) underscores the importance of distinguishing lipedema from other conditions like lymphedema and obesity through careful clinical evaluation. Additionally, family history plays a critical role, as lipedema shows a genetic predisposition, with many patients reporting a family member with similar symptoms. This genetic link not only aids in the diagnosis but also informs the patient and their family about the hereditary nature of the condition, guiding future assessments and interventions. Therefore, a meticulous approach to history taking and clinical examination is essential in identifying lipedema, facilitating early intervention, and tailoring management strategies to individual patient needs.

The physical examination is a critical component of the diagnostic process for conditions like lipedema, requiring meticulous inspection and palpation techniques to accurately assess the patient's condition. During the examination, healthcare professionals focus on evaluating the symmetry of adipose tissue distribution, the texture of the affected areas, and the sensitivity to pain upon palpation. Inspection involves visually assessing the lower and, sometimes, upper extremities for signs of disproportionate fat accumulation, noting any presence of skin changes or varicosities. Palpation is then employed to discern the texture of the adipose tissue, which may feel nodular or rubbery in lipedema, and to evaluate pain sensitivity, which is a distinctive feature of the condition. The symmetry of the fatty deposits, particularly their bilateral and symmetrical nature, differentiates lipedema from other disorders such as lymphedema. Documentation of physical findings is paramount, providing a detailed record of the clinical assessment that supports the diagnosis and guides the management plan. This documentation should include descriptions of the fat distribution, texture, and pain response, as well as any notable findings such as the Stemmer sign, which remains negative in lipedema unlike in lymphedema. Through a thorough physical examination, clinicians can gather essential information that aids in the accurate diagnosis of lipedema, facilitating appropriate treatment and management strategies.

Differentiating lipedema from similar conditions such as lymphedema and obesity is crucial for accurate diagnosis and appropriate management. Lipedema is characterized by symmetrical accumulation of painful fat in the legs and arms, sparing the feet and hands, which distinguishes it from lymphedema where swelling often includes the feet or hands and may not be symmetrical. The Stemmer sign, a diagnostic test where the inability to pinch and lift the skin at the base of the second toe or finger indicates lymphedema, is negative in patients with lipedema, providing a clear diagnostic distinction. Unlike obesity, which is characterized by generalized fat accumulation that can be influenced by diet and exercise, lipedema fat is resistant to these measures and has a distinct pattern of accumulation. Furthermore, lipedema often presents with pain and bruising, symptoms not typically associated with obesity. Other differential diagnoses include lipohypertrophy, which lacks the pain and bruising seen in lipedema, and venous insufficiency, where symptoms are primarily related to the venous circulation rather than adipose tissue distribution. Recognition of these distinctions underscores the importance of comprehensive clinical evaluation—and, when indicated, the use of imaging and lymphoscintigraphy—to accurately distinguish lipedema from clinically similar disorders.

Imaging plays a vital role in the diagnosis of lipedema, providing valuable insights that complement clinical evaluation. Ultrasound examination is a commonly used modality that helps differentiate lipedema from other conditions by assessing the echogenicity and structure of subcutaneous tissue, which appears more fibrous in lipedema compared to normal adipose tissue. A study published in the *Journal of Ultrasound in Medicine* highlights the utility of ultrasound in identifying characteristic patterns of subcutaneous fat and tissue edema, aiding in the diagnosis of lipedema. Magnetic resonance imaging (MRI) offers a more detailed view, enabling the visualization of the subcutaneous fat layer's architecture and the distribution of fat deposits, which are distinct in lipedema. MRI can also help rule out other pathologies, such as lymphedema, by showing the absence of significant fluid accumulation. Other relevant imaging techniques include lymphoscintigraphy, particularly useful in excluding lymphedema by assessing the lymphatic system's functionality. While not routinely used for diagnosing lipedema, lymphoscintigraphy can provide critical differential diagnostic information when lymphedema is a consideration. Collectively, these imaging techniques enhance diagnostic accuracy, facilitating the differentiation of lipedema from similar conditions and guiding treatment planning.

In the diagnostic process for lipedema, laboratory and other diagnostic tests play an essential role in excluding other conditions and understanding the underlying pathophysiology. Blood tests can be utilized to identify biomarkers indicative of inflammation or coagulation disorders, which may be present in lipedema or contribute to its symptoms. For instance, a study in the *International Journal of Obesity* suggested that individuals with lipedema might exhibit elevated levels of certain inflammatory markers, distinguishing it from typical obesity. Assessment of lymphatic and vascular function is crucial, given that lipedema can be confused with lymphedema. Tests such as lymphoscintigraphy or Doppler ultrasound can evaluate the lymphatic system's integrity and venous flow, respectively, helping to rule out lymphatic or venous insufficiency. The importance of excluding other conditions cannot be overstated, as lipedema shares symptoms with a variety of disorders. Comprehensive diagnostic testing, including hormone levels to exclude endocrine disorders and imaging to rule out venous disease, ensures a correct diagnosis. This approach allows for targeted management strategies that address the specific needs of individuals with lipedema, avoiding treatments that may be effective for other conditions but not for lipedema.

The staging of lipedema is critical for tailoring treatment approaches and understanding the progression and prognosis of the condition. Lipedema is typically classified into four stages based on physical characteristics and clinical findings. Stage 1 is characterized by a smooth skin surface with an enlarged subcutaneous fat layer, while stage 2 shows the fat layer becoming lumpy and nodular. In stage 3, large extrusions of fat begin to form, and there may be significant skin overhang. Stage 4 involves the presence of lymphedema, termed lipolymphedema. The clinical significance of staging lies in its ability to guide treatment decisions and provide insight into the condition's progression. Early stages might be managed with conservative treatments such as manual lymphatic drainage and compression therapy, whereas later stages may require more invasive interventions, such as liposuction. A study in the *Journal of Vascular Surgery* highlighted that early diagnosis and intervention could slow the progression of lipedema and improve quality of life. The progression from one stage to the next can vary significantly among individuals and may be influenced by factors such as weight management and physical activity. Understanding the stage of lipedema is essential for setting realistic expectations, planning treatment strategies, and monitoring disease progression, emphasizing the importance of early and accurate diagnosis.

The psychosocial assessment of patients with lipedema is a crucial aspect of comprehensive care, given the significant impact the condition can have on mental health and quality of life. Lipedema is not only a physical but also an emotional burden, often leading to issues such as body image dissatisfaction, depression, anxiety, and social isolation due to the visible and progressive nature of the disease. Evidence underscores the importance of evaluating these psychosocial factors; for instance, a study published in the *British Journal of Dermatology* found that individuals with lipedema reported higher levels of psychological distress and lower quality of life compared to the general population. This highlights the need for psychological support as an integral part of the diagnostic and treatment process for lipedema. Incorporating mental health professionals into the care team can facilitate early identification of psychological distress, provide counseling or therapy to address mental health issues, and offer strategies to improve coping mechanisms. The aim is to support the patient holistically, acknowledging that addressing the psychological aspects of living with lipedema is as important as managing the physical symptoms. This approach not only aids in improving the overall well-being of individuals with lipedema but also enhances their engagement with and adherence to treatment plans, ultimately contributing to better outcomes.

Diagnosing lipedema presents significant challenges, often resulting in common misdiagnoses and delays that can adversely affect patient outcomes. The condition is frequently mistaken for obesity or lymphedema due to similarities in physical appearance, such as the disproportionate accumulation of fat in the limbs. This confusion is compounded by a lack of awareness and understanding of lipedema within the medical community, as evidenced by a study published in the *Archives of Dermatological Research*, which highlighted the condition's underrepresentation in medical literature and training. Furthermore, the variability in clinical presentation and the absence of universally accepted diagnostic criteria contribute to the diagnostic challenges. Barriers to accurate diagnosis in clinical practice include the subjective nature of the physical examination and the limited use of advanced imaging techniques, which are not routinely employed due to cost and accessibility issues. These factors lead to a reliance on clinical judgment, which, without specific training and awareness of lipedema, can result in misdiagnosis or dismissal of symptoms as merely obesity or lifestyle-related issues. Consequently, many individuals with lipedema experience significant delays in receiving an accurate diagnosis, impacting their access to appropriate treatment and support and exacerbating the psychological burden of living with an unrecognized and misunderstood condition.

The multidisciplinary approach to the diagnosis of lipedema involves the collaboration of various specialists, ensuring a comprehensive assessment that addresses the complexity of the condition. This collaborative model typically includes vascular surgeons, dermatologists, physiotherapists, dietitians, and mental health professionals, among others. The involvement of these specialists facilitates a holistic evaluation of the patient, integrating different perspectives and expertise to accurately diagnose lipedema and distinguish it from conditions with similar presentations, such as lymphedema and obesity. For instance, vascular surgeons and dermatologists can assess the physical and functional aspects of lipedema, while physiotherapists focus on mobility and lymphatic drainage issues. Dietitians offer nutritional guidance tailored to the patient's condition, and mental health professionals address the psychological impact of lipedema.

A study published in the *European Journal of Vascular and Endovascular Surgery* emphasizes the importance of this multidisciplinary approach in improving diagnostic accuracy and patient outcomes by ensuring that all aspects of the condition are considered. Coordinating care among these specialists is crucial for a comprehensive assessment, allowing for the development of a personalized treatment plan that addresses the multifaceted needs of patients with lipedema, thereby enhancing their quality of life and minimizing the progression of the disease.

The accurate and timely diagnosis of lipedema is paramount in the effective management of this often misunderstood and underdiagnosed condition. An early and precise identification of lipedema not only facilitates the initiation of appropriate interventions but also prevents the progression to more severe stages, thereby significantly impacting patient outcomes. The evidence underscores the necessity of distinguishing lipedema from other conditions with similar presentations, such as obesity and lymphedema, to avoid misdiagnoses that can lead to ineffective treatments and further psychological distress for patients. The implementation of a multidisciplinary approach in the diagnostic process ensures a comprehensive evaluation, encompassing the physical, nutritional, and psychological aspects of the condition, thereby enabling personalized treatment strategies. These strategies may include conservative measures such as manual lymphatic drainage, compression therapy, and dietary modifications, as well as more invasive options like liposuction for advanced cases. Ultimately, the goal is to improve the quality of life for individuals with lipedema by alleviating physical symptoms, enhancing mobility, and addressing the psychosocial challenges associated with the condition. The implications of accurate and timely diagnosis extend beyond immediate treatment outcomes, contributing to a broader understanding of lipedema, increasing awareness among healthcare providers, and advocating for patient support and research into more effective management and treatment options.

Differential Diagnosis

In this chapter, we explore disorders associated with subcutaneous adipose tissue (SAT), where fat within this compartment abnormally grows in amount or structure, frequently causing pain and discomfort. SAT, comprised of loose connective tissue or adipofascia, is the most prevalent connective tissue in vertebrates and involves components such as blood vessels, lymphatic vessels, immune cells, mesenchymal stem cells, fascia, and the interstitial matrix organ.

The conditions under discussion include lipedema, predominantly affecting women, and four rare adipose tissue diseases (RAD): familial multiple lipomatosis (FML), angiolipomatosis, Dercum's disease, and Madelung's disease. These diseases are characterized by adipose tissue that is notably resistant to reduction through conventional methods such as significant dietary modifications or physical exercise, often leading to what is referred to as persistent fat tissue. This resistance is also observed in individuals with diabetes and/or obesity, who may exhibit a mix of normal and resistant fat, underscoring the importance of clinician awareness in managing SAT diseases effectively. Furthermore, persistent fat is commonly found in scenarios where adipose tissue proliferation is triggered, such as during infections, autoimmune diseases, hypermobile joint disorders, or exposure to environmental toxins.

Subcutaneous adipose tissue, alongside the gastrointestinal tract, is considered one of the largest endocrine organs in the body. It hosts various immune cells like monocytes/macrophages, mast cells, and lymphocytes, which contribute to the hormonal activity of fat tissue. An increased presence of fat and immune cells fosters an inflammatory response that can induce insulin resistance and diminish the efficiency of lymphatic vessels, potentially prolonging inflammation.

Clinically, patients, particularly women, may experience slowed blood and lymphatic flow in fat-rich areas such as the abdomen or the gynoid region (hips, thighs, and buttocks). This impaired circulation leads to the accumulation of fluid, cellular waste, proteins, and other metabolic products in the extracellular matrix (ECM) surrounding adipocytes and other components of the adipofascia, creating a hypoxic environment that furthers cellular distress. Adipocytes in these conditions may

G. Laur, *Lipoedema*, https://doi.org/10.1007/978-981-96-8939-2_15

signal for additional immune cell recruitment, perpetuating inflammation and tissue degradation. The connective tissue may replace the degraded areas through a process known as fibroplasia or fibrosis, which, if unchecked, can lead to extensive ECM remodeling and irreversible scar tissue formation, obstructing proper flow through the adipose tissue.

Obesity is a primary contributor to the densification of fascia and the development of fibrosis within loose connective tissue. The resultant fibrotic network surrounding adipocytes and fat lobules, known as adisopathy, heightens the risk of metabolic diseases. Moreover, fibrotic adipose tissue shows less responsiveness to reduction efforts via diet, exercise, weight loss medications, or bariatric surgery. Understanding why SAT diseases develop such fibrotic and adisopathic characteristics is crucial to prevent their progression and to develop effective treatments.

Lipedema, often mischaracterized as common obesity, presents distinct clinical features that set it apart from typical obesity, underscoring the necessity for accurate diagnosis and appropriate management. Women with lipedema may not necessarily meet the BMI criteria for obesity, yet they experience a unique set of symptoms related to their condition that are not present in conventional obesity. These include tenderness of the affected tissue and easy bruising over areas where lipedema fat accumulates, which are notably absent in women with common obesity.

A distinction in lipedema is the pain associated with fat tissue, which varies widely among patients. While some women with lipedema experience significant pain in the affected tissues, others report little to no pain. This variance raises questions about whether the presence or absence of pain indicates different subtypes or stages of the disease. Importantly, pain in lipedema can often be managed effectively through comprehensive treatment strategies. Women who adhere to low-inflammatory diets, avoiding processed sugars and starches, engage in regular exercise, and use compression garments can experience substantial relief from pain. This suggests that the inflammatory response within lipedema fat tissue can be modulated by lifestyle factors.

The diagnostic process for lipedema should include a thorough medical history to document any history of pain and assess the distribution of adipose tissue. Unlike common obesity, which tends to distribute fat more uniformly or centralizes in the abdominal area, lipedema is characterized by a disproportionate accumulation of fat in the lower extremities compared to the trunk (Fig. 1). Additionally, a lack of significant fat loss from the lower limbs despite weight loss efforts, and a family history of similar symptoms, can further support a diagnosis of lipedema.

Moreover, when lipedema coexists with obesity, and particularly when interventions such as bariatric surgery or medical weight loss are applied, patients may lose significant weight. However, they often cannot effectively reduce lipedema fat to the same extent, leading to residual adipose tissue and subsequent excess skin formation in these areas. This underscores the resistant nature of lipedema fat to typical weight loss strategies.

The interplay between lipedema and conditions like obesity and polycystic ovary syndrome (PCOS) exacerbates the complexity of managing lipedema. The increase in adipokines such as tumor necrosis factor alpha (TNF-α) and leptin, commonly

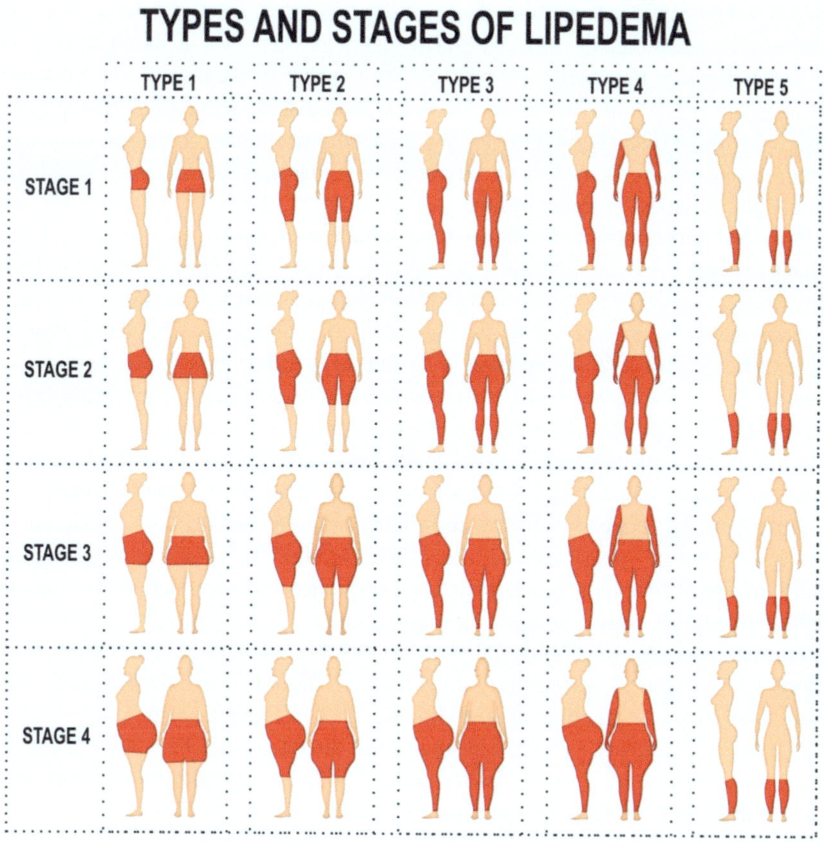

Fig. 1 Diagram combining the different types and stages of lpedema

observed in obesity and PCOS, can worsen the severity of lipedema. These conditions promote inflammatory processes and may contribute to venous dysfunction, a factor that aggravates both lipedema and potential lymphedema by causing fluid to leak back into the tissues.

Thus, distinguishing lipedema from common obesity is crucial not only for effective management but also for understanding the pathophysiological mechanisms underlying the disease. An informed approach that includes recognizing the unique distribution of fat, sensitivity to pain, and familial patterns, coupled with an understanding of how associated conditions can intensify symptoms, is essential for advancing care for women with lipedema.

Women with lipedema face a significantly heightened risk of developing lymphedema, particularly as the condition progresses from stage 1 to more advanced stages. This progression not only complicates the management of lipedema but also introduces the potential for severe secondary health issues such as cellulitis and chronic wounds.

These complications arise due to impaired lymphatic drainage, which can lead to fluid buildup and increased susceptibility to infections and delayed wound healing. The integration of manual lymphatic drainage and deeper tissue therapies, including instrument-assisted techniques like Astym therapy and the Graston technique, as well as manual therapies such as myofascial release, is critical in managing this risk. Following these therapies with consistent compression and targeted reduction of obese adipofascia can further mitigate the progression to lymphedema, enhancing both physical health outcomes and the patient's quality of life.

Psychosocial challenges are notably significant in women with lipedema, deeply impacting their mental health and societal interactions. The stigma associated with body image, exacerbated by pervasive cultural ideals of thinness and the widespread dissemination of highly edited images in media, contributes to a range of emotional and psychological distress. Women with lipedema often experience appearance-related distress and depression, conditions that can lead to disordered eating behaviors in an attempt to conform to societal standards of body size and shape. Alarmingly, the psychological burden can be so severe that, as research in Germany indicates, there is a noted prevalence of suicide attempts among these women.

Moreover, the reduced mobility commonly associated with both lipedema and obesity can severely restrict social interactions, leading to isolation and diminished quality of life. These factors necessitate a comprehensive approach to the management of lipedema, which includes not only addressing the physical symptoms but also providing robust psychological support. Assessing and treating associated conditions such as anxiety, particularly prevalent in individuals with hypermobile joint disorders—which often coincide with lipedema—must be a priority.

Lipedema, a complex and often misdiagnosed disorder characterized by disproportionate fat accumulation, can coexist with other conditions, complicating its identification and management. One such coexisting condition is Dercum's disease, leading to what can be considered a mixed disorder. This overlap presents significant challenges in differentiating the two conditions due to their shared and unique symptoms.

Distinguishing lipedema from Dercum's disease involves a careful clinical evaluation, as individuals with Dercum's disease often exhibit a broader spectrum of pain disorders, including higher pain scores, fibromyalgia, abdominal pain, and migraines. Additionally, they frequently present with lipomas, cognitive dysfunction, and shortness of breath. In contrast, women with lipedema typically display more fibrotic tissue, easy bruising, hypermobility in joints, venous disease, and edema of the feet. These distinguishing features, while helpful, require a nuanced understanding to effectively separate and manage these conditions in clinical practice.

The co-occurrence of other medical conditions with lipedema further complicates diagnosis and management. Notably, hypothyroidism is prevalent in a significant percentage of women with lipedema. Misdiagnosis is common, as symptoms such as persistent lower body fat can mimic or obscure underlying endocrine disorders. Women with lipedema often seek treatment for what they suspect to be thyroid-related weight issues, leading to potential frustrations in patient-provider interactions, especially if comprehensive thyroid testing is denied despite normal initial thyroid function tests.

For clinicians, recognizing the potential for lipedema in patients presenting with symptoms typical of other disorders is crucial. This recognition can be transformative, both for patient outcomes and for the therapeutic relationship. Effective diagnosis of lipedema involves taking a thorough medical history that scrutinizes eating habits, exercise patterns, and the timeline of symptom development, particularly noting any hormonal transitions such as puberty, pregnancy, or menopause. A detailed family history is also essential, as lipedema often runs in families and primarily affects female members.

During physical examination, the assessment should start with visual inspections to determine the disproportionality of body fat distribution, particularly between the upper and lower body, and measuring the waist-to-hip ratio to evaluate for central obesity. Palpation of fat tissues should be performed to assess for the pain and fibrosis characteristic of lipedema, with special attention to common areas like the upper arms and legs. Such comprehensive evaluations not only aid in diagnosing lipedema but also in distinguishing it from similar conditions like Dercum's disease and other comorbidities, enabling targeted and effective management strategies that significantly enhance the quality of life for affected individuals.

Familial multiple lipomatosis (FML) is a rare adipose disorder characterized by the development of multiple lipomas across subcutaneous fat layers. This condition, which varies significantly within affected families, shows a perplexing pattern of unequal penetrance where some individuals may have just a few lipomas while others develop hundreds to thousands. The reason behind this variable expression remains a topic of scientific inquiry. Typically, these lipomas are non-painful and benign but may become tender or itchy, particularly when they are growing or if they are situated in areas subjected to regular pressure or trauma.

The distinction between FML and similar conditions such as Dercum's disease is crucial yet challenging. Dercum's disease is typically marked by painful lipomas, known as lipoma dolorosa, which can complicate diagnoses in FML patients who also experience pain. It has been noted in the literature that while some cases of painful lipomas in FML families may resemble Dercum's disease, they are distinct conditions and should be regarded as FML with painful lipomas, particularly when a familial history of FML is present.

Interestingly, gender-related patterns have been observed in FML, where males predominantly develop lipomas and females exhibit symptoms resembling lipedema, suggesting a potential genetic or hormonal interplay affecting fat distribution and disorder manifestation.

The prevalence of FML is estimated at about 1 in 50,000, indicating its rarity. Genetic studies have revealed that FML often follows an autosomal-dominant inheritance pattern, with no significant gender disparity in incidence rates. Genes implicated in FML include HMGA2 and PALB2, the latter of which is also associated with an increased risk of several cancers, including breast and ovarian cancers, underlining the genetic susceptibility and potential systemic implications of FML. This association with cancer risk highlights the importance of genetic counseling and screening for FML patients, especially since FML may serve as a clinical marker for underlying genetic abnormalities.

FML has been linked to various genetic conditions and mutations in tumor suppressor genes, suggesting that FML could be a phenotypic manifestation of broader genetic dysregulations. Associations have been made with conditions such as MEN-1, retinoblastoma, and Cowden's disease, all of which involve mutations that may predispose individuals to both lipomatosis and malignant conditions. The identification of these genetic links has profound implications for patient management, suggesting a need for comprehensive genetic screening and possibly proactive surveillance for associated malignancies.

Furthermore, the development of multiple lipomas has been observed following chemotherapy, pointing to the potential influence of environmental factors or treatment-induced genetic changes on the expression of FML. This observation underscores the complexity of FML as a condition influenced by both intrinsic genetic factors and external medical interventions.

Angiolipomatosis, classified under the broader category of adipose disorders, is a rare condition predominantly affecting men postpuberty, though isolated cases in children suggest potential hereditary aspects. This disorder is characterized by the presence of multiple angiolipomas—lipomas with a significant vascular component, containing between 10 and 90% blood vessels. These lipomas vary widely in size, from as small as a rice grain to as large as a marble, and typically manifest along the trunk and limbs, rarely appearing on the head, hands, or feet.

The distinctive feature of angiolipomas compared to traditional lipomas is their painfulness, which can range from mild to intense. This pain is not always consistent and may vary based on the lipoma's size, location, and the individual's pain threshold. Pathologically, angiolipomas are noted for their unique composition, integrating adipose cells, fibrotic tissue, and an abundance of blood vessels filled with fibrin clots. These features not only contribute to the distinctive bluish hue visible through the skin but also to the texture and feel of the growths, which can sometimes be palpated as small, raised areas when they extend into the epidermis.

The pathogenesis of angiolipomas is thought to be linked to the fascia—the densely woven, connective tissue layer that surrounds muscles, blood vessels, and nerves. Fascia is richly innervated and highly sensitive to inflammation, which can lead to significant pain. This suggests that angiolipomas may originate from fascial layers, where inflammation and subsequent angiogenesis—the formation of new blood vessels—play critical roles.

The presence of microthrombi within these growths, leading to localized necrosis of blood vessels and adipocytes, supports a hypothesis where limited blood flow and fibrotic tethering could damage nerves, further exacerbating pain.

Developmentally, the genesis of angiolipomas may be tied to hormonal changes during puberty, which stimulate the differentiation of adipogenic precursors found within the adipofascia into mature adipocytes closely associated with blood vessels. Trauma to the fascia may induce repeated cycles of injury and repair, promoting vascular proliferation and the eventual formation of angiolipomas. While these growths are typically benign, there is an ongoing debate regarding their potential neoplastic nature. Research indicating chromosomal deletions, particularly involving tumor suppressor genes like the retinoblastoma gene on chromosome 13,

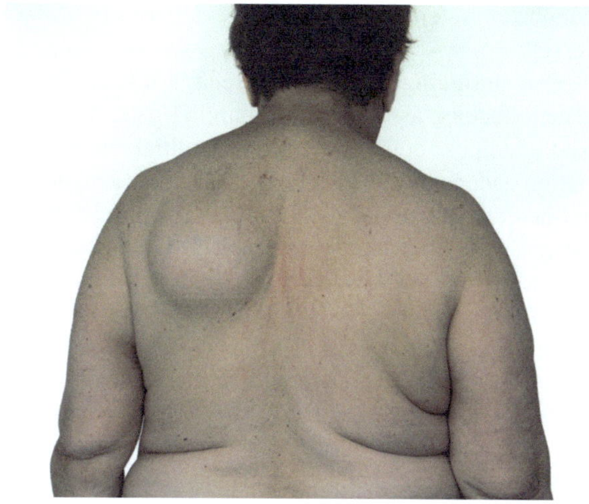

Fig. 2 Picture of a patient with angiolipomatosis

suggests a possible neoplastic transformation in some cases. This raises significant clinical implications, as individuals with extensive angiolipomatosis (Fig. 2) might require evaluation for neoplastic transformation and consideration of antineoplastic therapies if conventional treatments prove ineffective.

Dercum's disease (DD), also known as adiposis dolorosa, is a complex condition characterized by extremely painful adipofascial tissue, which notably resists weight loss through conventional means such as diet and exercise and responds poorly to analgesics. The challenge in diagnosing and managing Dercum's disease stems from its symptomatic overlap with other conditions characterized by chronic pain and obesity, such as fibromyalgia. The ambiguity in the literature about the precise definition and classification of Dercum's disease complicates the clinical understanding and differentiation from other adipose disorders. Historical and contemporary classifications have struggled to adequately distinguish Dercum's disease due to a focus on phenotypic descriptions without a comprehensive evaluation of the disease's history and progression.

The onset of Dercum's disease is frequently associated with metabolic disturbances, leading to the development of painful adipose masses. This is particularly evident in cases where patients initially diagnosed with lipedema progress to develop obesity and/or lymphedema, potentially transforming their metabolic state and exacerbating the growth of painful adipose tissue. The etiology of these painful masses often involves inflammation, which is believed to impair lymphatic functioning and encourage adipogenesis through the accumulation of pre-lymph fluid in the extracellular matrix.

Additionally, Dercum's disease exhibits a range of systemic symptoms that mirror those found in fibromyalgia and other chronic pain conditions. These include chronic pain, fatigue, cognitive disturbances such as brain fog, gastrointestinal distress, and cardiovascular symptoms like tachycardia. The broad spectrum of symptoms suggests a systemic inflammatory process possibly linked to an altered lymphatic system, which may be evidenced by irregular and thickened lymphatic vessels.

One intriguing aspect of Dercum's disease is its potential relationship with genetic factors, as observed in familial patterns where multiple members develop painful adipose conditions such as familial multiple lipomatosis (FML). This association underscores the necessity for further genetic research to elucidate the potential hereditary components of Dercum's disease and related disorders. Moreover, the presence of painful masses in FML suggests a possible overlap or spectrum where Dercum's disease may represent a variant or progression of FML characterized by significant pain and systemic symptoms.

Given these complexities, it is critical for the medical community to refine the diagnostic criteria for Dercum's disease to better identify and treat affected individuals. This involves a detailed patient history that considers the onset, progression, and familial occurrence of symptoms, combined with a thorough physical examination focused on identifying painful adipose masses and associated systemic features. An accurate diagnosis can significantly impact the management approach, which should be tailored to address both the painful adipose symptoms and any underlying metabolic or systemic conditions.

The management of Dercum's disease remains a challenge due to its resistance to conventional therapies. Treatment strategies should therefore be comprehensive, potentially including the management of obesity and metabolic syndrome, pharmacological approaches to control pain and inflammation, and possibly surgical interventions for severe cases. Additionally, exploring the role of manual lymphatic drainage and compression therapy may offer symptomatic relief and improve quality of life for these patients. As research progresses, a deeper understanding of the pathophysiological mechanisms underlying Dercum's disease will be essential for developing targeted therapies and improving patient outcomes.

Multiple symmetric lipomatosis (MSL), also known as Madelung's disease or Launois-Bensaude syndrome, represents a rare and complex clinical entity characterized by the symmetrical distribution of adipose tissue. Since its first description by Brodie in 1846 and the more detailed account by Launois and Bensaude in 1898, the understanding of MSL has evolved significantly. Originally observed predominantly in men with a history of alcoholism, it is now recognized that MSL can affect individuals irrespective of alcohol consumption, including women and children, indicating a broader epidemiological spread.

MSL is notably characterized by the growth of multiple lipomas, particularly around the neck, shoulders, and upper body, leading to distinctive physical appearances such as the "buffalo hump." The growths associated with MSL are typically non-painful, though they can occasionally cause discomfort if located in areas subjected to frequent pressure or strain. This disorder is not benign as previously thought, as it can lead to serious complications, including tracheal or esophageal compression, resulting in superior vena cava syndrome, and even more severe outcomes due to the encroachment of fatty growths into other critical anatomical areas.

From a genetic standpoint, MSL has been linked with mutations in mitochondrial DNA, particularly the MERRF tRNA(Lys) A>G(8344) mutation, though not all cases exhibit these mutations. Research also suggests a connection with the LIPE gene, which encodes for hormone-sensitive lipase, implicating disruptions in lipid metabolism as a contributory factor. Additionally, mutations in the MFN2 gene, which is crucial for mitochondrial fusion and function, have been associated with MSL, suggesting a mitochondrial dysfunction component to the disease.

Pathophysiologically, two hypotheses have been proposed to explain the development of MSL. The first hypothesis revolves around the transformation of adipose tissue, particularly brown adipose tissue, which may contribute to the unusual fat distributions observed in MSL. This is supported by findings of altered adipogenesis and mitochondrial function in affected tissues. The second hypothesis suggests that systemic inflammation, potentially exacerbated by alcohol consumption, plays a critical role. This inflammation could impair the normal function of the lymphatic system, leading to abnormal fat deposition and progression of MSL.

The involvement of the lymphatic system is particularly intriguing in the context of MSL, as dysfunctions in this system can lead to significant medical complications. The altered lymphatic architecture in MSL could result in inefficient lymphatic drainage, contributing to the persistence and expansion of adipose tissue. Given that MSL often presents with systemic symptoms such as dyslipidemia, metabolic syndrome, and even cardiovascular issues, understanding the interplay between lymphatic function, inflammation, and adipose tissue pathology is crucial for effective management.

In summary, multiple symmetric lipomatosis is a multifaceted disorder with significant genetic, metabolic, and inflammatory components. Its management requires a comprehensive approach that addresses not only the cosmetic concerns associated with excessive fat deposition but also the potential metabolic, cardiovascular, and respiratory complications. Ongoing research into the genetic and pathophysiological underpinnings of MSL is essential to develop targeted therapies that can effectively address the complex manifestations of this challenging condition.

Adipofascial diseases, characterized by the proliferation of fibrotic adipofascial tissue resistant to lifestyle modifications, pose significant challenges in both diagnosis and management. The pathophysiological complexity of these disorders often necessitates surgical intervention as a primary treatment modality, especially when conservative measures fail to achieve desired outcomes. The intricate overlap among various adipofascial diseases further complicates the clinical landscape, making accurate diagnosis a complex endeavor that is heavily reliant on nuanced understanding of each condition's unique features.

The current state of knowledge underscores a critical need for advancements in the understanding of these disorders at a molecular and genetic level. As the field progresses, the discovery of specific genes and biomarkers associated with adipofascial diseases could revolutionize diagnostic processes, allowing for more precise identification and differentiation among conditions that currently present with similar phenotypes. Such advancements are imperative not only for enhancing diagnostic accuracy but also for developing targeted therapies that could address the underlying mechanisms of these disorders rather than merely managing their symptoms. While the management of adipofascial diseases currently leans heavily on surgical interventions, the future holds potential for significant advances. With ongoing research aimed at unraveling the genetic and molecular bases of these conditions, there is hope for the development of more effective, less invasive treatment modalities. Until then, the medical community must rely on existing diagnostic tools and treatment strategies, continuously seeking to refine and enhance them in light of new research findings. The goal is to improve patient outcomes through more personalized and precise medical care, tailored to the specific pathophysiological profiles of each adipofascial disorder.

Suggested Reading

Herbst KL. Rare adipose disorders (RADs) masquerading as obesity. Acta Pharmacol Sin 2012; 33:155-172. doi: 1 https://doi.org/10.1038/aps.2011.1153.

Luong Q, Huang J, Lee KY. Deciphering White Adipose Tissue Heterogeneity. Biology (Basel) 2019; 8(2).biology8020023. doi: 80200 10.8023390/biology8020023.

Hussain I, Patni N, Garg A. Lipodystrophies, dyslipidaemias and atherosclerotic cardiovascular disease. Pathology 2019; 51:202-212. doi: 2 https://doi.org/10.1016/j.pathol.2018.1011.1004. Epub 2018 Dec 1027.

Akinci B, Sahinoz M, Oral E. Lipodystrophy Syndromes: Presentation and Treatment. In: Feingold KR AB, Boyce A, Chrousos G, Dungan K, Grossman A, Hershman JM, Kaltsas G, Koch C, Kopp P, Korbonits M, McLachlan R, Morley JE, New M, Perreault L, Purnell J, Rebar R, Singer F, Trence DL, Vinik A, Wilson DP, ed. Endotext [Internet]. South Dartmouth (MA): MDText.com, Inc.; 2000–2018.

Hogan S, Velez MW, Kaminer MS. Updates on the understanding and treatment of cellulite. Semin Cutan Med Surg 2018; 37:242–246. doi: 2 https://doi.org/10.12788/j.sder.12018.12056. [CrossRef]

van der Valk ES, van den Akker ELT, Savas M, Kleinendorst L, Visser JA, Van Haelst MM, Sharma AM, van Rossum EFC. A comprehensive diagnostic approach to detect underlying causes of obesity in adults. Obes Rev 2019; 20:795–804. doi: 7 https://doi.org/10.1111/obr.12836. Epub 12019 Mar 12831. [CrossRef]

Kyrou I, Randeva HS, Tsigos C, Kaltsas G, Weickert MO. Clinical Problems Caused by Obesity. In: Feingold KR AB, Boyce A, Chrousos G, Dungan K, Grossman A, Hershman JM, Kaltsas G, Koch C, Kopp P, Korbonits M, McLachlan R, Morley JE, New M, Perreault L, Purnell J, Rebar R, Singer F, Trence DL, Vinik A, Wilson DP, ed. Endotext [Internet]. South Dartmouth (MA): MDText.com, Inc.; 2000–2018.

Gruzdeva O, Borodkina D, Uchasova E, Dyleva Y, Barbarash O. Localization of fat depots and cardiovascular risk. Lipids Health Dis 2018; 17:218. doi: 2 10.1186/s12944-12018-10856–12948.

Ahlman H. Nilsson. The gut as the largest endocrine organ in the body. Ann Oncol. 2001;12:S63–68.

Coelho M, Oliveira T, Fernandes R. Biochemistry of adipose tissue: an endocrine organ. Archives of medical science. AMS. 2013;9:191–200.

Chung KJ, Nati M, Chavakis T, Chatzigeorgiou A. Innate immune cells in the adipose tissue. Rev Endocr Metab Disord 2018; 19:283–292. doi: 2 https://doi.org/10.1007/s11154-11018-19451-11156.

Del Corno M, Conti L, Gessani S. Innate Lymphocytes in Adipose Tissue Homeostasis and Their Alterations in Obesity and Colorectal Cancer. Front Immunol 2018; 9:2556.: https://doi.org/10.3389/fimmu.2018.02556. eCollection 02018.

Chen Y, Rehal S, Roizes S, Zhu HL, Cole WC, von der Weid PY. The pro-inflammatory cytokine TNF-alpha inhibits lymphatic pumping via activation of the NF-kappaB-iNOS signaling pathway. Microcirculation. 2017;24(3)

Arngrim N, Simonsen L, Holst JJ, Bulow J. Reduced adipose tissue lymphatic drainage of macromolecules in obese subjects: a possible link between obesity and local tissue inflammation? Int J Obes (Lond) 2013; 37:748–750. doi: 7 https://doi.org/10.1038/ijo.2012.1098. Epub 2012 Jul 1033.

Blaak EE, van Baak MA, Kemerink GJ, Pakbiers MT, Heidendal GA, Saris WH. Beta-adrenergic stimulation and abdominal subcutaneous fat blood flow in lean, obese, and reduced-obese subjects. Metabolism. 1995;44:183–187.

L'Hermitte F, Behar A, Paries J, Cohen-Boulakia F, Attali JR, Valensi P. Impairment of lymphatic function in women with gynoid adiposity and swelling syndrome. Metabolism. 2003;52:805–809.

Kumar V, Abbas AK, Fausto N. Tissue renewal and repair: regeneration, healing, and fibrosis. In: Abbas VKAK, Fausto N, eds. Pathologic Basis of Disease. Philadelphia, PA, USA: Elsevier Saunders; 2005.

Usunier B, Benderitter M, Tamarat R, Chapel A. Management of fibrosis: the mesenchymal stromal cells breakthrough. Stem Cells Int 2014; 2014:340257.: https://doi.org/10.1155/2014/340257. Epub 342014 Jul 340214.

Sun K, Tordjman J, Clement K, Scherer PE. Fibrosis and adipose tissue dysfunction. Cell Metab 2013; 18:470–477. doi: 4 https://doi.org/10.1016/j.cmet.2013.1006.1016. Epub 2013 Aug 1015.

Crewe C, An YA, Scherer PE. The ominous triad of adipose tissue dysfunction: inflammation, fibrosis, and impaired angiogenesis. J Clin Invest 2017; 127:74–82. doi: https://doi.org/10.1172/JCI88883. Epub 82017 Jan 88883.

Chabot K, Gauthier MS, Garneau PY, Rabasa-Lhoret R. Evolution of subcutaneous adipose tissue fibrosis after bariatric surgery. Diabetes Metab 2017; 43:125–133. doi: 1 https://doi.org/10.1016/j.diabet.2016.1010.1004. Epub 2016 Nov 1011.

Bel Lassen P, Charlotte F, Liu Y, Bedossa P, Le Naour G, Tordjman J, Poitou C, Bouillot JL, Genser L, Zucker JD, Sokolovska N, Aron-Wisnewsky J, Clement K. The FAT Score, a Fibrosis Score of Adipose Tissue: Predicting Weight-Loss Outcome After Gastric Bypass. J Clin Endocrinol Metab 2017; 102:2443–2453. doi: 24 https://doi.org/10.1210/jc.2017-00138.

Allen EV, Hines EAJ. Lipedema of the legs: A syndrome characterised by fat legs and orthostatic edema. Proc Staff Meet Mayo Clin. 1940;15:184–187.

Fife CE, Maus EA, Carter MJ. Lipedema: a frequently misdiagnosed and misunderstood fatty deposition syndrome. Adv 2010; 23:81–92; quiz 93-84.

Beltran K, Herbst KL. Differentiating lipedema and Dercum's disease. Int J Obes (Lond). 2017;41:240–245.

Herbst K, Mirkovskaya L, Bharhagava A, Chava Y, Te CH. Lipedema Fat and Signs and Symptoms of Illness, Increase with Advancing Stage. Archives of Medicine. 2015;7:1–8.

Meier-Vollrath I, Schmeller W. Lipoedema – current status, new perspectives. Journal der Deutschen Dermatologischen Gesellschaft. 2004;2:181–186.

Wold LE, Hines EA Jr, Allen EV. Lipedema of the legs; a syndrome characterized by fat legs and edema. Ann Intern Med. 1951;34:1243–1250.

Coppel T, Cunneen J, Fetzer S, Gordon K, Hardy D, Jones J, McCarroll A, O'Neill C, Smith S, White C, Williams A. Best Practice Guidelines: The management of lipoedema. Wounds UK 2017;13(1). http://www.wounds-uk.com/best-practice-statements/best-practice-guidelines-the-management-of-lipoedema.

Herpertz U. Krankheitsspektrum des Lipödems an einer Lymphologischen Fachklinik – Erscheinungsformen, Mischbilder und Behandlungsmöglichkeiten. vasomed 1997:301–307.

Forner-Cordero I, Szolnoky G, Forner-Cordero A, Kemény L. Lipedema: an overview of its clinical manifestations, diagnosis and treatment of the disproportional fatty deposition syndrome – systematic review. Clinical Obesity. 2012;2:86–95.

Histopathology

Lipedema is a condition characterized by the accumulation of excess adipose tissue in the subcutaneous layer of the body, primarily in the lower extremities. The histopathology of lipedema tissue shows several distinct features, which can help to confirm the diagnosis. One of the key features of lipedema tissue is the presence of hypertrophied adipocytes, or fat cells. These cells are larger than normal and have a characteristic "signet-ring" appearance, with a small nucleus pushed to one side of the cell by a large lipid droplet. This is in contrast to normal adipocytes, which have a round nucleus and a smaller lipid droplet. In addition to the hypertrophied adipocytes, lipedema tissue may also show signs of inflammation and fibrosis. There may be an increase in the number of macrophages and other immune cells in the tissue, as well as fibrosis and thickening of the collagen fibers that support the adipose tissue. Lymphatic abnormalities are also commonly observed in lipedema tissue, including dilation of lymphatic vessels and lymphatic capillaries, and accumulation of lymphatic fluid in the interstitial spaces. These changes may contribute to the swelling and edema that are characteristic of the condition. Finally, studies have suggested that there may be alterations in the expression of certain genes in lipedema tissue, which could contribute to the development and progression of the condition. These include genes involved in adipocyte differentiation, inflammation, and lymphatic function.

Overall, the histopathology of lipedema tissue reflects the complex interplay between adipose tissue hypertrophy, inflammation, lymphatic dysfunction, and other factors. Further research is needed to fully understand the mechanisms underlying this condition and develop more effective treatments.

G. Laur, *Lipoedema*, https://doi.org/10.1007/978-981-96-8939-2_16

Macroscopically

The normal histology of fat involves the development and structure of adipocytes (fat cells) and their organization within the body. Fat cells begin to appear embryologically after 5 months of gestation as spindle-shaped, lipid-free precursor cells, eventually developing into young adipocytes with multiple cytoplasmic droplets. These stages represent different phases of lipoblast development, as observed in in vitro studies.

Fat cells originate from fibroblasts, which may come from perivascular sheath cells or spindle cells. The initial sign of fat cell differentiation is the emergence of small cytoplasmic vacuoles in these fibroblasts. Lipogenesis, or fat creation, leads to the expansion and merging of these vacuoles into a single large lipid droplet within mature fat cells, characterized by a large central lipid droplet and a peripherally located nucleus. These unilocular adipocytes serve as efficient long-term energy storage units.

When existing fat cells near their capacity, the body generates new fat cells from mesenchymal precursor cells, resembling immature fibroblasts. During periods of excessive dietary fat, extra triglycerides are stored in these newly formed adipocytes or lipoblasts. Conversely, when an adipocyte loses its intracellular fat, it appears vacuous and similar to a fibroblast.

Adipocytes possess receptors for various hormones and cytokines, influencing processes like lipolysis and capillary dilation. Histological techniques show an abundance of nerves around these cells, typically located near blood vessels.

Other types of fat cells include multilocular adipocytes found in fetuses and newborns, containing many small lipid droplets and functioning in heat production, similar to brown fat in hibernating animals.

The vascularity of fat is evident through special staining techniques, revealing each adipocyte's direct contact with one or more capillaries. The capillary bed in adipose tissue is denser compared to striated muscle, with blood flow in adipose tissue varying based on resting or dilated states and influenced by the size of the fat cells.

Subcutaneous fat consists of three layers: the apical layer, the mantle layer, and the deep compartment layer, each with distinct characteristics. The apical layer is a thin layer contiguous with the reticular dermis, extending upward into the dermis. It includes peri adnexal fat and fat around the vascular arcade and lymphatic plexus. The mantle layer, a superficial row of vertically oriented fat pearls, varies in thickness across the body and serves protective, cushioning, and insulating functions. The deep compartment layer, present in obese infants and children, becomes more prominent after puberty and varies based on genetic predisposition and obesity levels.

The hierarchical architecture of fat includes adipose tissue septa, which are fibrous sheets partitioning and supporting adipocyte groupings. These septa range from very thin, almost invisible structures surrounding fat lobules to thicker ones that separate larger fat compartments. The individual adipocyte, with its characteristic signet-ring appearance, is the smallest unit in this hierarchy. Factors like age, gender, and anatomical location influence fat cell size and number, with a maximum size limit per cell. Adipose tissue grows through cell multiplication rather than continuous expansion of individual cells.

Fat lobules, the next level in the hierarchy, consist of a group of adipocytes partitioned by thin fibrous septa, with small blood vessels and nerves interspersed. These lobules resemble compound fruits like raspberries. Fat pearls, visible when subcutaneous fat is transected, contain clusters of these lobules and vary in size depending on the body part.

Larger structures, fat sections and compartments, are conglomerations of many fat pearls and are the largest entities in the architectural hierarchy of subcutaneous fat. They determine the differences in surface anatomy between males and females and are named for specific body areas like the hips, thighs, and abdomen.

Tangential and oblique septa are two types of fibrous tissue sheets that structure the fat. Tangential planes are dense connective tissue sheets parallel to muscle fasciae, while oblique planes are thinner sheets that intersect tangential planes at angles, aiding in the partitioning of fat. This complex architecture contributes to the functional and aesthetic aspects of human fat, including its role in energy storage, insulation, protection, and shaping the body's contours. The structure and arrangement of these fat cells and their supporting tissues also have implications for conditions like cellulite, where the irregular distribution of mechanical forces on tethered skin leads to visible dimpling. This is due to the interaction of fibrous septa with the skin and deeper tissues.

In summary, the normal histology of fat in the human body is a sophisticated and dynamic system, consisting of various types of adipocytes and a hierarchical organization of fat cells, lobules, pearls, sections, and compartments. This system is supported by a network of fibrous tissue septa and is closely associated with blood vessels and nerves, playing critical roles in metabolic regulation, physical protection, and thermal insulation. The understanding of this intricate structure is crucial for medical fields dealing with obesity, metabolic disorders, cosmetic procedures, and reconstructive surgeries.

Fundamentals of Adipose Tissue Histology

From an anatomical standpoint, an organ is characterized as a collection of tissues that collaboratively carry out one or more interrelated functions (Fig. 1). The adipose organ meets this criteria because it consists of two types of tissues, white and brown adipose tissues, which work together to distribute the energy stored in lipids between thermogenesis and other metabolic processes. The adipose organ in rats and mice comprises many subcutaneous and visceral depots. The depots include both brown adipose tissue, which appears dark, and white adipose tissue, which appears white. The quantity of brown adipocytes present in white regions fluctuates depending on age, animal strain, and environmental circumstances. The progenitors

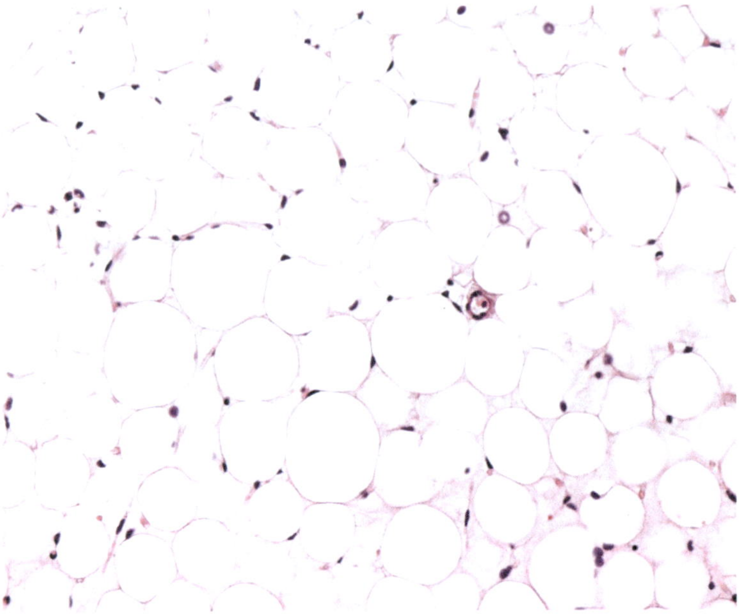

Fig. 1 White adipose tissue stained with HE. Adipocytes (fat cells) contain a large lipid droplet surrounded by a thin layer of cytoplasm. The nucleus is flattened and located on the periphery

of brown and white adipocytes exhibit distinct morphological differences. Brown areas are extensively innervated by noradrenergic nerve fibers, in addition to having a well-developed vascular system. The macroscopic structure and microscopic composition of the organ exhibit significant variations under different physiological conditions (cold acclimation, warm acclimation, fasting) and pathological conditions like obesity. Additionally, the expression of crucial genes, such as leptin and uncoupling protein-1, differs greatly between the two cell types. It is important to consider these fundamental principles while studying the physiological processes and therapy of obesity.

Adipose tissue is divided into two types: white adipose tissue (WAT) and brown adipose tissue (BAT). These tissues have distinct physiological differences, leading to specialized tissue functions. White adipose tissue is crucial for energy storage, endocrine communication, and insulin sensitivity and is the largest AT volume in most mammals, including humans. On the other hand, brown adipose tissue is largely present in mammals postnatally and during hibernation, using energy for non-shivering heat production, which is essential for body temperature maintenance. BAT was initially thought to only be present in infant humans, but studies have shown metabolically active BAT in adult regions. BAT activity is inversely correlated with age and BMI, with higher activity in winter and lower in summer. In healthy humans, BAT activity contributes to whole-body fat oxidation and diet-induced thermogenesis, supporting a physiological role for this AT depot in adults.

Brown and white adipocytes differ in shape, size, and intracellular structure of their organelles. White adipocytes are spherical and contain a large, single lipid droplet, while brown adipocytes have multiple lipid droplets dispersed throughout a more ellipsoidal-shaped cell enriched with iron-containing mitochondria. The thermogenic activity of brown adipocytes is conferred by the presence of numerous mitochondria containing uncoupling protein 1 (UCP-1), a proton transporter that short-circuits the ATP-generating proton gradient and allows for concurrent heat production.

Two new adipocyte hues, beige and pink, have been identified. Beige adipocytes, which are characterized by brown and white fat cells, develop within subcutaneous fat tissue (WAT) from preadipocytes or transdifferentiated white adipocytes. They were initially observed in rodents due to cold exposure but have since been found to be inducible in diet, exercise, pre- and post-biotics, pharmaceutical agents, plant-based bioactives, and adipokines. Pink adipocytes, first described in 2014, appear in the subcutaneous WAT of female mice during pregnancy and lactation. They derive from white adipocytes that take on epithelial-like features to form milk-secreting alveoli, giving the tissue a pink hue. Although reversible transdifferentiation is responsible for the development and disappearance of pink adipocytes in rodents, it remains uncertain whether they form in humans.

Further research into adipocyte plasticity could help identify novel therapeutic targets to combat obesity and its pathological consequences, as well as cancer.

Adipose tissue stores body fat as neutral TAGs and is the primary energy reservoir in mammals. Adipocytes, the largest cell types in whole AT, are characterized by their large unilocular central lipid droplets (cLDs). However, the biogenesis of unilocular LDs in adipocytes is poorly understood due to the fragile nature of WAT. Live-cell imaging and fluorescent labeling techniques have been used to investigate the cytoarchitecture of unilocular adipocytes and the spatiotemporal dynamics of lipid droplet formation. Cytoplasmic nodules containing micro LDs appear on the surface of fat cells, pushing them to the edges by the large cLD. Exogenously added lipids are rapidly taken up by the fat cell and esterified to TAG before being absorbed by mLDs.

Adipocytes accumulate lipid through two processes: taking up dietary lipids from the circulation in the form of FFA's liberated from circulating TAGs via lipoprotein lipase (LPL) and secreting LPL, which is transported to the adjacent capillary lumen to catalyze the hydrolysis of FFA's from circulating triglyceride-containing lipoproteins. Adipocytes also take up glucose, which is converted to glycerol and serves as the backbone for the sequential esterification of fatty acids for form TAG. The final step in TAG synthesis, re-esterification of circulating free fatty acids, is mediated by diacylglycerol acyltransferase (DGAT).

De novo lipogenesis (DNL) within adipocytes involves both de novo synthesis of fatty acids from acetyl-coenzyme A (acetyl-CoA) and the esterification of these fatty acids to a glycerol backbone producing TAGs. De novo lipogenesis can occur in fasting and fed states, with excess glucose oxidation yielding elevated levels of acetyl-CoA that become substrate to generate fatty acids.

Lipolysis is a catabolic process that breaks down adipocytes' total adipose tissue (TAG) into diacylglycerols (DAGs) and monoacylglycerols (MAGs) through the action of adipocyte triglyceride lipase (ATGL), hormone-sensitive lipase (HSL), and monoacylglycerol lipase (MGL). This process can occur in all tissues but is most prevalent in AT, where the bulk of TAG is stored. Lipolysis is controlled by sympathetic nervous system input and various hormones, including catecholamine noradrenaline (NA), which stimulates β-adrenergic receptors, which in turn stimulate protein kinase A (PKA) via adenylyl cylase (AC)-mediated production of cyclic AMP (cAMP). PKA activates the lipolytic action of ATGL and HSL by different mechanisms. Non-adrenergic lipolytic stimuli include glucocorticoids, natriuretic peptides, growth hormone, and tumor necrosis factor alpha (TNFα).

Postprandial increase in circulating insulin suppresses lipolysis by increasing the activity of phosphodiesterase 3 (PDE3B) and decreasing cAMP levels. Exercise is another major pro-lipolytic stimulus in humans, with growth hormone, NA, adrenaline, and cortisol increasing with exercise intensity while insulin levels decrease. When AT becomes insulin resistant, insulin's ability to inhibit adipocyte lipolysis and reduce serum levels of FFA and glycerol is impaired, leading to excessive lipolysis leading to increased FFA levels in both the fasted and fed state. Ectopic lipids impair insulin signaling, and insulin resistance at the level of adipocyte via increased lipolysis may be a major contributor to whole body insulin resistance.

In addition to potent anti-lipolytic action, insulin also stimulates lipogenesis by activating LPL and increasing the transcription of lipogenic enzymes. Growth hormone antagonizes insulin by promoting lipolysis and inhibiting lipogenesis. Both AT lipogenesis and lipolysis are attractive targets for pharmaceutical intervention. However, the balance between lipid storage, mobilization, and utilization is homeostatically regulated through a complex interaction of hormonal signaling, neurological input, and nutrient flow.

Adipocytes and other atherosclerotic cells secrete various mediators, including exosomes, miRNA, lipids, inflammatory cytokines, and peptide hormones, which have both paracrine and endocrine effects. Three endocrine hormones, leptin, adiponectin, and resistin, are almost exclusively produced in adipocytes and regulate food intake, reproductive axis, insulin sensitivity, and immune responses. Dysregulation of these hormones can contribute to systemic metabolic dysfunction, chronic metabolic diseases, and some types of cancer. Leptin was the first discovered endocrine hormone of adipocyte origin. In 1949, obese offspring in a nonobese mouse colony were found to be homozygous for a recessive mutation, leading to hyperglycemia and hyperinsulinemia. In the 1950s, parabiosis experiments were conducted to compare the effects of these hormones on obesity and other metabolic diseases.

The ob/ob gene product, a circulating factor, was found to inhibit weight gain in ob/ob mice when parabiosed with nonobese littermates. This led to improved hyperglycemia, hyperinsulinemia, and insulin sensitivity in lean animals. In the 1990s, leptin, derived from the Greek word "leptos" meaning "thin," was identified as the product of the ob gene. Its primary source was adipocytes, and its function was observed to be on food intake. Leptin levels in mice and men strongly correlate with fat mass and play a key role in body-weight homeostasis. The diabetes or db/db mouse, another spontaneously arising mutant mouse, developed obesity and type 2 diabetes. Parabiosis of db/db mice to wild-type littermates did not improve body weight or diabetes but resulted in unhealthy weight loss in lean littermates. The db gene was identified to encode the leptin receptor (LR) almost 5 years later.

The LR is a class 1 cytokine receptor that mediates the actions of many cytokines and lacks intrinsic kinase activity. It has six isoforms, with LRb being the best characterized. Leptin-regulated circuits involved in energy homeostasis are mapped to distinct brain regions expressing the long form of the LR. Increased central leptin signaling inhibits food intake and elevates energy expenditure, while leptin deficiency has opposite effects. Leptin levels strongly correlate with fat mass in mice and men, acting as a sensor of energy stores and regulating adipose reserves. However, during obesity, the negative feedback loop between increasing leptin levels and inhibiting food intake becomes disrupted due to leptin resistance. The physiological causes of leptin resistance are not well understood, but hyperleptinemia is required for its development.

Leptin, a hormone that regulates glucose and lipid metabolism, has been found to have various effects on various tissues, including skeletal muscle, liver, and intestines. When leptin levels are clamped to low levels, mice still develop obesity on high-fat diets (HFD), but they do not become leptin resistant. This resistance is a result of selective impairment of leptin's ability to reduce food intake while preserving its capacity to raise energy expenditure. The molecular basis for this phenomenon is still under investigation. Leptin also has central nervous system effects, including modulating reproduction and thermoregulation. Its mediating responses in peripheral tissues are complex due to its six receptor isoforms, differential expression across tissues, the pleiotropic nature of leptin's effects, and the complexity of signaling pathways involved. Adiponectin, a unique and extensively studied adipocyte-derived hormone, was discovered in 1995 and 1996 by three different research groups.

Adiponectin, secreted by adipocytes, has high circulating levels in humans, reaching 2–20 ug/ml. Its anti-hyperglycemic, anti-atherogenic, and anti-inflammatory effects make it an attractive therapeutic target for obesity and insulin resistance treatment. However, its complex structure and regulation have hindered efforts to develop therapies targeting adiponectin function. Adipocytes secrete different forms of adiponectin, including low-molecular weight trimers, medium-molecular weight hexamers, and high-molecular weight oligomers. The HMW oligomer is associated with enhanced insulin sensitivity and reduced glucose levels. Adiponectin signaling is complex and incompletely understood, with three adiponectin receptors identified: AdipoR1 and AdipoR2, which bind the LMW and globular forms, and T-cadherin, which binds HMW adiponectin. Both receptors can modulate insulin sensitivity and metabolic gene expression in insulin-responsive tissues and have demonstrated roles in insulin resistance and type 2 diabetes.

T-cadherin is the primary effector of cardioprotection by adiponectin, which enhances fatty acid oxidation through activation of AMP-activated kinase (AMPK). This inhibits acetyl CoA carboxylase, reducing malonyl-CoA production and enhancing fatty acid oxidation. Adiponectin can activate AMPK through two independent pathways and modulate lipid metabolism by increasing mitochondrial density and DNA content. It has diverse effects in various tissues, including bone and cartilage, and can act in an autocrine or paracrine manner in AT and other tissues. Adiponectin's insulin-sensitizing effects are most fully characterized at the mechanistic level in liver and muscle. The liver plays a critical role in maintaining normal blood glucose levels, but its ability to reduce glucose output when demand is low is often impaired with obesity and insulin resistance.

Adiponectin plays a crucial role in regulating glucose output in the liver, with studies showing that genetic deletion or overexpression of adiponectin can impair or enhance hepatic insulin sensitivity. Thiazolidinediones (TZDs) increase adiponectin levels, which improve insulin sensitivity and glucose tolerance. Adiponectin also promotes hepatocyte survival, inhibits fibrosis and inflammation, stimulates fatty acid oxidation, and modulates fatty acid uptake and metabolism. Low plasma adiponectin levels are associated with the progression of nonalcoholic fatty liver disease (NAFLD) and nonalcoholic steatohepatitis in insulin-resistant patients. Skeletal muscle, responsible for up to 80% of insulin-mediated glucose uptake, can also benefit from adiponectin. Defective adiponectin signaling in skeletal muscle may contribute to insulin resistance. Adiponectin is also cardioprotective, with low circulating levels correlated with coronary artery disease and a risk factor for cardiovascular diseases like hypertension, coronary artery disease, and restenosis.

Adiponectin, a hormone found in adipocytes, has significant therapeutic potential in treating obesity-associated metabolic diseases like diabetes, cardiovascular disease, and nonalcoholic fatty liver disease (NAFLD). Its cardioprotective effects are mediated by the vascular endothelium, which activates AMPK and eNOS. Small molecule AdipoR agonists, such as AdipoRon, have shown anti-hyperglycemia effects in diet-induced obese mice and a genetic mouse model for diabetes. Recent studies have shown that AdipoRon can decrease ceramides, lipotoxicity, and mitigate diabetic nephropathy. Resistin, a major adipocyte-derived hormone, was independently identified by two laboratories and has been shown to inhibit adipocyte differentiation. However, elucidating resistin's role in physiology remains challenging, as it is expressed in both white and brown fat in mice and has varying expression patterns in different depots and blood types.

Resistin, a hormone that produces similar metabolic and inflammatory effects in humans and mice, is primarily secreted from macrophages, not adipocytes. The complex regulation of resistin expression and differences in resistin biology between species make it difficult to fully understand its functions and mechanisms of action in humans. Resistin interacts with two known receptors: the toll-like receptor 4 (TLR4) and adenylyl cyclase-associated protein 1 (CAP1). TLR4 contributes to monocyte recruitment and chemokine expression, while CAP1 mediates pro-inflammatory effects. Resistin has been shown to regulate fasting blood glucose levels in mice, and its effects on insulin resistance have been observed in both human and mouse models. The humanized resistin mouse model addresses this issue by introducing the macrophage-expressed human resistin gene, allowing for a more comprehensive understanding of resistin's functions and mechanisms.

The study found that humanized resistin, similar to murine adipocyte-derived resistin, can cause systemic insulin resistance, inflammation, and elevated circulating free fatty acids in mice fed high-fat diets. In humans, resistin plays a role in metabolic dysfunction and related pathologies, with elevated serum levels during obesity and associated with atherosclerosis, coronary heart disease, congestive heart failure, and inflammatory conditions. The effectiveness of resistin interventions in treating metabolic or cardiovascular diseases in humans remains uncertain.

The AT stromal vascular fraction (SVF) is a complex network of non-adipocyte cell types that contribute to systemic metabolic regulation. It is important to understand the complex interactions between these cells and how they are altered by metabolic disease states. The SVF produces hormones and cytokines that can act paracrinely on adjacent adipocytes, such as TNF alpha, which is produced in adipose tissue macrophages (ATMs) during conditions of obesity and type 2 diabetes.

Adipogenesis is the process by which precursor cells differentiate and become committed to storing lipid and maintaining energy homeostasis as adipocytes. Adipogenesis is regulated by hundreds of factors, including nutrients, cellular signaling pathways, miRNAs, cytoskeletal proteins, and endocrine hormones. Pro-inflammatory cytokines generally inhibit adipogenesis, while cytoskeletal proteins, ECM proteins, microRNAs, and long noncoding RNAs differentially modulate adipogenesis.

The transcription factor peroxisome proliferator-activated receptor gamma (PPARg) is considered the principal adipogenesis regulator. Its discovery substantially enhanced our understanding of the adipocyte and its role in metabolic disease. Synthetic TZDs induce weight gain in humans and rodents by increasing fat mass, more so in the subcutaneous adipose depot, which is associated with improved metabolic outcomes. However, this weight gain is also considered a negative side effect of TZD treatment, especially in the typical patient with preexisting obesity.

Several selective PPARg modulators (SPPARMs) have been identified to act as partial PPARg agonists, alter specific posttranslational modifications of PPARg, and preserve anti-hyperglycemia effects while minimizing or eliminating the adipogenic effect that leads to increased fat mass via activation of distinct gene profiles that may be cell and tissue specific. Interestingly, the TZD, rosiglitazone, is capable of improving glucose homeostasis even in the absence of PPARg in mature adipocytes, suggesting that its adipogenic effects may also be important for its anti-hyperglycemic action.

PPARg binds endogenous lipophilic molecules, including long chain fatty acids (LCFAs), oxidized or nitrated FAs, prostaglandins, and arachidonic acid derivatives. Serotonin (5-hydroxytryptamine, 5-HT) has also been shown to be a high-affinity agonist for PPARg. Many endogenous PPARg ligands enhance adipocyte differentiation and regulate fat cell functions through PPARg-dependent and independent methods.

In conclusion, understanding the complex interactions between AT, adipogenesis, and CCAAT/enhancer-binding proteins is crucial for improving our understanding of AT development and function under both physiological and pathophysiological conditions.

The signal transducer and activator of transcription (STAT) family of transcription factors has been identified over 20 years ago and plays a crucial role in adipogenesis. STATs regulate gene expression during adipogenesis, with the expression of STATs 1, 3, 5A, and 5B induced during differentiation of murine and human preadipocytes. Sterol response element binding proteins (SREBP-1a, SREBP-1c, and SREBP-2) are three isoforms of STATs that regulate lipogenesis genes and cholesterol biosynthesis genes.

The early B cell factor (EBF) family of transcription factors is characterized for their ability to modulate islet beta-cell maturation and neural development. EBFs 1 and 2 can promote adipogenesis, while EBF2 can also play roles in determining brown versus white adipocyte identity in vivo and the beiging process of adipose tissue in mice.

The interferon-regulatory factor (IRF) family of transcription factors has functionally diverse roles in the immune system but also plays a role in adipocyte development. All nine IRF family members are regulated to different degrees during adipogenesis in vitro, and some members can repress adipogenesis and contribute to insulin resistance. Wingless-related integration site (Wnt) proteins regulate development and cell fate through both autocrine and paracrine signaling using three well-characterized pathways: the canonical Wnt signaling and the planar cell polarity and Wnt/calcium pathways, which are noncanonical.

The GATA family of transcription factors is named based on their ability to bind the DNA sequence GATA. Only GATAs 2 and 3 are expressed in preadipocytes residing in white AT, and both are repressed during adipogenesis. GATA2 can directly bind to the PPARγ promoter to suppress its activity, while GATA3 expression is driven by the canonical Wnt signaling pathway.

The Krüppel-like transcription factors (KLFs) include 17 members that can either activate or repress transcription. KLFs 4, 5, 6, 9, and 15 can promote adipogenesis, while KLFs 2, 3, and 7 repress adipocyte development. AP-1 transcription factors, including Jun proteins, Fos proteins, ATF, and JDP family members, can positively and negatively regulate adipogenesis.

Many zinc finger proteins (ZFPs) function as transcription factors, with several contributing to adipocyte determination and/or adipogenesis. Zfp423 and Zfp467 can promote adipocyte differentiation by enhancing PPARγ expression and activity, while Zfp521 can inhibit Zfp423 to reduce adipocyte development.

The transforming growth factor beta (TGF-β) superfamily encompasses a large number of proteins, including bone morphogenetic proteins (BMPs), which have been reported to be involved in both adipocyte commitment and differentiation.

While BMPs are known to promote adipogenesis, in vitro and in vivo studies demonstrated that TGF-β primarily inhibits fat cell differentiation.

Steroids play a crucial role in the development and distribution of atherosclerosis (AT) and are expressed in adipocytes. Steroid hormone receptors, such as estrogen and androgen receptors, are essential for transcriptional regulation of adipogenesis. Estrogens, such as ERα and ERβ, are expressed in rat and human preadipocytes, mature adipocytes, and other AT cells. These hormones inhibit adipocyte differentiation and the adipogenic action of PPARγ. Aromatase, an enzyme found in several tissues, including AT, aromatizes androgens into estrogens, suggesting that both estrogen and its receptor can reduce adipocyte development.

Androgen receptors (AR) are also expressed in rodents and human AT. Studies show contradictory actions of androgens on the differentiation and function of adipocytes, emphasizing the importance of accounting for sex-, depot-, and organism-specific effects. Testosterone and dihydrotestosterone, two non-aromatizable androgens, inhibit differentiation of preadipocytes obtained from subcutaneous and omental depots of both men and women. Overall, most studies indicate that androgens exert inhibitory effects on adipogenesis.

Glucocorticoids (GCs) are well-known promoters of adipocyte development, promoting adipocyte hypertrophy and differentiation of central fat depots that can lead to abdominal obesity and insulin resistance. In vitro adipogenesis studies include the wide use of the synthetic GC, dexamethasone. GCs induce expression of C/EBPs beta and δ and coordinate with C/EBPδ to induce PPARg expression and adipogenesis.

The glucocorticoid receptor (GR) is an enzyme highly expressed in AT and liver that converts inactive cortisone to the active hormone cortisol. 11β-hydroxysteroid dehydrogenase type 1 (11 beta HSD1) is an enzyme highly expressed in AT and liver that in AT converts inactive cortisone to the active hormone cortisol. GCs promote adipocyte development by suppression of anti-adipogenic factors, anti-proliferative effects on preadipocytes, and sensitizing or "priming" human preadipocytes to insulin action. Recent attention has focused on the potential contributions of environmental pollutants known as endocrine disrupting chemicals (EDCs) in the development of metabolic diseases.

In addition to regulating water and salt homeostasis, mineralocorticoid aldosterone and its receptor (MR) have been shown to play a role in the regulation of adipocyte development. Aldosterone promotes adipogenesis in an MR-dependent manner, and a MR antagonist can inhibit adipogenesis. However, there could be depot differences in the relative importance of MR and GR in cortisol-induced adipogenesis.

Vitamin D is another steroid hormone with strong experimental evidence that it can regulate adipogenesis. Its receptor (VDR) and 1α-hydroxylase (CYP27B1) are expressed in human AT, primary preadipocytes and newly differentiated adipocytes. Vitamin D represses adipocyte differentiation and can block adipogenesis by inhibiting C/EBPβ expression. Vitamin D and VDR also play a role in the inhibition of adipogenesis of bone marrow stromal cells, in part by suppressing the expression of inhibitors of the canonical Wnt/β-catenin signaling pathway.

The role of vitamin D in adipocyte development in humans is controversial and contradictory. A systematic review and meta-analysis of 23 studies between 2002 and 2014 found that overweight or obese subjects exhibit a higher prevalence of vitamin D deficiency. In two double-blind, placebo-controlled randomized clinical trials, vitamin D-supplemented individuals with healthy overweight or obesity lost significantly more fat mass than the placebo group when fed either a calorie-restriction (289) or weight-maintenance (290) diet for 12 weeks. While decreased fat mass may result from vitamin D-induced inhibition of adipogenesis, this hypothesis was not directly tested in the studies. Two other longer-term studies demonstrated no change in fat mass with vitamin D supplementation between 14,000 and 20,000 IU per week.

The relationship between adipocyte development and thyroid hormones has been recognized since 1888. The most biologically active form of thyroid hormone, T3, can induce brown adipocyte differentiation. Hyperthyroidism in rodents induces adipocyte hyperplasia, whereas hypothyroidism impedes AT development. Studies on the involvement of thyroid hormones in AT development are controversial.

In adipose tissue (AT), pools of adipose stem/progenitor cells (APs) exist that can differentiate into mature adipocytes. At least two distinct progenitor populations give rise to adipocytes: developmental APs and adult APs. Our understanding of the molecular characteristics of APs has dramatically increased in recent years.

Adipose tissue continues to generate new adipocytes throughout the lifespan, with a median adipocyte turnover rate of 8.3 years. Adult APs have been found in the SVF of AT depots in both rodents and humans and are thought to represent an AP pool that contributes to this adipocyte renewal. Flow cytometry techniques have helped identify stromal cells that can undergo adipogenesis, and bone marrow-derived adipocytes (BMDAs) from the myeloid lineage can also be recruited to AT where they become adipocytes.

Most of the information regarding AP proliferation in obesity comes from rodent models. In mice fed high-fat diets to induce obesity, APs form new adipocytes primarily in the visceral depot. However, convincing evidence for depot-specific AP populations in humans has emerged. Subcutaneous APs were shown to have a higher growth rate and adipogenic potential than visceral APs, giving rise to more functional adipocytes.

The adipose extracellular matrix (ECM) plays a crucial role in the development and function of adipocytes. During adipogenesis, there is increased synthesis of laminar ECM constituents and maintenance of peri-adipocyte fibrillar collagens, which allows adipocytes to embed themselves in the basal lamina. In the growth phase of adipogenesis, adipocytes require ECM-mediated traction forces to properly accumulate lipids and increase in size. A number of inhibitors, enzymes, and modifiers contribute to adipocyte ECM maintenance and renewal, which consume a large amount of energy in the mature fat cell.

In obesity, the ECM expands to accommodate adipocyte hypertrophy and hyperplasia and subsequent tissue growth, induced by the increased demand for lipid storage. This process appears to occur in both animal models and humans. Adipose tissue expansion during obesity, coupled with immune cell accumulation and hypoxia, can lead to AT fibrosis. Fibrosis is the excessive accumulation of ECM components, such as collagens, that typically results from an imbalance of the synthesis and degradation of ECM components.

Ultimately, adipocyte dysfunction will result from the decreased ECM flexibility conferred by the accumulation of fibrillar ECM components.

Abnormal ECM collagen deposition is associated with immune cell infiltration, which can worsen fibrosis and contribute to AT dysfunction that often occurs in obesity. The removal of collagen VI, a major AT ECM component, improves adipocyte function and metabolism in obese mice by both decreasing AT immune cell infiltration and "weakening" the ECM, which allows uninhibited adipocyte hypertrophy. In humans, AT collagen VI expression is increased in obesity, and subjects with higher collagen VI have increased macrophage content and AT inflammation. Endotrophin, an adipocyte-derived cleavage product of collagen VI, directly stimulates AT fibrosis and macrophage accumulation and can lead to systemic insulin resistance.

Accumulation of ECM components and increased ECM receptor signaling are associated with insulin resistance in obesity thought to be mediated by several possible mechanisms. Excess ECM components can also increase AT inflammation by interactions with their cell surface receptors (CD44, CD36, and integrins), which can induce adipocyte death, inhibit angiogenesis, and promote macrophage infiltration and inflammation in adipose tissue, thereby driving insulin resistance.

The ECM has clear roles in the normal development and function of adipocytes but in excess can also play roles in obesity development and metabolic dysfunction. More research is needed to better understand how ECM components and their interactions can directly influence AT physiology and pathophysiology.

In humans, fat deposition in the upper body, mainly the visceral and subcutaneous abdominal depot, is linked to a higher risk of metabolic dysfunction, while lower body adiposity in the subcutaneous gluteal and femoral regions is associated with lower risk and may even be protective. Rodent studies reveal that surgical removal of visceral fat pads improves insulin action, glucose tolerance, and longevity, while the removal of subcutaneous fat pads can cause metabolic syndrome. However, human studies have shown that the removal of small amounts of omental AT in individuals with obesity provided no metabolic health benefits. Liposuction of subcutaneous AT in humans neither harmed nor improved the cardio-metabolic profile.

Studies of depot-specific expression patterns have enhanced our understanding of the mechanisms underlying abdominal versus gluteal and femoral adiposity. Unique expression patterns in different adipose tissue depots in mice indicate substantial difference in the expression of homeobox (HOX) developmental genes. Structural and hormonal regulators, including collagen VI and glucocorticoids, that influence fat distribution are similarly associated with AT expansion in both rodents and humans.

Similar to humans, female rodents have a higher percentage fat mass relative to males but remain more insulin sensitive. However, there are many notable sex differences in rodent versus human depots. The inguinal depots of female mice contain mammary glands, and the gonadal fat pad is near reproductive tissue, which is not the case in humans. High-fat diet-induced obesity affects men and women alike, but females are resistant HFD obesity in many strains of mice. Lower body AT has been shown to secrete more metabolically favorable adipokines such as adiponectin.

Lipolysis can be stimulated in rodents and humans under similar physiological conditions, but important biological differences in AT lipolysis among these species have been suggested.

Dermal adipose tissue (dWAT) is a distinct adipose depot that differs from subcutaneous fat. It can alter its cellular characteristics and have high turnover rates, and its organization is unique. In rodents, dWAT forms several adipocyte layers between the dermis and muscle layer, while in humans, it is present as individual units called dermal cones. These cones are concentrated around pilosebaceous units that interact to form the dWAT structure.

DWAT has distinct roles in insulation, barrier protection from skin infection, and hair follicle cycling. It slows down to provide an effective layer of insulation when exposed to cold temperatures, unlike brown adipose tissue (BAT), which rapidly responds to cold temperature challenges by mobilizing lipids for heat generation. However, dWAT can also thicken or expand over days to provide an effective layer of insulation.

Epicardial atrophy (EAT) has recently emerged as an important player in the development of cardiovascular disorders. EAT is distinct from pericardial fat and lies between the visceral pericardium and the myocardium, sharing a blood supply with the coronary arteries. The adipocytes in EAT are smaller than those in other visceral or subcutaneous depots and are outnumbered by preadipocytes. The gene expression and adipokine secretion profiles of EAT are unique from those of other depots.

In normal physiological conditions, EAT behaves like BAT and serves to protect the coronary vessels and myocardium against hypothermia. In pathologies such as coronary artery disease and type 2 diabetes, EAT can display an extensive pro-inflammatory signature. Macrophages and mast cells have been shown to infiltrate EAT, undergo activation, and facilitate lipid accumulation in atherosclerotic plaques. Pro-inflammatory adipokine secretion from EAT has also been shown to induce atrial fibrosis. Insulin sensitivity and EAT thickness are inversely correlated, while fasting glucose and EAT size are positively correlated, with enlarged EAT depots often found in individuals with type 2 diabetes.

White adipose tissue (AT) has the ability to expand during adult life to accommodate chronic excess caloric intake. AT expansion is characterized by adipocytes accumulating lipid and growing in size or number, either hypertrophy or hyperplasia or adipogenesis. The capacity of subcutaneous AT to expand and the manner of expansion can influence cardiometabolic health, which is thought to underlie the benefits of thiazolidinedione (TZD) medications, which are approved for the treatment of type 2 diabetes. These PPARγ agonists stimulate preadipocyte differentiation and the proliferation of adipocytes, especially in subcutaneous depots as compared to visceral adipose tissue, which leads to increased adiponectin levels and improved insulin sensitivity.

However, the presence of enlarged, hypertrophic adipocytes, a lack of hyperplasia, and development of AT inflammation and fibrosis reflect impaired AT expansion and is associated with metabolic derangements. These observations support the "AT expandability hypothesis," which postulates that a lack of adipogenesis (or hyperplasia) results in the limited capacity of AT to expand and store lipid, causing ectopic fat accretion and "lipotoxicity" in non-adipose tissues such as skeletal muscle and liver. The degree of ectopic lipid deposition in the liver and skeletal muscle is a significant determinant of metabolic syndrome (MetS) and the development of T2D and CVD.

Other findings do not support the AT expandability hypothesis and indicate that higher adipogenesis does not necessarily denote improvements in metabolic health. Studies report a higher population of small adipocytes in the AT of individuals with insulin resistance and T2D (403–406) and in those with more visceral AT and liver fat (406,407). Experimental overfeeding intervention studies have shown that individuals with smaller adipocytes at baseline have poorer metabolic health outcomes in response to substantial weight gain than those with larger adipocytes (408,409). In addition, one in vivo analysis in humans demonstrated that increased hyperplastic expansion correlated with an increased number of metabolic syndrome components (410). Collectively, these data imply an alternative model of impaired AT expansion, as compared to the mechanisms proposed by the AT expandability hypothesis, suggesting that there is not a deficiency in hyperplasia but an abundance of adipocytes with a limited capacity to adequately expand and accommodate lipid, whether large or small. This inability to store excess lipid in AT is thought to be a key feature that leads to metabolic dysfunction.

AT inflammation is considered a major contributor to the metabolic dysfunction associated with obesity. During nutrient excess as AT expandability reaches its limit, a strong association exists between adipocyte size and adipocyte death. In response to adipocyte death, pro-inflammatory macrophages surround dead and dying cells and remove debris from the damaged area, producing inflammatory cytokines that often fail to resolve, becoming chronic, and leading to impaired adipocyte insulin signaling, further inflammation, and a continued worsening of AT dysfunction. Evidence also indicates adaptive and homeostatic roles for pro-inflammatory signaling in AT expansion and function.

Metabolically healthy (MHO) versus metabolically unhealthy (MUO) obesity is characterized by normal insulin sensitivity, normal fasting glucose levels, low incidence of hypertension, and blood lipid profiles in the healthy range. Factors that distinguish individuals with MHO from MUO highlight the premise that metabolic health risk is not solely dependent on body weight. Understanding these characteristics and potential mechanisms underlying the MHO and the perceived healthy metabolic state of these individuals is an important area of ongoing research.

Ectopic lipid accumulation in both the liver and skeletal muscle is significant as part of the "lipotoxicity" hypothesis and may impact the varying health risk of metabolically obese (MHO) vs. metabolically obese (MUO) individuals. Extramyocellular lipid (EMCL) and intramyocellular lipid (IMCL) are postulated to cause defects in insulin signaling and reduce insulin-stimulated skeletal muscle glucose uptake, which are strong correlates of insulin resistance and are increased in individuals with type 2 diabetes. Intrahepatic lipid accumulation strongly associates with impaired insulin-induced suppression of hepatic glucose production, even independently of visceral AT amount, and the development of type 2 diabetes. Ectopic fat in both the liver and skeletal muscle has been shown to be lower in MHO than MUO individuals.

The differential secretion of pro-inflammatory adipokines has also been proposed as a mechanism underlying the MHO phenotype. However, studies show reduced macrophage infiltration in MHO, supporting a reduced inflammatory state in these individuals. Intriguing data implicating potential genetic differences among MHO vs. MUO indicate that specific polymorphisms in genes, including the adiponectin receptor 1 and hepatic lipase, may be associated with the MHO phenotype. Genes encoding some pro-inflammatory cytokines can be more highly expressed in the adipose tissue of MUO compared with MHO individuals.

A lingering question remains unanswered: whether MHO subjects will sustain a healthy metabolic state throughout their lifespan or if they will eventually become MUO. Additionally, the length of time for follow-up assessments of MHO individuals is an important factor that may have considerable effects on the observed outcomes. A major obstacle in advancing the understanding of the MHO phenotype is the manner by which metabolic health is described, including the parameters used to define insulin sensitivity and metabolic syndrome.

Lipodystrophy is a condition characterized by the deficiency of athrostrophin and reduced levels of leptin and adiponectin. Leptin plays a crucial role in body weight regulation and energy metabolism, and low levels can impact glucose metabolism, appetite, and excessive caloric intake in patients with lipodystrophy. Transgenic animal models have shown that fatless rodents display hypertriglyceridemia and ectopic lipid accumulation, along with severe insulin resistance. However, transplanting AT from leptin-deficient mice did not improve metabolic abnormalities in fatless mice, while leptin administration ameliorated insulin resistance and hepatic steatosis in humans with total lipodystrophy.

Adiponectin has insulin-sensitizing and anti-inflammatory effects, and low levels of this adipokine have also been observed in patients with lipodystrophies. Recombinant adiponectin, adiponectin analogues, and compounds that upregulate endogenous adiponectin (TZDs) have all been proposed as treatment approaches for lipodystrophy. In a fatless mouse model, treatment with the globular domain of adiponectin significantly improved the hyperglycemia and hyperinsulinemia characteristic of lipoatrophic diabetic mice. Insulin resistance observed in these mice was completely ameliorated by treatment with both adiponectin and leptin, suggesting that both adiponectin and leptin deficiency may contribute to the insulin resistance in humans with lipodystrophy.

Too little AT, as seen in lipodystrophy, appears to be just as deleterious as too much AT. Patients with lipodystrophy may have reduced survival and high mortality at an early age, predominantly due to cardiometabolic complications. Lipodystrophy has no cure, so the primary treatment option is to improve metabolic outcomes via physical activity and dietary and pharmacological interventions. Conventional insulin-sensitizing agents, such as metformin and TZDs, are often used, and leptin replacement is also an approved therapy for total congenital lipodystrophy.

Leptin and adiponectin are the most investigated adipokines as mediators of reproductive health and pathology. Receptors for both leptin and adiponectin have been identified in all major reproductive tissues, including the testes, placenta, ovaries, oviducts, and endometrium. Obese mice that are deficient in leptin or the leptin receptor are unable to reproduce. In humans, leptin levels increase during pregnancy and rapidly fall in the postpartum period, and other reports suggest that adiponectin may influence gestational weight gain and weight maintenance postpartum.

Adiponectin plasma levels were shown to be significantly lower in overweight patients than normal weight women during pregnancy and negatively correlated with progressive gestational age and weight gain.

Insufficient or excessive adipose tissue (AT) can have detrimental effects on reproductive health, with women with lipodystrophy disorders often experiencing infertility due to AT and leptin deficiency. Anorexia nervosa is an eating disorder characterized by low AT mass and amenorrhea, which affects approximately 38% of women affected by anorexia. Leptin deficiency is common in these patients and may lead to disruptions in downstream neuroendocrine signaling. Estrogen deficiency in these women results in major implications for bone health, contributing to increased osteopenia or osteoporosis.

Body weight has been shown to predict testosterone levels in men, and obesity, specifically central adiposity, is associated with low testosterone levels. Increased AT also leads to elevated estradiol, resulting in reduced circulating testosterone through feedback inhibition of gonadotrophs. A common medical condition in women at the crossroads of dysfunctional AT and reproduction is polycystic ovary syndrome (PCOS), which in roughly 50% of affected women is associated with increased central obesity and metabolic health risk. Studies of PCOS generally show that adiponectin levels are lower in these patients.

Excessive AT and reproductive malignancies are another area of research, as obesity increases the risk of breast, uterine, cervical, and prostate cancers. Studies have reported inverse relationships between leptin and adiponectin levels with breast, endometrial, ovarian, and prostate cancers.

Adipocyte biology is a critical area of research, with the focus shifting toward recognizing neglected AT depots, the expanding types of adipocytes, and the complex developmental and sex-regulated origins of adipocytes. Adipocytes are critical secretory cells that contribute a variety of circulating proteins, including endocrine hormones, and can release genetic material with profound systemic functions. Much remains to be discovered about the types of nerves present in fat tissue and how they vary according to AT type and location. Recent advances in whole tissue AT imaging and studies on brain-adipose communication suggest we are just beginning to uncover the capabilities and function of AT nerves.

Exercise on adipocyte function is another developing area of fat cell biology. Recent studies have shown that transplantation of subcutaneous AT from exercise-trained mice improves glucose tolerance and insulin sensitivity in recipient, non-exercised mice, suggesting that exercise favorably remodels AT to improve systemic metabolic health. A new discovered pathway shows that lipids can be released by adipocytes in the form of exosome-sized, lipid-filled vesicles, independent of canonical lipolytic pathways.

AT is now considered an important endocrine organ and site of inflammatory cell signaling that governs not only survival but also plays critical roles in reproduction and glucometabolic homeostasis. As scientific methods for studying AT continue to rapidly evolve, so does our understanding regarding the metabolic, biomechanical, immune, and secretory functions of AT in normal physiology and metabolic disease.

Comparative Histological Analysis of Normal Adipose Tissue, Lipedema

Normal adipose tissue exhibits a homogeneity in adipocyte size. In contrast, lipedema is characterized by a significant variation in adipocyte size, including hypertrophic cells, which are also observed in obese individuals. However, this heterogeneity is not exclusive to lipedema, as similar patterns are seen in obese and nonobese control groups. This finding suggests that adipocyte size variation alone may not be a definitive marker for diagnosing lipedema.

An increase in macrophages is noted in both obese and nonobese individuals with lipedema, indicative of an inflammatory response. This parallels observations in obesity, where macrophage presence is linked to adipose tissue inflammation. The presence of crown-like structures (CLS), typically associated with metabolically poor tissue, further emphasizes the inflammatory aspect of lipedema fat.

Notably, lipedema exhibits increased angiogenesis, as evidenced by the proliferation of blood vessels in the dermal layers. This angiogenesis is independent of obesity and suggests a unique vascular component in lipedema pathophysiology. Conversely, in normal adipose tissue, angiogenesis is less pronounced and does not exhibit the same patterns of vessel proliferation and dilation.

Lipedema also displays changes in lymphatic vessel morphology, particularly in obese individuals, where increased lymphatic vessel size is noted. This contrasts with the relatively stable lymphatic vessel architecture in nonobese lipedema and normal fat tissue, highlighting a potential link between obesity and lymphatic alterations in lipedema.

The study also examines various molecular markers, including vascular endothelial growth factor (VEGF), associated with angiogenesis and lymphangiogenesis. Elevated VEGF levels in patients with lipedema, compared to controls, align with the observed histological vascular changes. This differential expression of angiogenic markers further supports the distinct vascular remodeling in lipedema.

Interestingly, when comparing lipedema with secondary lymphedema and lipohypertrophy, each condition displays unique histological and molecular features. Secondary lymphedema shows pronounced vascular and lymphatic changes, while lipohypertrophy differs significantly in its lack of inflammatory and lymphatic alterations, suggesting it may represent a distinct pathological entity rather than a preliminary stage of lipedema.

Inflammatory Markers and Pathophysiological Mechanisms in Lipedema

Lipedema, a condition marked by the expansion of subcutaneous adipose tissue (SAT) in the lower extremities, presents a unique pathological profile distinct from common obesity. This chapter focuses on the inflammatory markers and pathophysiological mechanisms underlying lipedema, exploring adipocyte dysfunction, tissue inflammation, altered extracellular matrix (ECM) components, and microvascular dysfunctions contributing to its etiology.

The expansion of SAT in lipedema primarily occurs due to adipocyte hypertrophy, which is distinct from the fat distribution in obesity. This hypertrophic expansion is coupled with evidence of adipogenesis, indicated by the proliferation of adipose-derived stem cells (ASCs). In lipedema, ASCs, particularly CD34+ and Ki67+ types, colocalize with areas of macrophage residency and adipocyte necrosis, suggesting a complex interaction between adipocyte development and inflammation.

Lipedema tissue exhibits significant immune cell infiltration, notably macrophages, which form adipose crown-like structures around hypertrophic adipocytes. This is similar to the persistent inflammation observed in lymphedema, albeit with less T cell involvement. The presence of CD45+ lymphocytes and CD68+ macrophages in both lipedema adipose tissue and skin highlights the inflammatory nature of this condition.

The ECM in lipedema exhibits a fibrotic pathology, characterized by increased fibrosis and altered composition. This change in the ECM contributes to adipose tissue dysfunction and potentially elevated tissue sodium content. An intriguing aspect of lipedema pathogenesis is the possible uncoupling of the MMP-14-CAV1 axis in adipocytes, leading to abnormal matrix processing and, consequently, hypertrophic SAT expansion. Studies have shown variations in expressions of MMPs and ECM components like fibronectin and collagen in lipedema, compared to controls. These changes in the ECM might be linked to clinical symptoms such as joint hypermobility and reduced skin and aortic elasticity in some patients with lipedema.

Another aspect of lipedema's pathophysiology is the interstitial fluid accumulation resulting from microvascular dysfunction. Disruption in tissue volume homeostasis, including increased interstitial fluid and tissue sodium, points toward compromised lymphatic bulk transport in lipedema. This is further supported by clinical evidence of lymphatic disease in patients with lipedema. Elevated levels of platelet factor 4 (PF4) and VEGF-C in patients with lipedema suggest lymphatic dysfunction. However, unlike lymphedema, changes to lymphatic architecture are not predominantly observed in lipedema. Instead, there is substantial evidence of a blood capillary component, as indicated by patient reports of frequent hematoma, imaging studies showing vascular permeability, and observed capillary fragility. Histological studies have revealed an increased number of dilated blood capillaries in lipedema SAT, supporting the notion of blood and lymphatic microvascular contributions to the condition.

The inflammatory markers and pathophysiological mechanisms in lipedema highlight a complex interplay between adipocyte dysfunction, inflammation, ECM remodeling, and microvascular changes. Understanding these mechanisms is crucial for developing targeted therapies and effective management strategies for lipedema. The distinct nature of lipedema's inflammatory profile, compared to conditions like obesity and lymphedema, underscores the need for specific diagnostic criteria and treatment approaches tailored to this unique condition. Further research is necessary to elucidate the full spectrum of inflammatory and pathophysiological processes at play in lipedema.

Suggested Reading

Cuthbertson D, Tompsett S. The degree of unsaturation of the fats of human adipose tissue in relation to depth from skin surface. Biochem. J. 1933;27(4):1103–1106.

Cook KS, Min HY, Johnson D, Chaplinsky RJ, Flier JS, Hunt CR, Spiegelman BM. Adipsin: a circulating serine protease homolog secreted by adipose tissue and sciatic nerve. Science. 1987;237(4813):402–405.

Cianflone K, Maslowska M, Sniderman AD. Acylation stimulating protein (ASP), an adipocyte autocrine: new directions. Semin. Cell Dev. Biol. 1999;10(1):31–41.

Saleh J, Al-Wardy N, Farhan H, Al-Khanbashi M, Cianflone K. Acylation stimulating protein: a female lipogenic factor? Obes. Rev. 2011;12(6):440–448.

Zhang Y, Proenca R, Maffei M, Barone M, Leopold L, Friedman JM. Positional cloning of the mouse obese gene and its human homologue. Nature. 1994;372(6505):425–432.

Chlouverakis C. Insulin resistance of parabiotic obese-hyperglycemic mice (obob). Horm. Metab. Res. 1972;4(3):143–148.

Cava A, La, Matarese G. The weight of leptin in immunity. Nat. Rev. Immunol. 2004;4(5):371–379.

Carobbio S, Pellegrinelli V, Vidal-Puig A. Adipose tissue function and expandability as determinants of lipotoxicity and the metabolic syndrome. In: Obesity and Lipotoxicity. Springer, Cham; 2017:161–196.

Cancers Associated with Overweight and Obesity Make up 40 percent of Cancers Diagnosed in the United States | CDC Online Newsroom | CDC. Available at: https://www.cdc.gov/media/releases/2017/p1003-vs-cancer-obesity.html. Accessed January 21, 2019.

Hales CM, Carroll MD, Fryar CD, Ogden CL. Prevalence of obesity among adults and youth: United States, 2015–2016. NCHS data brief, no 288. Hyattsville, MD: National Center for Health Statistics; 2017. Available at: https://www.cdc.gov/nchs/products/databriefs/db288.htm. Accessed February 27, 2019.

Hruby A, Hu FB. The epidemiology of obesity: A big picture. Pharmacoeconomics. 2015;33(7):673–689.

Nedergaard J, Bengtsson T, Cannon B. Unexpected evidence for active brown adipose tissue in adult humans. Am. J. Physiol. Metab. 2007;293(2):E444–E452.

Zingaretti MC, Crosta F, Vitali A, Guerrieri M, Frontini A, Cannon B, Nedergaard J, Cinti S. The presence of UCP1 demonstrates that metabolically active adipose tissue in the neck of adult humans truly represents brown adipose tissue. FASEB J. 2009;23(9):3113–3120.

Cypess AM, Lehman S, Williams G, Tal I, Rodman D, Goldfine AB, Kuo FC, Palmer EL, Tseng Y-H, Doria A, Kolodny GM, Kahn CR. Identification and importance of brown adipose tissue in adult humans. N. Engl. J. Med. 2009;360(15):1509–1517.

Au-Yong ITH, Thorn N, Ganatra R, Perkins AC, Symonds ME. Brown adipose tissue and seasonal variation in humans. Diabetes. 2009;58(11):2583–7.

Hibi M, Oishi S, Matsushita M, Yoneshiro T, Yamaguchi T, Usui C, Yasunaga K, Katsuragi Y, Kubota K, Tanaka S, Saito M. Brown adipose tissue is involved in diet-induced thermogenesis and whole-body fat utilization in healthy humans. Int. J. Obes. (Lond). 2016;40(11):1655–1661.

de Sá PM, Richard AJ, Hang H, Stephens JM. Transcriptional regulation of adipogenesis. In: Comprehensive Physiology. Vol 7. Hoboken, NJ, USA: John Wiley & Sons, Inc.; 2017:635–674.

Cinti S. The adipose organ at a glance. Dis. Model. Mech. 2012;5(5):588–594.

Wu J, Boström P, Sparks LM, Ye L, Choi JH, Giang A-H, Khandekar M, Virtanen KA, Nuutila P, Schaart G, Huang K, Tu H, van Marken Lichtenbelt WD, Hoeks J, Enerbäck S, Schrauwen P, Spiegelman BM. Beige adipocytes are a distinct type of thermogenic fat cell in mouse and human. Cell. 2012;150(2):366–376.

Barbatelli G, Murano I, Madsen L, Hao Q, Jimenez M, Kristiansen K, Giacobino JP, De Matteis R, Cinti S. The emergence of cold-induced brown adipocytes in mouse white fat depots is determined predominantly by white to brown adipocyte transdifferentiation. Am. J. Physiol. Metab. 2010;298(6):E1244–E1253.

Himms-Hagen J, Melnyk A, Zingaretti MC, Ceresi E, Barbatelli G, Cinti S. Multilocular fat cells in WAT of CL-316243-treated rats derive directly from white adipocytes. Am. J. Physiol. Physiol. 2000;279(3):C670–C681.

Young P, Arch JRS, Ashwell M. Brown adipose tissue in the parametrial fat pad of the mouse. FEBS Lett. 1984;167(1):10–14.

Loncar D, Afzelius BA, Cannon B. Epididymal white adipose tissue after cold stress in rats. I. Nonmitochondrial changes. J. Ultrastruct. Mol. Struct. Res. 1988;101(2–3):109–122.

Wang S, Pan M-H, Hung W-L, Tung Y-C, Ho C-T. From white to beige adipocytes: therapeutic potential of dietary molecules against obesity and their molecular mechanisms. Food Funct. 2019;10:1263–1279.

Mika A, Macaluso F, Barone R, Di Felice V, Sledzinski T. Effect of exercise on fatty acid metabolism and adipokine secretion in adipose tissue. Front. Physiol. 2019;10(26):1–7.

Reynés B, Palou M, Rodríguez AM, Palou A. Regulation of adaptive thermogenesis and browning by prebiotics and postbiotics. Front. Physiol. 2018;9:1–15.

Kaisanlahti A, Glumoff T. Browning of white fat: agents and implications for beige adipose tissue to type 2 diabetes. J. Physiol. Biochem. 2019;75(1):1–10.

Ikeda K, Maretich P, Kajimura S. The common and distinct features of brown and beige adipocytes. Trends Endocrinol. Metab. 2018;29(3):191–200.

Giordano A, Smorlesi A, Frontini A, Barbatelli G, Cinti S. MECHANISMS IN ENDOCRINOLOGY: White, brown and pink adipocytes: the extraordinary plasticity of the adipose organ. Eur. J. Endocrinol. 2014;170(5):R159–R171.

Cinti S. Pink Adipocytes. Trends Endocrinol. Metab. 2018:1–16.

Apostoli AJ, Skelhorne-Gross GEA, Rubino RE, Peterson NT, Di Lena MA, Schneider MM, SenGupta SK, Nicol CJB. Loss of PPARγ expression in mammary secretory epithelial cells creates a pro-breast tumorigenic environment. Int. J. Cancer. 2014;134(5):1055–1066.

Chu M, Sampath H, Cahana DY, Kahl CA, Somwar R, Cornea A, Roberts CT, Varlamov O. Spatiotemporal dynamics of triglyceride storage in unilocular adipocytes. Gruenberg JE, ed. Mol. Biol. Cell 2014;25(25):4096–4105.

Kersten S. Physiological regulation of lipoprotein lipase. Biochim. Biophys. Acta - Mol. Cell Biol. Lipids. 2014;1841(7):919–933.

Fielding BA, Frayn KN. Lipoprotein lipase and the disposition of dietary fatty acids. Br. J. Nutr. 1998;80(6):495–502.

Frayn K. Adipose tissue as a buffer for daily lipid flux. Diabetologia. 2002;45(9):1201–1210.

Luo L, Liu M. Adipose tissue in control of metabolism. J. Endocrinol. 2016;231(3):R77–R99.

Harris CA, Haas JT, Streeper RS, Stone SJ, Kumari M, Yang K, Han X, Brownell N, Gross RW, Zechner R, Farese R V Jr. DGAT enzymes are required for triacylglycerol synthesis and lipid droplets in adipocytes. J. Lipid Res. 2011;52(4):657–667.

Smith SJ, Cases S, Jensen DR, Chen HC, Sande E, Tow B, Sanan DA, Raber J, Eckel RH, Farese R V. Obesity resistance and multiple mechanisms of triglyceride synthesis in mice lacking Dgat. Nat. Genet. 2000;25(1):87–90.

Song Z, Xiaoli AM, Yang F. Regulation and metabolic significance of de novo lipogenesis in adipose tissues. Nutrients. 2018;10(1383):1–22.

Swierczynski J, Goyke E, Wach L, Pankiewicz A, Kochan Z, Adamonis W, Sledzinski Z, Aleksandrowicz Z. Comparative study of the lipogenic potential of human and rat adipose tissue. Metabolism. 2000;49(5):594–599.

Letexier D, Pinteur C, Large V, Fréring V, Beylot M. Comparison of the expression and activity of the lipogenic pathway in human and rat adipose tissue. J. Lipid Res. 2003;44(11):2127–2134.

A, Chinkes D, Wolfe RR. Hepatic and whole-body fat synthesis in humans during carbohydrate overfeeding. Am. J. Clin. Nutr. 1997;65(6):1774–1782.

Kawahito S, Kitahata H, Oshita S. Problems associated with glucose toxicity: Role of hyperglycemia-induced oxidative stress. World J. Gastroenterol. 2009;15(33):4137.

Crewe C, Zhu Y, Paschoal VA, Joffin N, Ghaben AL, Gordillo R, Oh DY, Liang G, Horton JD, Scherer PE. SREBP-regulated adipocyte lipogenesis is dependent on substrate availability and redox modulation of mTORC1. JCI Insight. 2019;4(15)

Herman MA, Peroni OD, Villoria J, Schön MR, Abumrad NA, Blüher M, Klein S, Kahn BB. A novel ChREBP isoform in adipose tissue regulates systemic glucose metabolism. Nature. 2012;484(7394):333–338.

Vijayakumar A, Aryal P, Wen J, Syed I, Vazirani RP, Moraes-Vieira PM, Camporez JP, Gallop MR, Perry RJ, Peroni OD, Shulman GI, Saghatelian A, McGraw TE, Kahn BB. Absence of carbohydrate response element binding protein in adipocytes causes systemic insulin resistance and impairs glucose transport. Cell Rep. 2017;21(4):1021–1035.

Shimano H, Shimomura I, Hammer RE, Herz J, Goldstein JL, Brown MS, Horton JD. Elevated levels of SREBP-2 and cholesterol synthesis in livers of mice homozygous for a targeted disruption of the SREBP-1 gene. J. Clin. Invest. 1997;100(8):2115–2124.

Lodhi IJ, Wei X, Semenkovich CF. Lipoexpediency: de novo lipogenesis as a metabolic signal transmitter. Trends Endocrinol. Metab. 2011;22(1):1–8.

Smith U, Kahn BB. Adipose tissue regulates insulin sensitivity: role of adipogenesis, de novo lipogenesis and novel lipids. J. Intern. Med. 2016;280(5):465–475.

Zhou P, Santoro A, Peroni OD, Nelson AT, Saghatelian A, Siegel D, Kahn BB. PAHSAs enhance hepatic and systemic insulin sensitivity through direct and indirect mechanisms. J. Clin. Invest. 2019;129(10):4138–4150.

Yore MM, Syed I, Moraes-Vieira PM, Zhang T, Herman MA, Homan EA, Patel RT, Lee J, Chen S, Peroni OD, Dhaneshwar AS, Hammarstedt A, Smith U, McGraw TE, Saghatelian A, Kahn BB. Discovery of a class of endogenous mammalian lipids with anti-diabetic and anti-inflammatory effects. Cell. 2014;159(2):318–32.

Eissing L, Scherer T, Tödter K, Knippschild U, Greve JW, Buurman WA, Pinnschmidt HO, Rensen SS, Wolf AM, Bartelt A, Heeren J, Buettner C, Scheja L. De novo lipogenesis in human fat and liver is linked to ChREBP-β and metabolic health. Nat. Commun. 2013;4:1528.

Bruss MD, Khambatta CF, Ruby MA, Aggarwal I, Hellerstein MK. Calorie restriction increases fatty acid synthesis and whole body fat oxidation rates. Am. J. Physiol. Metab. 2010;298(1):E108–E116.

Mottillo EP, Balasubramanian P, Lee Y-H, Weng C, Kershaw EE, Granneman JG. Coupling of lipolysis and de novo lipogenesis in brown, beige, and white adipose tissues during chronic β3-adrenergic receptor activation. J. Lipid Res. 2014;55(11):2276–2286.

Braun K, Oeckl J, Westermeier J, Li Y, Klingenspor M. Non-adrenergic control of lipolysis and thermogenesis in adipose tissues. J. Exp. Biol. 2018;221:1–14.

Kuriyama H, Shimomura I, Kishida K, Kondo H, Furuyama N, Nishizawa H, Maeda N, Matsuda M, Nagaretani H, Kihara S, Nakamura T, Tochino Y, Funahashi T, Matsuzawa Y. Coordinated regulation of fat-specific and liver-specific glycerol channels, aquaporin adipose and aquaporin 9. Diabetes. 2002;51(10):2915–2921.

Sztalryd C, Brasaemle DL. The perilipin family of lipid droplet proteins: Gatekeepers of intracellular lipolysis. Biochim. Biophys. acta. Mol. cell Biol. lipids. 2017;1862 10 Pt B:1221–1232.

Nielsen TS, Jessen N, Jorgensen JOL, Moller N, Lund S. Dissecting adipose tissue lipolysis: molecular regulation and implications for metabolic disease. J. Mol. Endocrinol. 2014;52(3):R199–R222.

Greenberg AS, Egan JJ, Wek SA, Garty NB, Blanchette-Mackie EJ, Londos C. Perilipin, a major hormonally regulated adipocyte-specific phosphoprotein associated with the periphery of lipid storage droplets. J. Biol. Chem. 1991;266(17):11341–11346.

Strålfors P, Björgell P, Belfrage P. Hormonal regulation of hormone-sensitive lipase in intact adipocytes: identification of phosphorylated sites and effects on the phosphorylation by lipolytic hormones and insulin. Proc. Natl. Acad. Sci. U. S. A. 1984;81(11):3317–3321.

Garton AJ, Campbell DG, Cohen P, Yeaman SJ. Primary structure of the site on bovine hormone-sensitive lipase phosphorylated by cyclic AMP-dependent protein kinase. FEBS Lett. 1988;229(1):68–72.

Anthonsen MW, Rönnstrand L, Wernstedt C, Degerman E, Holm C. Identification of novel phosphorylation sites in hormone-sensitive lipase that are phosphorylated in response to isoproterenol and govern activation properties in vitro. J. Biol. Chem. 1998;273(1):215–221.

Lass A, Zimmermann R, Haemmerle G, Riederer M, Schoiswohl G, Schweiger M, Kienesberger P, Strauss JG, Gorkiewicz G, Zechner R. Adipose triglyceride lipase-mediated lipolysis of cellular fat stores is activated by CGI-58 and defective in Chanarin-Dorfman Syndrome. Cell Metab. 2006;3(5):309–319.

Granneman JG, Moore H-PH, Krishnamoorthy R, Rathod M. Perilipin controls lipolysis by regulating the interactions of AB-hydrolase containing 5 (Abhd5) and adipose triglyceride lipase (Atgl). J. Biol. Chem. 2009;284(50):34538–34544.

Jensen MD. Gender differences in regional fatty acid metabolism before and after meal ingestion. J. Clin. Invest. 1995;96(5):2297–303.

Gjedsted J, Gormsen LC, Nielsen S, Schmitz O, Djurhuus CB, Keiding S, Ørskov H, Tønnesen E, Møller N. Effects of a 3-day fast on regional lipid and glucose metabolism in human skeletal muscle and adipose tissue. Acta Physiol. 2007;191(3):205–216.

Moro C, Pillard F, de Glisezinski I, Crampes F, Thalamas C, Harant I, Marques M-A, Lafontan M, Berlan M. Sex differences in lipolysis-regulating mechanisms in overweight subjects: effect of exercise intensity*. Obesity. 2007;15(9):2245–2255.

Morigny P, Houssier M, Mouisel E, Langin D. Adipocyte lipolysis and insulin resistance. Biochimie. 2016;125:259–266.

Czech MP. Mechanisms of insulin resistance related to white, beige and brown adipocytes. Mol. Metab. 2020. in press. doi:https://doi.org.

Czech MP. Insulin action and resistance in obesity and type 2 diabetes. Nat. Med. 2017;23(7):804–814.

Gandotra S, Le Dour C, Bottomley W, Cervera P, Giral P, Reznik Y, Charpentier G, Auclair M, Delépine M, Barroso I, Semple RK, Lathrop M, Lascols O, Capeau J, O'Rahilly S, Magré J, Savage DB, Vigouroux C. Perilipin deficiency and autosomal dominant partial lipodystrophy. N. Engl. J. Med. 2011;364(8):740–8.

Rubio-Cabezas O, Puri V, Murano I, Saudek V, Semple RK, Dash S, Hyden CSS, Bottomley W, Vigouroux C, Magré J, Raymond-Barker P, Murgatroyd PR, Chawla A, Skepper JN, Chatterjee VK, Suliman S, Patch A-M, Agarwal AK, Garg A, Barroso I, Cinti S, Czech MP, Argente J, O'Rahilly S, Savage DB. LD Screening Consortium LS. Partial lipodystrophy and insulin resistant diabetes in a patient with a homozygous nonsense mutation in CIDEC. EMBO Mol. Med. 2009;1(5):280–7.

Zhou L, Park S-Y, Xu L, Xia X, Ye J, Su L, Jeong K-H, Hur JH, Oh H, Tamori Y, Zingaretti CM, Cinti S, Argente J, Yu M, Wu L, Ju S, Guan F, Yang H, Choi CS, Savage DB, Li P. Insulin resistance and white adipose tissue inflammation are uncoupled in energetically challenged Fsp27-deficient mice. Nat. Commun. 2015;6:5949.

Czech MP, Tencerova M, Pedersen DJ, Aouadi M. Insulin signalling mechanisms for triacylglycerol storage. Diabetologia. 2013;56(5):949–964.

Fasshauer M, Blüher M. Adipokines in health and disease. Trends Pharmacol. Sci. 2015;36(7):461–470.

INGALLS AM. DICKIE MM, SNELL GD. Obese, a new mutation in the house mouse. J. Hered. 1950;41(12):317–318.

Lindström P. The physiology of obese-hyperglycemic mice. ScientificWorldJournal. 2007;7:666–85.

Hausberger FX. Parabiosis and transplantation experiments in hereditary obese mice. Anat Rec 1958;130:313 abstr.

Friedman JM, Halaas JL. Leptin and the regulation of body weight in mammals. Nature. 1998;395(6704):763–770.

Hummel KP, Dickie MM, Coleman DL. Diabetes, a new mutation in the mouse. Science. 1966;153(3740):1127–1128.

Coleman DL. Obese and diabetes: two mutant genes causing diabetes-obesity syndromes in mice. Diabetologia. 1978;14(3):141–148.
Harris RB. Loss of body fat in lean parabiotic partners of ob/ob mice. Am. J. Physiol. 1997;272(6 Pt 2):R1809–R1815.
Harris RBS. Parabiosis between db/db and ob/ob or db/+ mice. Endocrinology. 1999;140(1):138–145.
Bahary N, Leibel RL, Joseph L, Friedman JM. Molecular mapping of the mouse db mutation. Proc. Natl. Acad. Sci. U. S. A. 1990;87(21):8642–8646.
Tartaglia LA, Dembski M, Weng X, Deng N, Culpepper J, Devos R, Richards GJ, Campfield LA, Clark FT, Deeds J, Muir C, Sanker S, Moriarty A, Moore KJ, Smutko JS, Mays GG, Wool EA, Monroe CA, Tepper RI. Identification and expression cloning of a leptin receptor, OB-R. Cell. 1995;83(7):1263–1271.
Peelman F, Zabeau L, Moharana K, Savvides SN, Tavernier J. 20 years of leptin: insights into signaling assemblies of the leptin receptor. J. Endocrinol. 2014;223(1):T9–23.
Münzberg H, Morrison CD. Structure, production and signaling of leptin. Metabolism. 2015;64(1):13–23.
Wauman J, Tavernier J. Leptin receptor signaling: pathways to leptin resistance. Front. Biosci. (Landmark Ed. 2011;16:2771–2793.
Guo K, McMinn JE, Ludwig T, Yu Y-H, Yang G, Chen L, Loh D, Li C, Chua S, Zhang Y. Disruption of peripheral leptin signaling in mice results in hyperleptinemia without associated metabolic abnormalities. Endocrinology. 2007;148(8):3987–3997.
Frederich RC, Hamann A, Anderson S, Löllmann B, Lowell BB, Flier JS. Leptin levels reflect body lipid content in mice: Evidence for diet-induced resistance to leptin action. Nat. Med. 1995;1(12):1311–1314.
Maffei M, Halaas J, Ravussin E, Pratley RE, Lee GH, Zhang Y, Fei H, Kim S, Lallone R, Ranganathan S, Kern PA, Friedman JM. Leptin levels in human and rodent: Measurement of plasma leptin and ob RNA in obese and weight-reduced subjects. Nat. Med. 1995;1(11):1155–1161.
Enriori PJ, Evans AE, Sinnayah P, Jobst EE, Tonelli-Lemos L, Billes SK, Glavas MM, Grayson BE, Perello M, Nillni EA, Grove KL, Cowley MA. Diet-induced obesity causes severe but reversible leptin resistance in arcuate melanocortin neurons. Cell Metab. 2007;5(3):181–194.
Knight ZA, Hannan KS, Greenberg ML, Friedman JM. Hyperleptinemia Is Required for the Development of Leptin Resistance. Stadler K, ed. PLoS One 2010;5(6):e11376.
Balland E, Cowley MA. New insights in leptin resistance mechanisms in mice. Front. Neuroendocrinol. 2015;39:59–65.
Friedman J. 20 years of leptin: leptin at 20: an overview. J. Endocrinol. 2014;223(1):T1–8.
Denroche HC, Huynh FK, Kieffer TJ. The role of leptin in glucose homeostasis. J. Diabetes Investig. 2012;3(2):115–129.
Ducy P, Amling M, Takeda S, Priemel M, Schilling AF, Beil FT, Shen J, Vinson C, Rueger JM, Karsenty G. Leptin inhibits bone formation through a hypothalamic relay: a central control of bone mass. Cell. 2000;100(2):197–207.
Dalamaga M, Chou SH, Shields K, Papageorgiou P, Polyzos SA, Mantzoros CS. Leptin at the intersection of neuroendocrinology and metabolism: current evidence and therapeutic perspectives. Cell Metab. 2013;18(1):29–42.
Chen XX, Yang T. Roles of leptin in bone metabolism and bone diseases. J. Bone Miner. Metab. 2015;33(5):474–485.
Sáinz N, Barrenetxe J, Moreno-Aliaga MJ, Martínez JA. Leptin resistance and diet-induced obesity: central and peripheral actions of leptin. Metabolism. 2015;64(1):35–46.

Prognosis

Lipedema is a chronic and progressive condition characterized by the symmetrical buildup of adipose tissue, predominantly in the legs and arms, leading to pain, swelling, and mobility issues. Unlike typical fat distribution, lipedema fat is not responsive to diet and exercise, making it a particularly challenging condition to manage. The importance of prognostic assessment in lipedema cannot be overstated, as it provides crucial insights into the likely course and outcome of the condition for an individual patient. Early and accurate diagnosis, combined with a comprehensive assessment of the disease's stage, the patient's symptoms, and their impact on quality of life, is essential for developing an effective management strategy. Prognostic assessment helps in tailoring treatment plans to individual needs, which may include a combination of lifestyle modifications, physical therapy, compression therapy, and surgical options like liposuction. It also facilitates a better understanding of the potential progression of lipedema, enabling patients and healthcare providers to set realistic expectations and goals for treatment. Ultimately, a thorough prognostic evaluation empowers patients with lipedema to make informed decisions about their care, potentially improving their long-term outcomes and quality of life.

The natural progression of lipedema is typically categorized into stages, reflecting the severity and distribution of adipose tissue accumulation, and the presence of symptoms such as pain and mobility impairment. These stages range from stage 1, where there is a smooth surface with an enlarged subcutaneous fat layer, to stage 4, characterized by the presence of large masses of tissue (lipolymphedema). The typical progression pattern of lipedema involves an initial accumulation of fat in the lower extremities, extending from the hips to the ankles, sparing the feet. Over time, without intervention, the condition can progress to involve the arms and potentially lead to increased pain, mobility issues, and the development of secondary health conditions, including lymphedema and joint problems.

Factors influencing the progression of lipedema include genetic predisposition, hormonal changes (notably during puberty, pregnancy, and menopause), and lifestyle factors such as diet and physical activity.

G. Laur, *Lipoedema*, https://doi.org/10.1007/978-981-96-8939-2_17

Additionally, obesity can exacerbate the condition, although lipedema can occur in individuals of all body sizes. The rate of progression varies widely among individuals; some may experience a slow progression over many years, while others may see a rapid advancement in a shorter period. Early diagnosis and intervention are crucial in managing lipedema's progression. Treatments aimed at controlling symptoms and improving quality of life, such as compression therapy, manual lymphatic drainage, and in some cases, liposuction, can help manage the condition effectively and slow its progression. Understanding the natural progression of lipedema is essential for healthcare providers and patients alike to adopt proactive management strategies and mitigate the impact of this chronic condition.

The impact of early detection and intervention in lipedema cannot be understated, as it significantly influences the trajectory of the condition and the patient's overall quality of life. Early diagnosis of lipedema is pivotal, as it allows for the timely implementation of treatment strategies that can slow the progression of the disease, alleviate symptoms, and prevent complications. Initiating treatment in the early stages of lipedema, including lifestyle modifications, compression therapy, manual lymphatic drainage, and exercise, can markedly reduce the accumulation of lipedematous fat, minimize pain and swelling, and improve mobility. Furthermore, early intervention has a profound effect on long-term outcomes by potentially delaying or reducing the need for surgical interventions, such as liposuction, which may be considered in more advanced stages of the disease. Strategies for early recognition of lipedema include increasing awareness among healthcare professionals and the general public, incorporating screening for lipedema into routine physical examinations for individuals presenting with disproportionate lower body fat accumulation, and advocating for further research into the genetic and environmental factors contributing to the condition. By emphasizing the importance of early detection and intervention, there is a greater chance of managing lipedema effectively, enhancing the patient's quality of life, and mitigating the physical and psychological burden of the condition.

The influence of lifestyle and management strategies on lipedema prognosis underscores the critical role of diet, nutrition, and exercise in mitigating the condition's progression and impact. A well-balanced diet, rich in anti-inflammatory foods and low in processed and high-fat foods, can help manage inflammation and potentially reduce lipedema pain. Nutrition plays a role in maintaining overall health and supporting the body's lymphatic system while also aiding in weight management. Weight management and physical activity are particularly important, as excessive weight gain can exacerbate lipedema symptoms and progression. Regular, low-impact exercises such as swimming, walking, and cycling are recommended to improve lymphatic drainage, enhance mobility, and prevent the accumulation of lipedematous fat. These lifestyle modifications can significantly influence the prognosis of lipedema by slowing disease progression, reducing symptom severity, and improving quality of life. Implementing and maintaining these lifestyle changes require a comprehensive and individualized approach, often involving collaboration with healthcare professionals specializing in lipedema management. Through such collaborative efforts, individuals with lipedema can achieve better control over their symptoms, highlighting the profound effect of lifestyle and management strategies on the condition's prognosis.

The outcomes of medical and surgical treatments for conditions like lipedema significantly depend on the efficacy of pharmacological approaches and the long-term success of surgical interventions, underlining the importance of consistent and comprehensive management.

Pharmacological treatments, while limited in directly targeting the pathological fat accumulation characteristic of lipedema, can offer symptomatic relief, particularly in managing pain and inflammation. However, the cornerstone of effectively altering the disease's course lies in surgical interventions, such as liposuction, which directly removes lipedematous fat and has shown promising results in improving both physical symptoms and quality of life. Long-term outcomes of these surgical procedures are generally positive, with many patients experiencing sustained relief from pain, improved mobility, and a more favorable body image. Nevertheless, these outcomes are maximized when surgery is part of an integrated approach that includes diet, nutrition, exercise, and possibly pharmacological support to manage comorbid conditions. The consistent application of comprehensive management strategies is crucial in preventing progression, managing symptoms, and improving the overall prognosis of lipedema. This holistic approach underscores the necessity of a multidisciplinary team to address the complex needs of patients with lipedema, ensuring that both the physical and psychological aspects of the condition are adequately managed.

Lipedema, a chronic condition marked by an abnormal accumulation of fat in the limbs, exerts a significant emotional and psychological toll on those affected, impacting their quality of life. The visible and physical manifestations of lipedema can lead to body image issues, low self-esteem, and social isolation, exacerbating the psychological burden. The role of social support is paramount in the prognosis and management of lipedema; a strong support system can mitigate the psychosocial impact, providing emotional comfort, practical assistance, and motivation for managing the condition. Strategies to improve quality of life include psychological counseling to address body image and self-esteem issues, support groups to foster a sense of community and shared experience, and patient education to empower individuals with knowledge about their condition and its management. These strategies, coupled with comprehensive medical and surgical interventions, aim to not only address the physical symptoms of lipedema but also to support the emotional well-being of patients, enhancing their overall quality of life and enabling them to lead more fulfilling lives despite the challenges posed by the condition.

Lipedema, a chronic condition marked by disproportionate fat distribution, is associated with a range of complications and comorbidities that can significantly impact prognosis and quality of life. Common complications include lymphedema, due to impaired lymphatic drainage; mobility issues and joint pain, as a result of the excess weight of lipedematous tissues; and psychological distress, including depression and anxiety, stemming from body image concerns and chronic pain. The presence of coexisting conditions such as obesity, cardiovascular disease, and venous insufficiency can further complicate the management of lipedema, potentially accelerating its progression and exacerbating symptoms. Preventing and managing these complications involves a comprehensive approach that includes regular monitoring for signs of progression, prompt treatment of comorbid conditions, and lifestyle modifications aimed at maintaining a healthy weight and promoting physical activity. Additionally, psychological support and social support networks play a crucial role in mitigating the emotional impact of the condition and enhancing overall well-being. Through early intervention and a holistic management strategy, it is possible to minimize the complications associated with lipedema, thereby improving the long-term prognosis and quality of life for those affected.

The role of genetics in lipedema is increasingly recognized as a critical factor influencing the prognosis and opening avenues for personalized medicine approaches. Research indicates that lipedema may have a hereditary component, with many patients reporting a family history of similar symptoms, suggesting a genetic predisposition to the condition. This genetic underpinning not only affects the prognosis by determining the severity and progression of lipedema but also highlights the potential for personalized treatment strategies tailored to an individual's genetic makeup. Personalized medicine in lipedema could involve genetic screening to identify those at higher risk, enabling earlier diagnosis and intervention, and the development of targeted therapies that address specific genetic pathways involved in fat accumulation and distribution. Future directions in genetic research aim to uncover the specific genes and molecular mechanisms responsible for lipedema, which could lead to groundbreaking advances in treatment, such as gene therapy or precision pharmacological interventions. By focusing on the genetic aspects of lipedema, there is the potential to significantly enhance our understanding of the condition, improve patient outcomes through more accurate prognoses, and develop personalized treatment plans that offer the promise of more effective management and potentially curative therapies.

Prognostication in the context of medical conditions, such as lipedema, is fraught with variability and uncertainty, presenting significant challenges for healthcare providers and patients alike. The prognosis for individuals with lipedema can be highly variable, influenced by a multitude of factors including disease stage at diagnosis, effectiveness of management strategies, and individual patient responses to treatment. A key limitation in current knowledge and research is the paucity of longitudinal studies and large-scale clinical trials that specifically address the long-term outcomes of lipedema treatments. This gap in research contributes to difficulties in predicting disease progression and response to treatment accurately. Furthermore, the heterogeneity of the condition, both in terms of clinical presentation and individual patient experiences, complicates the development of standardized prognostic models. Addressing these challenges requires a concerted effort to enhance the quality and scope of lipedema research, incorporating genetic studies, personalized medicine approaches, and the evaluation of comprehensive treatment modalities. By expanding our understanding of lipedema and its myriad presentations, the medical community can move toward more accurate and individualized prognostic assessments, ultimately improving patient care and outcomes.

Emerging trends and future perspectives in the field of lipedema research and treatment are promising, indicating significant advances in understanding and managing this complex condition. Recent years have seen a burgeoning interest in the pathophysiology of lipedema, with studies exploring genetic predispositions, hormonal influences, and the role of inflammation, offering new insights into its etiology and progression. These advances pave the way for the development of targeted therapies that could drastically improve prognosis for individuals with lipedema. Furthermore, the potential impact of new therapies, including pharmacological interventions aimed at reducing inflammation and fibrosis, as well as advanced surgical techniques that offer more precise fat removal with minimal trauma, hold promise for enhancing treatment outcomes and quality of life. Future directions in prognostic research are likely to focus on personalized medicine approaches, utilizing genetic profiling and biomarkers to tailor treatments to individual patient needs and disease characteristics.

Additionally, the integration of digital health technologies for monitoring disease progression and treatment response offers exciting possibilities for more dynamic and responsive lipedema management strategies. As our understanding of lipedema deepens, these emerging trends underscore the potential for significant improvements in prognosis, treatment efficacy, and patient well-being in the years to come.

In conclusion, the prognosis of lipedema is a complex and multifaceted issue, deeply influenced by early detection, comprehensive management strategies, and the evolving understanding of the condition's pathophysiology. Advances in the understanding and treatment of lipedema hold promising potential for improving long-term outcomes, emphasizing the critical role of holistic and individualized approaches in patient care. As research continues to uncover the genetic underpinnings and effective therapeutic interventions for lipedema, the potential for personalized medicine to tailor treatments to individual needs becomes increasingly apparent. The importance of incorporating diet, exercise, and psychosocial support alongside medical and surgical interventions cannot be overstated, addressing not only the physical symptoms but also the emotional and psychological impact of lipedema. Future directions in prognostic research are poised to refine our understanding of lipedema progression, offering hope for more accurate predictions of outcomes and the development of targeted therapies. Ultimately, a comprehensive approach that integrates the latest research findings with patient-centered care will be paramount in enhancing the quality of life and prognosis for individuals living with lipedema.

Suggested Reading

Földi M, Földi E, Strößenreuther R, Kubik S. *Urban & Fischer.* München, Germany: 2012. Lipedema Földi's textbook of lymphology: for physicians and lymphedema therapists third Edition; pp. 364–369.

Meier-Vollrath I, Schneider W, Schmeller W. Lipödem: Verbesserte Lebensqualität durch Therapiekombination. *Dtsch Arztebl.* 2005;102:A1061–A-1067.

Forner-Cordero I, Szolnoky G, Forner-Cordero A, Kemeny L. Lipedema: an overview of its clinical manifestations, diagnosis and treatment of the disproportional fatty deposition syndrome—systematic review. *Clin Obes.* 2012;2:86–95.

Peled AW, Kappos EA. Lipedema: diagnostic and management challenges. *Int J Womens Health.* 2016;8:389–395.

Deutsche Gesellschaft für Phlebologie D. S1-Leitlinie Lipödem. *AWMF.* 2015.

Buck DW second, Herbst KL. Lipedema: a relatively common disease with extremely common misconceptions. *Plast Reconstr Surg Glob Open.* 2016;4.

Allen EV, Hines EA. Lipedema of the legs: a syndrome characterized by fat legs and orthostatic edema. *Proc Staff Mayo Clinic.* 1940:184–187.

Bauer AT, von Lukowicz D, Lossagk K, et al. New insights on lipedema: the enigmatic disease of the peripheral fat. *Plast Reconstr Surg.* 2019;144:1475–1484.

Fife CE, Maus EA, Carter MJ. Lipedema: a frequently misdiagnosed and misunderstood fatty deposition syndrome. *Adv Skin Wound Care.* 2010;23:81–92. quiz 3–4.

Langendoen SI, Habbema L, Nijsten TE, Neumann HA. Lipoedema: from clinical presentation to therapy A review of the literature. *Br J Dermatol.* 2009;161:980–986.

Child AH, Gordon KD, Sharpe P, et al. Lipedema: an inherited condition. *Am J Med Genet A.* 2010;152a:970–976.

Herbst KL. Rare adipose disorders (RADs) masquerading as obesity. *Acta Pharmacol Sin.* 2012;33:155–172.

Szel E, Kemeny L, Groma G, Szolnoky G. Pathophysiological dilemmas of lipedema. *Med Hypotheses.* 2014;83:599–606.

Wiedner M, Aghajanzadeh D, Richter DF. Lipedema—basics and current hypothesis of pathomechanism. *Handchir Mikrochir Plast Chir.* 2018;50:380–385.

Suga H, Araki J, Aoi N, Kato H, Higashino T, Yoshimura K. Adipose tissue remodeling in lipedema: adipocyte death and concurrent regeneration. *J Cutan Pathol.* 2009;36:1293–1298.

Priglinger E, Wurzer C, Steffenhagen C, et al. The adipose tissue-derived stromal vascular fraction cells from lipedema patients: are they different? *Cytotherapy.* 2017;19:849–860.

Földi E, Földi M. Lipedema Foldi's textbook of lymphology. In: Földi E, Földi M, editors. 2. Munich, Germany Elsevier: 2006. pp. 417–427.

Prantl L, Schreml J, Gehmert S, et al. Transcription profile in sporadic multiple symmetric lipomatosis reveals differential expression at the level of adipose tissue-derived stem cells. *Plast Reconstr Surg.* 2016;137:1181–1190.

Bauer AT, von Lukowicz D, Lossagk K, et al. Adipose stem cells from lipedema and control adipose tissue respond differently to adipogenic stimulation in Vitro. *Plast Reconstr Surg.* 2019;144:623–632.

Al-Ghadban S, Diaz ZT, Singer HJ, et al. Increase in leptin and PPAR-gamma gene expression in lipedema adipocytes differentiated in vitro from adipose-derived stem cells. *Cells.* 2020;9.

Conservative Management

Diet

The role of diet in managing lipedema is an area of emerging interest within the medical community, offering potential avenues for symptom mitigation and quality of life improvements for patients. Lipedema, characterized by the symmetrical buildup of painful fatty tissue predominantly in the legs and arms, is often misdiagnosed and misunderstood, leading to an absence of standardized therapeutic protocols. However, dietary management is increasingly recognized for its adjunctive value in comprehensive care.

A diet low in inflammatory foods and refined carbohydrates, and rich in anti-inflammatory omega-3 fatty acids, antioxidants, and bioflavonoids, may contribute to the reduction of tissue inflammation and oxidative stress associated with lipedema. Furthermore, the adoption of a modified ketogenic diet, which emphasizes a higher intake of healthy fats and proteins with a restriction of carbohydrates, has been suggested to facilitate a metabolic shift that might alleviate lipedema symptoms due to the anti-inflammatory and potential lipolytic effects. Nonetheless, the paucity of large-scale, peer-reviewed studies necessitates caution, emphasizing personalized dietary plans crafted in collaboration with healthcare providers, taking into account individual patient responses and nutritional needs. It is crucial to underscore that while diet may serve as a supportive strategy, it is not a standalone cure and should be integrated into a multidisciplinary approach to lipedema management.

The intricate synergy between macronutrients and micronutrients is foundational to human nutrition and the sustaining of physiological processes. Macronutrients, which include carbohydrates, proteins, and fats, are required by the body in substantial amounts due to their role as the primary sources of energy and as critical building blocks for body tissues. Carbohydrates serve as the primary energy source, proteins are vital for growth and repair, and fats provide a concentrated energy source and are necessary for the absorption of fat-soluble vitamins. Conversely, micronutrients, encompassing vitamins and minerals, are required in smaller quantities but are essential in supporting biochemical reactions and maintaining cellular function. Vitamins such as A, C, D, E, and K, along with B complex vitamins, facilitate enzymatic reactions, support immune function, and play roles in bone health

G. Laur, *Lipoedema*, https://doi.org/10.1007/978-981-96-8939-2_18

and blood coagulation. Minerals like calcium, potassium, and iron contribute to bone structure, regulate fluid balance, and are involved in oxygen transport, respectively. Understanding the interaction between macronutrients and micronutrients is paramount; deficiencies or excesses in one can affect the absorption and functionality of the other, thus highlighting the need for a balanced and varied diet to optimize health and prevent disease. This interrelationship also underscores the complexity of nutritional science and the need for ongoing research to elucidate the precise mechanisms by which these nutrients influence human health at both the molecular and systemic levels.

Balanced nutrition is integral to maintaining health and preventing chronic diseases, as it ensures an adequate intake of essential nutrients necessary for the body's myriad functions. This balance encompasses a proportional intake of macronutrients—carbohydrates, proteins, and fats—which provide energy and serve as the building blocks for repairing and building tissues, as well as micronutrients, vitamins and minerals, which are crucial for metabolic pathways, enzymatic processes, and overall cellular function. The significance of a balanced diet extends beyond the mere prevention of nutrient deficiencies; it supports the optimization of body weight, enhances immune function, and contributes to the prevention of nutrition-related conditions such as obesity, type 2 diabetes, cardiovascular diseases, and certain cancers. Moreover, a balanced diet promotes mental well-being, influencing mood, cognitive function, and sleep quality. The intricate interplay of nutrients in growth, development, and aging also exemplifies the necessity for tailored nutrition across different life stages. Importantly, balanced nutrition should also factor in the diversity of individual dietary needs and cultural preferences, ensuring sustainability and adherence. In essence, balanced nutrition is not simply about food intake but about fostering a harmonious relationship with food that supports a healthy lifestyle and overall well-being.

Hydration plays a role in the management of lipedema, a chronic condition characterized by the abnormal accumulation of adipose tissue in the lower extremities.

Proper hydration is crucial in maintaining the body's homeostasis and facilitating the lymphatic system's function, which is often compromised in patients with lipedema. Adequate fluid intake ensures the dilution of the lymph, reducing its viscosity and promoting its flow, which can help mitigate the painful swelling associated with lipedema. Furthermore, hydration supports kidney function, enabling the efficient removal of waste products and excess fluids from the body, thus potentially alleviating the burden on the lymphatic system. From a cellular perspective, sufficient hydration is essential for maintaining the health of adipocytes and supporting cellular metabolism. It also plays a role in nutrient transport and biochemical reactions, which are fundamental in maintaining tissue integrity and mitigating inflammation. However, the role of hydration must be understood within a broader nutritional context, as the consumption of certain nutrients and electrolytes also influences fluid balance. Despite the intuitive benefits of hydration, empirical research specifically targeting lipedema is sparse, necessitating further studies to explore the depth of hydration's therapeutic impact on this condition. Nonetheless, current clinical practices often recommend hydration as a component of a multifaceted approach to lipedema management, emphasizing its importance alongside other lifestyle interventions.

The principles of an anti-inflammatory diet rest on the premise that dietary choices can modulate the body's inflammatory processes, with implications for chronic disease management and overall health. This dietary approach emphasizes the consumption of foods rich in antioxidants and phytochemicals, which possess natural anti-inflammatory properties. Central to this dietary pattern is the high intake of fruits and vegetables, whole grains, lean proteins—especially those from fish rich in omega-3 fatty acids like salmon and mackerel—and plant-based proteins such as legumes and nuts. These foods provide essential nutrients, including fiber, vitamins, minerals, and essential fats, which contribute to the reduction of inflammation markers in the body. Concurrently, an anti-inflammatory diet involves limiting the intake of processed foods, red meats, and refined sugars, which are known to provoke inflammatory responses, potentially exacerbating conditions such as cardiovascular disease, diabetes, and arthritis. Additionally, the diet encourages the use of spices and herbs like turmeric and ginger, known for their anti-inflammatory effects. It also recommends a moderate consumption of red wine and dark chocolate, in light of their polyphenolic compounds. By adhering to these principles, an anti-inflammatory diet aims to not only mitigate the symptoms associated with chronic inflammation but also to promote an overall healthier lifestyle, potentially reducing the risk of various inflammatory-related diseases. The scientific literature, while supportive of the benefits of anti-inflammatory nutrients, continues to explore the diet's comprehensive impact on long-term health outcomes.

The concept of the glycemic index (GI) has gained prominence in nutritional science as a tool for managing blood sugar levels through diet. Low-glycemic index (LGI) foods, which are digested and absorbed at a slower rate, produce a gradual rise in blood glucose and insulin levels, as opposed to high-GI foods that cause rapid spikes. This quality makes LGI foods particularly beneficial for individuals with diabetes or insulin resistance, as they can help in the maintenance of blood glucose within a desired range, reducing the risk of hyperglycemia. Foods typically classified as LGI include most fruits and vegetables, whole grains, legumes, nuts, and dairy products like yogurt and milk. These foods contribute to sustained energy release, satiety, and control of appetite, which can be advantageous for weight management. Moreover, the consumption of LGI foods has been linked to reduced risk of developing type 2 diabetes and has been associated with improvements in both lipid profiles and endothelial function, thus potentially offering protective cardiovascular benefits.

Despite the benefits, it is critical to recognize that the GI is not the sole factor determining a food's healthfulness or its effects on blood sugar. The overall nutritional content, preparation methods, and the presence of other macronutrients like fats and proteins also influence the glycemic response. Therefore, a comprehensive approach that considers the GI within the context of a balanced diet is essential for effective blood sugar control and overall health.

The incorporation of lean proteins, fruits, and vegetables into the diet is a cornerstone of healthful eating, underpinning numerous dietary guidelines and nutrition recommendations globally. Lean proteins, which include sources like poultry, fish, legumes, and tofu, are essential for their high-quality amino acids, which are the building blocks of muscle, enzymes, hormones, and other vital bodily components. They also have a reduced content of saturated fats compared to their fatty protein counterparts, thereby supporting cardiovascular health. Fruits and vegetables, rich in vitamins, minerals, fiber, and phytochemicals, contribute to a plethora of health benefits, including bolstering the immune system; reducing the risk of chronic diseases such as heart disease, hypertension, and certain cancers; and aiding in weight management due to their low calorie and high fiber content. The fiber found in these plant foods enhances digestive health and helps in maintaining stable blood glucose levels, making it beneficial for diabetes control. Additionally, the diverse array of bioactive compounds found in fruits and vegetables, such as flavonoids and carotenoids, exhibit antioxidant properties, combating oxidative stress and inflammation, which are underlying factors in the pathogenesis of many diseases. The importance of these food groups is not only grounded in their individual nutritional attributes but also in their combined synergistic effects that contribute to overall dietary patterns associated with improved health outcomes and longevity. As such, public health initiatives often promote a diet high in lean proteins, fruits, and vegetables to foster a healthy population and reduce the prevalence of nutrition-related health issues.

The dichotomy between healthy and unhealthy fats is pivotal in the discourse on dietary recommendations for cardiovascular health and overall wellness. Healthy fats, chiefly mono- and polyunsaturated fats, are found in foods such as avocados, nuts, seeds, and fatty fish and have been shown to support heart health by improving plasma lipid profiles. Specifically, they can lower low-density lipoprotein (LDL) cholesterol levels, thus reducing the risk of atherosclerosis and associated cardiovascular events. Polyunsaturated fats, including omega-3 and omega-6 fatty acids, are essential fats the body cannot synthesize and must be obtained through diet. Omega-3 fatty acids, in particular, exhibit anti-inflammatory properties and have been linked to a lower incidence of coronary heart disease. In contrast, unhealthy fats, primarily saturated and trans fats, are typically solid at room temperature and are found in high quantities in processed foods, certain meat products, and dairy. These fats can raise LDL cholesterol levels and have been associated with an increased risk of heart disease. Trans fats, which are largely produced by industrial hydrogenation, are especially deleterious, as they not only raise LDL cholesterol but also lower high-density lipoprotein (HDL) cholesterol, exacerbating cardiovascular risk. The understanding of the differential effects of various fats has led to a paradigm shift in nutritional guidelines, which now emphasize the quality of fat intake over mere quantity. This nuanced approach to dietary fats is fundamental in public health messaging, aiming to foster informed food choices conducive to long-term health.

The impact of fatty acids on lipedema, a chronic condition marked by the disproportionate accumulation of fat in the lower body, is an area of clinical interest due to the potential implications for disease management and patient quality of life.

Fatty acids, particularly the ratio of omega-3 to omega-6 polyunsaturated fatty acids (PUFAs) in the diet, are hypothesized to influence inflammation, which is a noted characteristic of lipedema. Omega-3 fatty acids, found in high concentrations in fish oil and flaxseeds, possess anti-inflammatory properties that could hypothetically benefit individuals with lipedema by attenuating inflammatory responses in adipose tissue. Conversely, an excess of omega-6 fatty acids, prevalent in the Western diet, might exacerbate inflammatory pathways. The altered lipid metabolism inherent in lipedema may also interact uniquely with dietary fatty acids, influencing their absorption and the subsequent fatty acid composition of the adipose tissue. While the theoretical benefits of modifying fatty acid intake in lipedema are grounded in our understanding of their roles in inflammation and fat metabolism, empirical evidence remains limited. Thus, further research is essential to delineate the effects of specific fatty acids on the pathophysiology of lipedema. Current perspectives on the condition suggest a holistic approach to management, with dietary strategies including an optimal balance of fatty acids as a potential component, pending robust scientific validation.

Managing dietary fat intake is crucial for maintaining optimal health and preventing diet-related chronic diseases. Dietary fats are a heterogeneous group of compounds essential for various bodily functions, including energy provision, cellular structure maintenance, and hormone synthesis. However, the type and quantity of fat consumed are vital considerations. Saturated and trans fats, predominantly found in animal products and processed foods, should be consumed sparingly due to their association with increased levels of LDL cholesterol and a heightened risk of cardiovascular disease. In contrast, unsaturated fats—particularly mono- and polyunsaturated fats present in plant oils, nuts, seeds, and fatty fish—contribute to the maintenance of healthy blood lipid profiles and are associated with reduced inflammation. Managing intake involves not only reducing the total amount of unhealthy fats but also replacing them with healthier alternatives, a practice which has been shown to confer cardiovascular benefits. The American Heart Association recommends that saturated fats constitute no more than 5–6% of total daily calories, while trans fat intake should be as low as possible. Additionally, the inclusion of omega-3 fatty acids is encouraged for their protective effects against heart disease. Nutrition labeling and dietary guidelines serve as tools for consumers to make informed choices, while public health initiatives aim to reduce trans fat content in commercial food products. Overall, the management of dietary fat intake requires a conscious effort to select nutrient-dense foods that align with recommendations for a balanced and heart-healthy diet.

Understanding caloric needs is fundamental to achieving and maintaining optimal health and body weight, a concept central to nutritional science and dietary management. Caloric needs vary significantly among individuals, influenced by factors such as age, sex, weight, height, and level of physical activity. These needs represent the balance of energy consumed through food and beverages against energy expended through basic physiological functions and physical activities. Basal metabolic rate (BMR) is the energy required for maintaining core physiological functions at rest and constitutes the largest portion of an individual's total energy expenditure. Additional energy is required for the digestion of food (thermic effect of food) and physical activities (exercise and non-exercise activity thermogenesis).

Calculating an individual's caloric needs involves estimating the BMR using equations such as the Harris-Benedict or Mifflin-St Jeor and then adjusting for activity level to derive the total daily energy expenditure (TDEE). This personalized approach allows for tailored dietary recommendations aimed at achieving specific health goals, whether for weight loss, gain, or maintenance.

Importantly, the quality of calories consumed—nutrient-dense foods versus empty calories—also plays a crucial role in health outcomes, highlighting the need for a holistic view of caloric intake that considers both quantity and quality. Understanding and applying these principles in dietary planning can significantly contribute to the prevention and management of obesity, malnutrition, and associated metabolic disorders.

Strategies for healthy weight loss or maintenance encompass a multifaceted approach that prioritizes sustainable changes to dietary habits, physical activity, and behavioral practices. Central to effective weight management is the creation of a balanced energy equation, where caloric intake does not exceed caloric expenditure. Dietary strategies emphasize the importance of a nutrient-dense diet rich in fruits, vegetables, whole grains, lean proteins, and healthy fats while reducing the consumption of processed foods, sugary beverages, and high-calorie, low-nutrient items. Portion control and mindful eating are crucial for recognizing hunger and satiety cues, preventing overeating. In addition to dietary modifications, increasing physical activity is paramount, with recommendations suggesting at least 150 minutes of moderate aerobic activity or 75 minutes of vigorous activity per week, coupled with muscle-strengthening exercises. Behavioral strategies, including goal setting, self-monitoring, and seeking social support, play a significant role in maintaining motivation and addressing psychological factors related to eating and physical activity. Importantly, weight management programs should advocate for gradual weight loss (about 1–2 pounds per week) to ensure sustainability and minimize the risk of nutritional deficiencies. Integrating these strategies requires a personalized approach, taking into account individual dietary preferences, lifestyle, and health status, thereby promoting adherence and improving long-term health outcomes.

The relationship between obesity and lipedema is complex and multifaceted, highlighting the intricacies of diagnosing and managing these distinct yet sometimes overlapping conditions. Lipedema is characterized by the pathological accumulation of adipose tissue, typically in the lower extremities, and is often misdiagnosed as obesity or lymphedema. Unlike obesity, which is a generalized increase in body fat due to an energy imbalance, lipedema fat is not significantly affected by caloric restriction or conventional weight loss strategies. This fundamental difference underscores the necessity for healthcare professionals to distinguish between the two conditions for appropriate management. Obesity can exacerbate the symptoms of lipedema, such as pain and mobility issues, due to the added mechanical stress and potential for increased inflammation from the excess adipose tissue. Conversely, the presence of lipedema can complicate the achievement and maintenance of a healthy weight, leading to a vicious cycle that can impact physical health and psychological well-being. Understanding the relationship between obesity and lipedema is crucial for developing effective treatment plans that address both conditions. Such plans may include a combination of diet, exercise, and possibly surgical interventions, tailored to the individual's needs and the specifics of their conditions. Moreover, this relationship emphasizes the importance of a nuanced approach to weight management in patients with lipedema, recognizing that traditional metrics of obesity treatment efficacy, such as body mass index (BMI), may not fully capture the complexities of the condition.

In the management of lipedema, a complex and often misunderstood adipose tissue disorder, the use of dietary supplements has emerged as a complementary strategy alongside conventional treatments such as compression therapy, manual lymphatic drainage, and, in some cases, liposuction.

Common supplements utilized by individuals with lipedema include bioflavonoids, such as rutin and quercetin, which are believed to strengthen blood vessels and improve lymphatic drainage, potentially reducing pain and inflammation associated with the condition. Omega-3 fatty acids, found in fish oil supplements, are another popular choice due to their anti-inflammatory properties, which may help in managing the chronic pain and swelling characteristic of lipedema. Furthermore, supplements containing selenium are sometimes recommended to support thyroid function and overall immune health, considering the potential link between lipedema and hormonal imbalances. Magnesium, known for its muscle relaxant properties, can also be beneficial in alleviating the muscle cramps and discomfort that some individuals with lipedema experience. It is imperative to note, however, that while these supplements may offer symptomatic relief and support overall well-being, they should not replace conventional medical treatments. The effectiveness of supplements can vary greatly among individuals, and there is a need for more rigorous, scientifically robust research to better understand their role in lipedema management. Patients are advised to consult with healthcare professionals before starting any new supplement regimen to ensure safety and appropriateness for their specific health condition.

The interaction between dietary supplements and medications is a critical consideration in clinical practice, necessitating vigilant management to optimize therapeutic outcomes and minimize adverse effects. Dietary supplements, including vitamins, minerals, herbal products, and amino acids, are widely used for various health benefits but can interact with medications through multiple mechanisms. These interactions may alter the pharmacokinetics of a drug—how it is absorbed, distributed, metabolized, and excreted by the body—or its pharmacodynamics, which refers to the drug's effects on the body. For instance, supplements such as St. John's Wort can induce the activity of enzymes responsible for drug metabolism, leading to decreased efficacy of medications like antidepressants, contraceptives, and anticoagulants. Conversely, supplements rich in vitamin K, such as green leafy vegetables, can antagonize the effects of warfarin, a blood thinner, increasing the risk of blood clots. Furthermore, certain minerals like calcium and magnesium can interfere with the absorption of a variety of drugs, including bisphosphonates and some antibiotics, by binding to the drug molecules in the gastrointestinal tract. Recognizing and managing these interactions requires a comprehensive understanding of both the patient's medication regimen and their supplement use. Healthcare professionals must meticulously review all substances their patients are taking and provide guidance on proper timing and administration to avoid interactions. Additionally, patient education on the potential for such interactions is essential to ensure adherence to prescribed therapies and to encourage reporting of all nonprescription supplement use. This holistic approach is fundamental in preventing adverse interactions and ensuring the safety and efficacy of treatment protocols.

Exploring gluten-free, dairy-free, and other restrictive diets has become increasingly prevalent in both clinical settings and public health discourse, driven by the recognition of food sensitivities, allergies, and specific chronic conditions that may benefit from dietary modifications. Gluten-free diets are essential for individuals with celiac disease, an autoimmune disorder triggered by gluten, a protein found in wheat, barley, and rye, leading to gastrointestinal distress and malabsorption of nutrients. Similarly, dairy-free diets cater to those with lactose intolerance or milk protein allergies, aiming to eliminate symptoms such as bloating, gas, and diarrhea. Beyond these medically indicated restrictions, such diets have also gained popularity in the wider population due to perceptions of health benefits, including weight management and improved digestion.

However, the adoption of restrictive diets without professional guidance can lead to nutritional deficiencies. For instance, eliminating gluten without adequate substitution can result in lower intakes of fiber, iron, and B vitamins, while avoiding dairy may decrease calcium and vitamin D intake, critical for bone health. Thus, when exploring restrictive diets, it is crucial to ensure balanced nutrition through alternative sources or supplementation as needed, emphasizing the importance of consultation with healthcare professionals. This approach helps in identifying genuine food sensitivities and managing dietary restrictions in a manner that supports overall health and well-being, tailoring interventions to individual nutritional needs and health objectives.

The roles of sodium and potassium in the human body exemplify the delicate balance required for optimal physiological function, particularly in maintaining fluid balance, nerve transmission, and muscle function. Sodium, predominantly ingested through salt (sodium chloride), plays a crucial role in fluid balance and blood pressure regulation. It operates alongside potassium in the sodium-potassium pump, a vital cellular mechanism that maintains the cell's electrical neutrality and enables nerve impulse transmission and muscle contraction. Despite its necessity, excessive sodium intake is linked to hypertension and cardiovascular disease, underscoring the importance of moderation. Potassium, on the other hand, aids in offsetting the hypertensive effects of sodium, promoting vasodilation and thus lowering blood pressure. It also plays a critical role in heart function, muscle contraction, and nerve transmission. A diet abundant in potassium—primarily sourced from fruits, vegetables, legumes, and nuts—has been consistently associated with a reduced risk of stroke, improved cardiovascular health, and better bone mineral density. Potassium plays a critical role in regulating blood pressure, maintaining fluid and electrolyte balance, and supporting neuromuscular function. Increasing dietary potassium intake, particularly through whole-food sources, may therefore offer protective effects against hypertension, osteoporosis, and related chronic conditions.

Strategies for reducing water retention focus on addressing its underlying causes, which range from high sodium intake, hormonal fluctuations, to certain health conditions. A primary approach involves dietary modifications to decrease sodium consumption, as excess sodium can lead to the body retaining extra fluid, particularly in the circulatory system and interstitial spaces. Increasing intake of potassium-rich foods, such as leafy greens, bananas, and avocados, can counterbalance sodium levels and support the natural elimination of excess fluid due to potassium's role in cellular fluid balance. Adequate hydration is also essential; paradoxically, consuming sufficient amounts of water can help reduce water retention by signaling the body to release stored water. Regular physical activity encourages the movement of fluids through the body and can stimulate sweat, through which the body can eliminate excess sodium. For hormonal-related water retention, such as that experienced premenstrually, strategies may include the management of hormonal fluctuations through lifestyle interventions or pharmacological means. Additionally, incorporating natural diuretics, such as dandelion or green tea, can support the kidneys in expelling unnecessary water. It is crucial, however, to approach the use of diuretics with caution and under medical advice, as excessive use can lead to dehydration and electrolyte imbalances. Addressing water retention effectively requires a comprehensive approach that considers dietary habits, lifestyle factors, and underlying health issues, ensuring interventions are tailored to individual needs and medical contexts.

Combining diet with physical activity represents a synergistic approach to achieving and maintaining optimal health, weight management, and chronic disease prevention. Nutrition and exercise are interrelated components of a healthy lifestyle, where dietary habits provide the necessary energy and nutrients to support physical activity, while exercise enhances metabolic health, contributing to more efficient use of nutritional intake.

A balanced diet ensures an adequate supply of macronutrients—carbohydrates, proteins, and fats—as well as essential vitamins and minerals to fuel physical activity, sustain energy levels, and facilitate recovery and muscle repair postexercise. Concurrently, engaging in regular physical activity increases muscle mass and improves insulin sensitivity, which can enhance nutrient partitioning and reduce the risk of obesity and metabolic diseases such as type 2 diabetes and cardiovascular disease. Furthermore, physical activity itself can act as a modulator of appetite and food preferences, potentially promoting a preference for more nutritious foods. The integration of diet and physical activity not only addresses the energy balance equation for weight management but also synergizes to improve overall physical fitness, mental health, and quality of life. Tailoring dietary intake to match physical activity levels, incorporating a variety of physical exercises, and ensuring adequate nutrient timing are key strategies in optimizing the combined benefits of diet and exercise. This holistic approach underscores the importance of comprehensive lifestyle interventions in public health strategies aimed at reducing the prevalence of lifestyle-related diseases.

Overcoming psychological barriers to dietary changes is a critical component of successful long-term adherence to healthier eating habits. These barriers, including emotional eating, food cravings, and resistance to change, often stem from deep-seated habits, cultural influences, and emotional associations with food. Strategies to surmount these challenges involve a multifaceted approach that includes cognitive-behavioral techniques, mindfulness practices, and support systems. Cognitive-behavioral therapy (CBT) can help individuals identify and reframe maladaptive thought patterns related to food, fostering a healthier relationship with eating. Mindfulness practices, such as mindful eating, encourage a more attuned eating experience, enhancing the awareness of hunger and satiety cues and reducing impulsive eating behaviors. Social support, whether from family, friends, or support groups, provides encouragement and accountability, which are essential in maintaining motivation and commitment to dietary changes. Additionally, setting realistic, incremental goals can help individuals build confidence and self-efficacy, reducing the perceived enormity of dietary modification. Education on the nutritional value of foods and the development of skills, such as meal planning and healthy cooking techniques, empower individuals to make informed food choices. Addressing psychological barriers requires recognizing the complex interplay between food, emotions, and behavior and adopting a compassionate, patient-centered approach that accommodates individual needs and preferences, facilitating a sustainable transition to healthier dietary patterns.

Building sustainable and healthy eating habits is an aspect of long-term health and wellness, requiring a nuanced understanding of both nutritional science and behavioral psychology. Sustainable eating habits are those that not only contribute to individual health and well-being but also consider environmental impact and can be maintained over a lifetime. Key strategies include emphasizing the consumption of whole foods, such as fruits, vegetables, whole grains, lean proteins, and healthy fats while minimizing processed and high-sugar foods. This approach not only ensures a high intake of essential nutrients and dietary fiber but also supports diverse and resilient agricultural practices. Integrating mindful eating practices, such as paying attention to hunger and satiety cues and eating without distraction, helps foster a healthy relationship with food and prevents overeating. Additionally, setting realistic, incremental goals and leveraging social support can enhance motivation and accountability. Education on meal planning and cooking skills can empower individuals to make healthful choices that align with their preferences and lifestyle, further enhancing sustainability.

Importantly, building healthy eating habits should also encompass flexibility and self-compassion, recognizing that occasional indulgences are part of a balanced diet and do not detract from overall health goals. Cultivating such habits requires time and patience, with a focus on long-term progress rather than short-term perfection, paving the way for lasting health improvements and a reduced risk of chronic diseases.

Addressing common dietary challenges in lipedema involves a multifaceted approach that takes into account the unique physiological and psychological aspects of the condition. Lipedema, characterized by the pathological accumulation of fat in the lower body, is often accompanied by pain, easy bruising, and a resistance to traditional weight loss strategies, posing significant dietary management challenges. A key strategy involves focusing on an anti-inflammatory diet, rich in omega-3 fatty acids, antioxidants, and phytonutrients found in fruits, vegetables, nuts, and seeds, to potentially alleviate inflammation and oxidative stress associated with lipedema. Incorporating a balanced intake of macronutrients with an emphasis on high-quality proteins and healthy fats can support satiety and muscle maintenance, while complex carbohydrates can provide steady energy. Given the tendency for weight gain and the difficulty in losing weight through conventional means, calorie awareness, without strict restriction, can help in managing energy intake. Moreover, addressing fluid retention through reduced sodium intake and increased consumption of foods with natural diuretic properties, like cucumber and asparagus, may offer symptomatic relief. Psychological challenges, including the frustration of limited weight loss despite dietary efforts, require compassionate support and counseling to foster a positive relationship with food and body image. Nutritional therapy in lipedema should be individualized, taking into consideration personal dietary preferences, nutritional deficiencies, and comorbid conditions, to enhance adherence and improve quality of life. Collaboration with healthcare professionals, including dietitians specialized in lipedema, can ensure that dietary strategies are both effective and sustainable, addressing the condition's complexity and the individual's holistic well-being.

Nutritional deficiencies occur when the body lacks essential vitamins or minerals necessary for its proper functioning, leading to a variety of health issues. These deficiencies can arise from inadequate intake, poor absorption, or higher bodily requirements not met by diet alone. Common deficiencies include iron, leading to anemia; vitamin D, affecting bone health; and vitamin B12, crucial for nerve function and blood cell formation. To avoid these, a balanced and varied diet is paramount. Incorporating a wide range of foods ensures the intake of a broad spectrum of nutrients. For example, leafy green vegetables, legumes, and fortified foods can provide iron; fatty fish, egg yolks, and fortified milk are good sources of vitamin D; and meat, dairy products, and fortified cereals can supply vitamin B12. For individuals with dietary restrictions or absorption issues, supplementation may be necessary, under medical guidance. Additionally, regular nutritional screenings can help identify deficiencies early, allowing for timely intervention. Education on food sources of different nutrients and how to combine foods to enhance nutrient absorption (such as vitamin C-rich foods with iron sources to improve iron absorption) is also beneficial. Ultimately, avoiding nutritional deficiencies requires a proactive approach to diet planning, emphasizing diversity in food choices and, when needed, appropriate supplementation, ensuring the body receives all necessary nutrients for optimal health.

Dietary strategies for managing lipedema emphasize the role of nutrition in alleviating symptoms and improving quality of life for individuals with this condition.

Given that lipedema is characterized by the abnormal accumulation of fat in the lower body, resistant to conventional weight loss methods, dietary approaches focus on anti-inflammatory foods, balanced macronutrient distribution, and careful management of caloric intake. An anti-inflammatory diet rich in omega-3 fatty acids, found in fatty fish, flaxseeds, and walnuts, alongside a high intake of fruits, vegetables, and whole grains, can help mitigate the inflammation associated with lipedema.

Adequate protein intake is crucial for maintaining muscle mass and supporting metabolism, while healthy fats are important for hormonal balance and satiety. Limiting processed foods, refined sugars, and excessive sodium can also reduce inflammation and fluid retention. Hydration plays a key role, with sufficient water intake supporting lymphatic drainage and overall fluid balance. While individual nutritional needs may vary, the goal is to support the body's natural processes, reduce symptoms, and prevent progression of the condition. Importantly, diet is a part of a comprehensive management strategy that may also include physical therapy, compression garments, and, in some cases, surgical interventions. Consulting with healthcare professionals, including dietitians familiar with lipedema, can tailor dietary recommendations to individual needs, ensuring they are both effective and sustainable. The emphasis on diet in the overall management of lipedema highlights its significance not only in symptom management but also in enhancing general well-being and quality of life for those affected by this challenging condition.

Suggested Reading

Buso G, Depairon M, Tomson D, Raffoul W, Vettor R, Mazzolai L. Lipedema: a call to action! *Obesity (Silver Spring)* 2019;27(10):1567–1576. doi: https://doi.org/10.1002/oby.22597.

Aksoy H, Karadag AS, Wollina U. Cause and management of lipedema-associated pain. Dermatol Ther. 2021;34(1):e14364.

Vyas A, Adnan G. Lipedema. StatPearls. Treasure Island (FL) ineligible companies. Disclosure: Ghufran Adnan declares no relevant financial relationships with ineligible companies. 2023.

Katzer K, Hill JL, McIver KB, Foster MT. Lipedema and the potential role of estrogen in excessive adipose tissue accumulation. Int J Mol Sci. 2021;22(21): 11720–11,732. https://doi.org/10.3390/ijms222111720 .

Chen SG, Hsu SD, Chen TM, Wang HJ. Painful fat syndrome in a male patient. *Br J Plast Surg.* 2004;57(3):282–286. doi: https://doi.org/10.1016/j.bjps.2003.12.020.

Giunta RE. Focus "liposuction in lipedema" *Handchir Mikrochir Plast Chir.* 2018;50(6):379.

Pereira de Godoy LM, Guerreiro Godoy MF, Pereira de Godoy JM. Lipedema in male progressing to subclinical and clinical systemic lymphedema. J Med Cases. 2022;13(6):249–52.

Child AH, Gordon KD, Sharpe P, Brice G, Ostergaard P, Jeffery S, et al. Lipedema: an inherited condition. *Am J Med Genet A.* 2010;152A(4):970–976. doi: https://doi.org/10.1002/ajmg.a.33313.

Paolacci S, Precone V, Acquaviva F, Chiurazzi P, Fulcheri E, Pinelli M, et al. Genetics of lipedema: new perspectives on genetic research and molecular diagnoses. *Eur Rev Med Pharmacol Sci.* 2019;23(13):5581–5594.

Szel E, Kemeny L, Groma G, Szolnoky G. Pathophysiological dilemmas of lipedema. *Med Hypotheses.* 2014;83(5):599–606. doi: https://doi.org/10.1016/j.mehy.2014.08.011.

Organization WH. Obesity and overweight. Available from: https://www.who.int/news-room/fact-sheets/detail/obesity-and-overweight.

Shavit E, Wollina U, Alavi A. Lipoedema is not lymphoedema: a review of current literature. *Int Wound J.* 2018;15(6):921–928. doi: https://doi.org/10.1111/iwj.12949.

Poojari A, Dev K, Rabiee A. Lipedema: insights into morphology, pathophysiology, and challenges. Biomedicines. 2022;10(12):3081–3114. https://doi.org/10.3390/biomedicines10123081.

Herbst KL, Kahn LA, Iker E, Ehrlich C, Wright T, McHutchison L, et al. Standard of care for lipedema in the United States. *Phlebology.* 2021;36(10):779–796. doi: https://doi.org/10.1177/02683555211015887.

Muscogiuri G, Verde L, Sulu C, Katsiki N, Hassapidou M, Frias-Toral E, et al. Mediterranean diet and obesity-related disorders: what is the evidence? *Curr Obes Rep.* 2022;11(4):287–304. doi: https://doi.org/10.1007/s13679-022-00481-1.

Welton S, Minty R, O'Driscoll T, Willms H, Poirier D, Madden S, et al. Intermittent fasting and weight loss: systematic review. *Can Fam Physician.* 2020;66(2):117–125.

Muscogiuri G, El Ghoch M, Colao A, Hassapidou M, Yumuk V, Busetto L, et al. European guidelines for obesity management in adults with a very low-calorie ketogenic diet: a systematic review and meta-analysis. *Obes Facts.* 2021;14(2):222–245. doi: https://doi.org/10.1159/000515381.

Forsythe CE, Phinney SD, Fernandez ML, Quann EE, Wood RJ, Bibus DM, et al. Comparison of low fat and low carbohydrate diets on circulating fatty acid composition and markers of inflammation. *Lipids.* 2008;43(1):65–77. doi: https://doi.org/10.1007/s11745-007-3132-7.

Sørlie V, De Soysa AK, Hyldmo AA, Retterstol K, Martins C, Nymo S. Effect of a ketogenic diet on pain and quality of life in patients with lipedema: the LIPODIET pilot study. Obes Sci Pract. 2022;8(4):483–93.

Cannataro R, Michelini S, Ricolfi L, Caroleo MC, Gallelli L, De Sarro G, Onorato A, Cione E. Management of lipedema with ketogenic diet: 22-month follow-up. Life (Basel). 2021;11(12)12):1402–1412. https://doi.org/10.3390/life11121402.

Wollina U. Lipedema-an update. Dermatol Ther. 2019;32(2):e12805.

Schwahn-Schreiber MMC. Prävalenz des Lipödems bei berufs-tätigen Frauen in Deutschland (Lipödem-3-Studie). 2011.

Buck DW 2nd, Herbst KL. Lipedema: a relatively common disease with extremely common misconceptions. Plast Reconstr Surg Glob Open. 2016;4(9):e1043.

Reich-Schupke S, Schmeller W, Brauer WJ, Cornely ME, Faerber G, Ludwig M, et al. S1 guidelines: lipedema. *J Dtsch Dermatol Ges.* 2017;15(7):758–767. doi: https://doi.org/10.1111/ddg.13036.

Kruppa P, Georgiou I, Biermann N, Prantl L, Klein-Weigel P, Ghods M. Lipedema-pathogenesis, diagnosis, and treatment options. *Dtsch Arztebl Int.* 2020;117(22–23):396–403.

Torre YS, Wadeea R, Rosas V, Herbst KL. Lipedema: friend and foe. Horm Mol Biol Clin Investig. 2018;33(1).

Halk AB, Damstra RJ. First Dutch guidelines on lipedema using the international classification of functioning, disability and health. *Phlebology.* 2017;32(3):152–159. doi: https://doi.org/10.1177/0268355516639421.

Hardy D, Williams A. Best practice guidelines for the management of lipoedema. Br J Community Nurs. 2017;22(Sup10):S44–S48. https://doi.org/10.12968/bjcn.2017.22.Sup10.S44.

Chakraborty A, Crescenzi R, Usman TA, Reyna AJ, Garza ME, Al-Ghadban S, Herbst KL, Donahue PMC, Rutkowski JM. Indications of peripheral pain, dermal hypersensitivity, and neurogenic inflammation in patients with lipedema. Int J Mol Sci. 2022;23(18):10313–10,328. https://doi.org/10.3390/ijms231810313.

Ratchford EV, Evans NS. Approach to lower extremity edema. *Curr Treat Options Cardiovasc Med.* 2017;19(3):16. doi: https://doi.org/10.1007/s11936-017-0518-6.

Hirschmann JV, Raugi GJ. Lower limb cellulitis and its mimics: part I. Lower limb cellulitis. J Am Acad Dermatol. 2012;67(2):163 e1–12; quiz 75–6. .

Hirsch T, Schleinitz J, Marshall M, Faerber G. Ist die differenzial diagnostik des lipödems mittels hochauflösender Sonografie möglich? Is the differential diagnosis of lipoedema by means of high-resolution ultrasonography possible? Phlebologie. 2018;47:182–7.

Birkballe S, Jensen MR, Noerregaard S, Gottrup F, Karlsmark T. Can tissue dielectric constant measurement aid in differentiating lymphoedema from lipoedema in women with swollen legs? *Br J Dermatol.* 2014;170(1):96–102. doi: https://doi.org/10.1111/bjd.12589.

Dietzel R, Reisshauer A, Jahr S, Calafiore D, Armbrecht G. Body composition in lipoedema of the legs using dual-energy X-ray absorptiometry: a case-control study. *Br J Dermatol.* 2015;173(2):594–596. doi: https://doi.org/10.1111/bjd.13697.

Romeijn JRM, de Rooij MJM, Janssen L, Martens H. Exploration of patient characteristics and quality of life in patients with lipoedema using a survey. *Dermatol Ther (Heidelb)* 2018;8(2):303–311. doi: https://doi.org/10.1007/s13555-018-0241-6.

Erbacher TBG. Lipödem—Mythen und Fakten Teil 2. *Phlebologie.* 2018;47:120–126. doi: https://doi.org/10.12687/phleb2418-3-2018.

Forner-Cordero I, Szolnoky G, Forner-Cordero A, Kemeny L. Lipedema: an overview of its clinical manifestations, diagnosis and treatment of the disproportional fatty deposition syndrome - systematic review. *Clin Obes.* 2012;2(3–4):86–95. doi: https://doi.org/10.1111/j.1758-8111.2012.00045.x.

Herbst KL. Rare adipose disorders (RADs) masquerading as obesity. *Acta Pharmacol Sin.* 2012;33(2):155–172. doi: https://doi.org/10.1038/aps.2011.153.

Dudek JE, Bialaszek W, Ostaszewski P, Smidt T. Depression and appearance-related distress in functioning with lipedema. *Psychol Health Med.* 2018;23(7):846–853. doi: https://doi.org/10.1080/13548506.2018.1459750.

Cornier MA, Despres JP, Davis N, Grossniklaus DA, Klein S, Lamarche B, et al. Assessing adiposity: a scientific statement from the American Heart Association. *Circulation.* 2011;124(18):1996–2019. doi: https://doi.org/10.1161/CIR.0b013e318233bc6a.

Jeziorek M, Szuba A, Kujawa K, Regulska-Ilow B. The effect of a low-carbohydrate, high-fat diet versus moderate-carbohydrate and fat diet on body composition in patients with lipedema. *Diabetes Metab Syndr Obes.* 2022;15:2545–2561. doi: https://doi.org/10.2147/DMSO.S377720.

Czerwinska M, Teodorczyk J, Hansdorfer-Korzon R. A scoping review of available tools in measurement of the effectiveness of conservative treatment in lipoedema. Int J Environ Res Public Health. 2022;19(12):7124–7135. https://doi.org/10.3390/ijerph19127124.

Herbst KL, Ussery C, Eekema A. Pilot study: whole body manual subcutaneous adipose tissue (SAT) therapy improved pain and SAT structure in women with lipedema. Horm Mol Biol Clin Investig. 2017;33(2).

Minetto MA, Pietrobelli A, Busso C, Bennett JP, Ferraris A, Shepherd JA, et al. Digital anthropometry for body circumference measurements: European phenotypic variations throughout the decades. J Pers Med. 2022;12(6).

Marra M, Sammarco R, De Lorenzo A, Iellamo F, Siervo M, Pietrobelli A, et al. Assessment of body composition in health and disease using bioelectrical impedance analysis (BIA) and dual energy X-ray absorptiometry (DXA): a critical overview. *Contrast Media Mol Imaging.* 2019;2019:3548284. doi: https://doi.org/10.1155/2019/3548284.

Reljic D, Zarafat D, Jensen B, Herrmann HJ, Neurath MF, Konturek PC, et al. Phase angle and vector analysis from multifrequency segmental bioelectrical impedance analysis: new reference data for older adults. J Physiol Pharmacol. 2020;71(4).

Di Renzo L, Cinelli G, Romano L, Zomparelli S, Lou De Santis G, Nocerino P, et al. Potential effects of a modified Mediterranean diet on body composition in lipoedema. Nutrients. 2021;13(2).

Kyle UG, Bosaeus I, De Lorenzo AD, Deurenberg P, Elia M, Manuel Gomez J, et al. Bioelectrical impedance analysis-part II: utilization in clinical practice. *Clin Nutr.* 2004;23(6):1430–1453. doi: https://doi.org/10.1016/j.clnu.2004.09.012.

Norman K, Stobaus N, Pirlich M, Bosy-Westphal A. Bioelectrical phase angle and impedance vector analysis–clinical relevance and applicability of impedance parameters. *Clin Nutr.* 2012;31(6):854–861. doi: https://doi.org/10.1016/j.clnu.2012.05.008.

Barrea L, Muscogiuri G, Pugliese G, Laudisio D, de Alteriis G, Graziadio C, et al. Phase angle as an easy diagnostic tool of meta-inflammation for the nutritionist. Nutrients. 2021;13(5).

Barrea L, Pugliese G, de Alteriis G, Colao A, Savastano S, Muscogiuri G. Phase angle: could be an easy tool to detect low-grade systemic inflammation in adults affected by Prader-Willi syndrome? Nutrients. 2020;12(7).

Barrea L, Muscogiuri G, Aprano S, Vetrani C, de Alteriis G, Varcamonti L, et al. Phase angle as an easy diagnostic tool for the nutritionist in the evaluation of inflammatory changes during the active stage of a very low-calorie ketogenic diet. *Int J Obes (Lond)* 2022;46(9):1591–1597. doi: https://doi.org/10.1038/s41366-022-01152-w.

Chawla A, Nguyen KD, Goh YP. Macrophage-mediated inflammation in metabolic disease. *Nat Rev Immunol.* 2011;11(11):738–749. doi: https://doi.org/10.1038/nri3071.

Crino A, Fintini D, Bocchini S, Grugni G. Obesity management in Prader-Willi syndrome: current perspectives. *Diabetes Metab Syndr Obes.* 2018;11:579–593. doi: https://doi.org/10.2147/DMSO.S141352.

Zatterale F, Longo M, Naderi J, Raciti GA, Desiderio A, Miele C, et al. Chronic adipose tissue inflammation linking obesity to insulin resistance and type 2 diabetes. *Front Physiol.* 2019;10:1607. doi: https://doi.org/10.3389/fphys.2019.01607.

Ward LC. Segmental bioelectrical impedance analysis: an update. *Curr Opin Clin Nutr Metab Care.* 2012;15(5):424–429. doi: https://doi.org/10.1097/MCO.0b013e328356b944.

Cornish BH, Jacobs A, Thomas BJ, Ward LC. Optimizing electrode sites for segmental bioimpedance measurements. *Physiol Meas.* 1999;20(3):241–250. doi: https://doi.org/10.1088/0967-3334/20/3/302.

Yamada Y, Masuo Y, Yokoyama K, Hashii Y, Ando S, Okayama Y, et al. Proximal electrode placement improves the estimation of body composition in obese and lean elderly during segmental bioelectrical impedance analysis. *Eur J Appl Physiol.* 2009;107(2):135–144. doi: https://doi.org/10.1007/s00421-009-1106-6.

Lontok E. Lipedema-Giving-Smarter-Guide. 2021.

Langendoen SI, Habbema L, Nijsten TE, Neumann HA. Lipoedema: from clinical presentation to therapy. A review of the literature. Br J Dermatol. 2009;161(5):980–6.

Szolnoky G, Nagy N, Kovacs RK, Dosa-Racz E, Szabo A, Barsony K, et al. Complex decongestive physiotherapy decreases capillary fragility in lipedema. *Lymphology.* 2008;41(4):161–166.

Szolnoky G, Varga E, Varga M, Tuczai M, Dosa-Racz E, Kemeny L. Lymphedema treatment decreases pain intensity in lipedema. *Lymphology.* 2011;44(4):178–182.

Wollina U, Heinig B, Schonlebe J, Nowak A. Debulking surgery for elephantiasis nostras with large ectatic podoplanin-negative lymphatic vessels in patients with lipo-lymphedema. Eplasty. 2014;14:e11.

Peprah K, MacDougall D. Liposuction for the treatment of lipedema: a review of clinical effectiveness and guidelines. CADTH rapid response reports. Ottawa (ON). 2019.

Baumgartner A, Hueppe M, Schmeller W. Long-term benefit of liposuction in patients with lipoedema: a follow-up study after an average of 4 and 8 years. Br J Dermatol. 2016;174(5):1061–1067. https://doi.org/10.1111/bjd.14289.

Dadras M, Mallinger PJ, Corterier CC, Theodosiadi S, Ghods M. Liposuction in the treatment of lipedema: a longitudinal study. *Arch Plast Surg.* 2017;44(4):324–331. doi: https://doi.org/10.5999/aps.2017.44.4.324.

Rapprich S, Dingler A, Podda M. Liposuction is an effective treatment for lipedema-results of a study with 25 patients. *J Dtsch Dermatol Ges.* 2011;9(1):33–40.

Falck J, Rolander B, Nygardh A, Jonasson LL, Martensson J. Women with lipoedema: a national survey on their health, health-related quality of life, and sense of coherence. *BMC Womens Health.* 2022;22(1):457. doi: https://doi.org/10.1186/s12905-022-02022-3.

Bertsch T, Erbacher G, Elwell R. Lipoedema: a paradigm shift and consensus. *J Wound Care.* 2020;29(Sup11b):1–51. doi: https://doi.org/10.12968/jowc.2020.29.Sup11b.1.

Dudek JE, Bialaszek W, Ostaszewski P. Quality of life in women with lipoedema: a contextual behavioral approach. *Qual Life Res.* 2016;25(2):401–408. doi: https://doi.org/10.1007/s11136-015-1080-x.

Organization WH. International statistical classification of diseases and related health problems (11th Revision). Available from: http://id.who.int/icd/entity/1172950828

Gregor MF, Hotamisligil GS. Inflammatory mechanisms in obesity. *Annu Rev Immunol.* 2011;29:415–445. doi: https://doi.org/10.1146/annurev-immunol-031210-101322.

Xu H. Obesity and metabolic inflammation. Drug Discov Today Dis Mech. 2013;10(1–2).

Wallach D, Kang TB, Kovalenko A. Concepts of tissue injury and cell death in inflammation: a historical perspective. *Nat Rev Immunol.* 2014;14(1):51–59. doi: https://doi.org/10.1038/nri3561.

Jeffery E, Wing A, Holtrup B, Sebo Z, Kaplan JL, Saavedra-Pena R, et al. The adipose tissue microenvironment regulates depot-specific adipogenesis in obesity. *Cell Metab.* 2016;24(1):142–150. doi: https://doi.org/10.1016/j.cmet.2016.05.012.

Ioannidou A, Fisher RM, Hagberg CE. The multifaceted roles of the adipose tissue vasculature. Obes Rev. 2022;23(4):e13403. https://doi.org/10.1111/obr.13403.

Hammarstedt A, Gogg S, Hedjazifar S, Nerstedt A, Smith U. Impaired adipogenesis and dysfunctional adipose tissue in human hypertrophic obesity. *Physiol Rev.* 2018;98(4):1911–1941. doi: https://doi.org/10.1152/physrev.00034.2017.

Felmerer G, Stylianaki A, Hagerling R, Wang A, Strobel P, Hollmen M, et al. Adipose tissue hypertrophy, an aberrant biochemical profile and distinct gene expression in lipedema. *J Surg Res.* 2020;253:294–303. doi: https://doi.org/10.1016/j.jss.2020.03.055.

Ishaq M, Bandara N, Morgan S, Nowell C, Mehdi AM, Lyu R, et al. Key signaling networks are dysregulated in patients with the adipose tissue disorder, lipedema. *Int J Obes (Lond)* 2022;46(3):502–514. doi: https://doi.org/10.1038/s41366-021-01002-1.

Ibarra M, Eekema A, Ussery C, Neuhardt D, Garby K, Herbst KL. Subcutaneous adipose tissue therapy reduces fat by dual X-ray absorptiometry scan and improves tissue structure by ultrasound in women with lipoedema and Dercum disease. *Clin Obes.* 2018;8(6):398–406. doi: https://doi.org/10.1111/cob.12281.

Suga H, Araki J, Aoi N, Kato H, Higashino T, Yoshimura K. Adipose tissue remodeling in lipedema: adipocyte death and concurrent regeneration. J Cutan Pathol. 2009;36(12):1293–8. https://doi.org/10.1111/j.1600-0560.2009.01256.x.

Shah JP, Danoff JV, Desai MJ, Parikh S, Nakamura LY, Phillips TM, et al. Biochemicals associated with pain and inflammation are elevated in sites near to and remote from active myofascial trigger points. *Arch Phys Med Rehabil.* 2008;89(1):16–23. doi: https://doi.org/10.1016/j.apmr.2007.10.018.

Olszewski WL, Ambujam PJ, Zaleska M, Cakala M. Where do lymph and tissue fluid accumulate in lymphedema of the lower limbs caused by obliteration of lymphatic collectors? *Lymphology.* 2009;42(3):105–111.

Ma W, Gil HJ, Escobedo N, Benito-Martin A, Ximenez-Embun P, Munoz J, et al. Platelet factor 4 is a biomarker for lymphatic-promoted disorders. JCI Insight. 2020;5(13).

Crescenzi R, Marton A, Donahue PMC, Mahany HB, Lants SK, Wang P, et al. Tissue sodium content is elevated in the skin and subcutaneous adipose tissue in women with lipedema. *Obesity (Silver Spring)* 2018;26(2):310–317. doi: https://doi.org/10.1002/oby.22090.

Al-Ghadban S, Cromer W, Allen M, Ussery C, Badowski M, Harris D, Herbst KL. Dilated blood and lymphatic microvessels, angiogenesis, increased macrophages, and adipocyte hypertrophy in lipedema thigh skin and fat tissue. J Obes. 2019;2019:8747461. https://doi.org/10.1155/2019/8747461.

Priglinger E, Wurzer C, Steffenhagen C, Maier J, Hofer V, Peterbauer A, et al. The adipose tissue-derived stromal vascular fraction cells from lipedema patients: are they different? *Cytotherapy.* 2017;19(7):849–860. doi: https://doi.org/10.1016/j.jcyt.2017.03.073.

Pereira de Godoy LM, Pereira de Godoy HJ, Pereira de Godoy Capeletto P, Guerreiro Godoy MF, Pereira de Godoy JM. Lipedema and the evolution to lymphedema with the progression of obesity. Cureus. 2020;12(12):e11854. 10.7759/cureus.11854.

Schmitt R, Lucas D, Buhmann S, Lanz U, Schindler G. Morphometry using computerized tomography of the wrist in idiopathic carpal tunnel syndrome. Comparison of pre- and postoperative findings. Handchir Mikrochir Plast Chir. 1988;20(1):41–6.

Keith L, Seo CA, Rowsemitt C, Pfeffer M, Wahi M, Staggs M, Dudek J, Gower B, Carmody M. Ketogenic diet as a potential intervention for lipedema. Med Hypotheses. 2021;146:110435. https://doi.org/10.1016/j.mehy.2020.110435.

Trimboli P, Castellana M, Bellido D, Casanueva FF. Confusion in the nomenclature of ketogenic diets blurs evidence. *Rev Endocr Metab Disord.* 2020;21(1):1–3. doi: https://doi.org/10.1007/s11154-020-09546-9.

Caprio M, Infante M, Moriconi E, Armani A, Fabbri A, Mantovani G, et al. Very-low-calorie ketogenic diet (VLCKD) in the management of metabolic diseases: systematic review and consensus statement from the Italian Society of Endocrinology (SIE) *J Endocrinol Invest.* 2019;42(11):1365–1386. doi: https://doi.org/10.1007/s40618-019-01061-2.

Goday A, Bellido D, Sajoux I, Crujeiras AB, Burguera B, Garcia-Luna PP, Oleaga A, Moreno B, Casanueva FF. Short-term safety, tolerability and efficacy of a very low-calorie-ketogenic diet interventional weight loss program versus hypocaloric diet in patients with type 2 diabetes mellitus. Nutr Diabetes. 2016;6(9):e230. https://doi.org/10.1038/nutd.2016.36.

Romano L, Marchetti M, Gualtieri P, Di Renzo L, Belcastro M, De Santis GL, Perrone MA, De Lorenzo A. Effects of a personalized VLCKD on body composition and resting energy expenditure in the reversal of diabetes to prevent complications. Nutrients. 2019;11(7):1526–39. https://doi.org/10.3390/nu11071526.

Castellana M, Conte E, Cignarelli A, Perrini S, Giustina A, Giovanella L, et al. Efficacy and safety of very low calorie ketogenic diet (VLCKD) in patients with overweight and obesity: a systematic review and meta-analysis. *Rev Endocr Metab Disord.* 2020;21(1):5–16. doi: https://doi.org/10.1007/s11154-019-09514-y.

Compression Stocking

Lipedema is a chronic condition characterized by the abnormal accumulation of fat in specific areas of the body, primarily in the legs and sometimes in the arms. This condition affects a significant number of individuals, predominantly women, and is often misunderstood and misdiagnosed. Lipedema is distinct from obesity and lymphedema, although it can coexist with these conditions, complicating its management. The fat distribution in lipedema is symmetrical, painful, and can lead to mobility issues, emotional distress, and a decreased quality of life.

The exact cause of lipedema is still under investigation, but it is believed to have a genetic component and hormonal influences. Its onset is often linked to periods of hormonal change such as puberty, pregnancy, or menopause. Despite its prevalence, lipedema remains under-recognized, leading to delays in diagnosis and treatment.

Management of lipedema is multifaceted, focusing on reducing symptoms, slowing the progression of the disease, and improving the patient's quality of life. Treatment strategies include lifestyle modifications, diet and exercise, manual lymphatic drainage, surgery (liposuction for fat removal), and the cornerstone of conservative management: compression therapy.

Compression therapy (Fig. 1) plays a critical role in the management of lipedema. It is a noninvasive treatment option that provides significant benefits in reducing symptoms and improving the quality of life for individuals with lipedema. Compression therapy involves wearing specially designed garments that apply gentle pressure to the affected areas.

These garments can be socks, stockings, sleeves, or full-body suits, depending on the areas affected by lipedema.

Compression therapy serves as an intervention for a spectrum of vascular and lymphatic ailments, notably lipedema, and is predicated on the strategic application of pressure to enhance circulatory and lymphatic dynamics (Fig. 2). The therapeutic benefits of this modality are particularly salient in the amelioration of symptoms attributable to venous insufficiency and lymphatic dysfunction, as observed in lipedema. Within this context, the mechanism of action of compression therapy is multifaceted, with the most salient being graduated compression. This technique

G. Laur, *Lipoedema*, https://doi.org/10.1007/978-981-96-8939-2_19

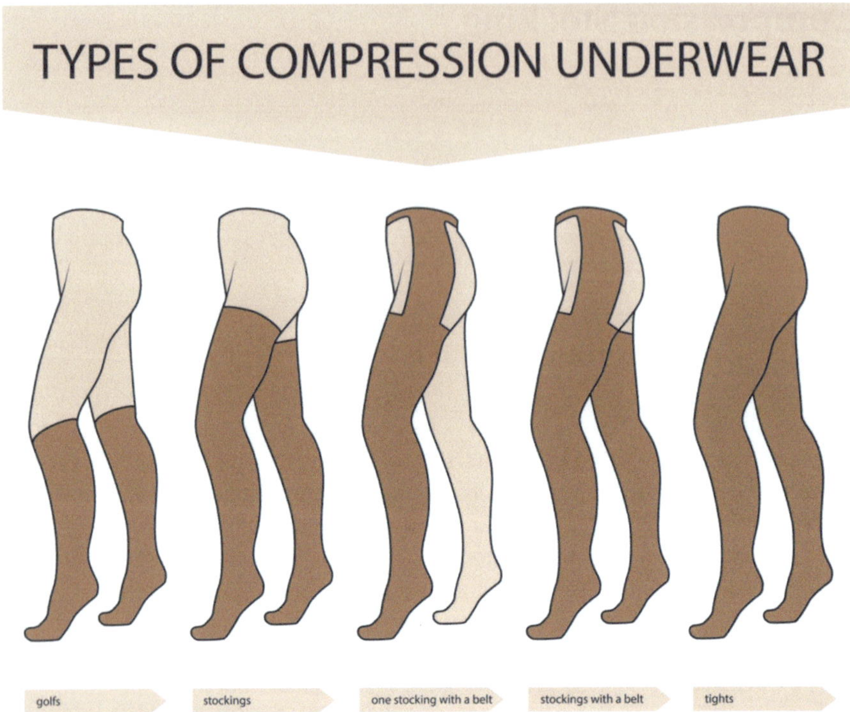

Fig. 1 Compression underwear. A special type of clothing designed to correct pathological processes and accelerate the recovery period

facilitates a pressure gradient, maximal at the ankle and diminishing proximally, bolstering both venous and lymphatic return, and mitigating interstitial fluid accumulation.

The application of this gradient pressure is crucial in augmenting venous return, especially in conditions marked by venous valve incompetence, and is instrumental in promoting the clearance of lymphatic fluid in lymphedema and lipedema. Furthermore, this modality is efficacious in edema reduction, providing symptomatic relief from the associated sensations of heaviness and discomfort.

In the specific context of lipedema, which is characterized by adipose deposition with symmetrical distribution, compression therapy exerts multiple physiological impacts. These include the alleviation of pain—which may be partly attributed to the reduction in edema—the enhancement of tissue microcirculation, and the stabilization of subcutaneous tissue structures.

Importantly, while not curative, the strategic use of compression therapy is vital in forestalling the progression of lipedema, maintaining functional mobility, and preempting secondary complications such as lymphedema or venous disorders.

In the domain of medical treatment for venous disorders, lymphedema, and lipedema, compression therapy is a critical intervention. The success of this

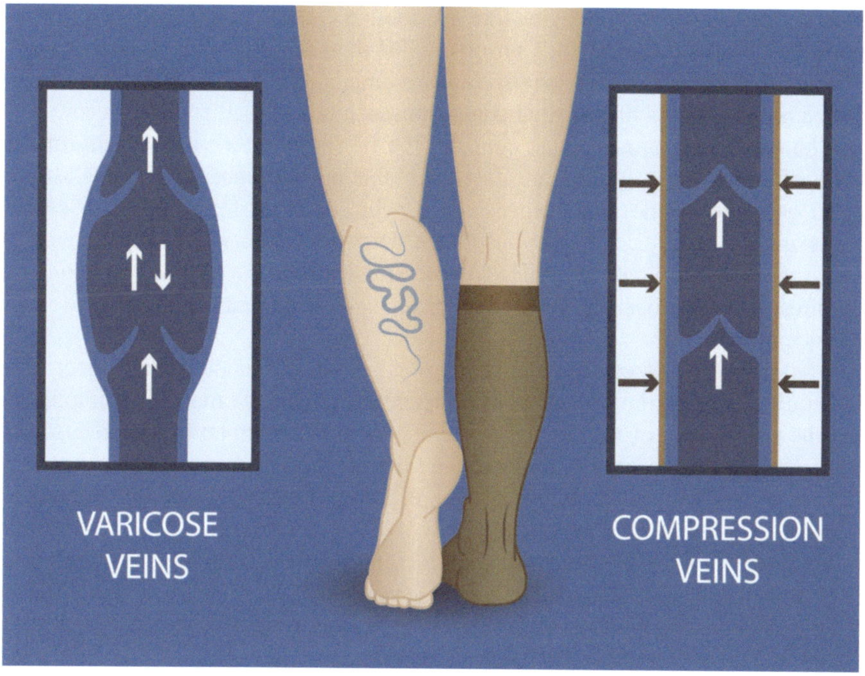

Fig. 2 Effect of compression stockings on varicose veins

therapeutic approach is closely linked to the appropriate selection of compression garments, which are engineered to deliver measured pressure to specific areas to enhance both blood and lymphatic circulation. This scholarly discussion delineates the various categories of compression garments available, such as graduated compression stockings, compression sleeves, and gloves, and evaluates the merits and considerations of custom-fitted versus standard off-the-shelf garments.

Graduated compression stockings are designed with a pressure gradient that diminishes from the ankle upward, facilitating venous return, mitigating the impact of gravitational forces, and ameliorating symptoms of venous stasis and edema. Such stockings are integral to the management of chronic venous insufficiency and prevention of deep vein thrombosis, as well as serving as a treatment modality for lymphedema and lipedema (Mosti & Partsch, 2018).

In contrast, compression sleeves and gloves cater to the upper extremities, providing targeted pressure to manage conditions such as lymphedema and aid recovery post-surgery, including mastectomy. These garments may also be designed with a graduated pressure system, although the specific gradient is contingent upon the garment's construction and the clinical condition addressed (International Lymphoedema Framework, 2012).

The debate between custom-fitted and off-the-shelf garments hinges on their therapeutic value. Custom-fitted garments are tailored to an individual's measurements, offering a precise fit for nonstandard limb dimensions and severe edematous states, which ensures optimal pressure distribution and can be adjusted over time as needed (Brizzio et al., 2010). Conversely, off-the-shelf garments provide a cost-effective and accessible solution for standard limb conformations or transient therapeutic needs, albeit with potential compromises in fit and therapeutic efficacy.

The choice of garment must consider the fit and comfort, the severity of the medical condition, and economic factors, including insurance coverage. Custom-fitted garments, while more expensive, may be indicated for complex or severe cases and potentially covered by insurance (Damstra & Partsch, 2013). In conclusion, the selection of an appropriate compression garment is a nuanced decision that requires careful consideration of clinical needs, patient comfort, and cost considerations.

The utilization of compression therapy constitutes a fundamental aspect of a holistic strategy for the management of lipedema, playing a crucial role in mitigating the progression of the condition and alleviating its symptoms. The determination of appropriate compression levels and the duration of garment use are critical factors that significantly influence the efficacy of this therapeutic approach. Compression levels, measured in millimeters of mercury (mmHg), are stratified into mild (15–20 mmHg), moderate (20–30 mmHg), firm (30–40 mmHg), and extra firm (>40 mmHg), each corresponding to the severity and stage of lipedema, ranging from early manifestations to severe cases necessitating rigorous medical oversight (International Society of Lymphology, 2013).

The recommended duration of wear is predominantly during waking hours, tailored to individual patient responses and the specific objectives of treatment, aiming to optimize therapeutic outcomes.

Lipedema progresses through distinct stages, necessitating a tailored approach to compression therapy that accommodates the unique characteristics and challenges presented at each stage. From the initial stage characterized by smooth skin and subcutaneous fat accumulation to more advanced stages marked by significant edema and mobility issues, the application of compression therapy must be meticulously adjusted to address the evolving needs of the patient.

Moreover, the integration of compression therapy within a multidisciplinary treatment framework enhances the overall efficacy of lipedema management. This comprehensive approach includes manual lymphatic drainage (MLD) to stimulate lymphatic circulation, low-impact exercises to promote lymphatic flow, nutritional guidance to manage weight, psychological support to address the emotional impact of lipedema, and surgical interventions for the removal of excess fat tissue, where compression therapy plays a vital role in post-surgical recovery and the maintenance of long-term outcomes (Warren Peled et al., 2018). Such an integrated treatment plan underscores the importance of a patient-centered approach that not only addresses the physical aspects of lipedema but also considers the psychological well-being of patients, thereby fostering more effective management and improved quality of life for individuals affected by this condition.

Compression therapy has garnered substantial evidence supporting its efficacy in managing various chronic conditions, such as venous disorders, lymphedema, and lipedema, highlighting its importance in both clinical settings and patient care strategies. Research and clinical experience have consistently demonstrated the benefits of compression therapy in improving patient outcomes, particularly in the reduction of pain, swelling, and the enhancement of mobility. Studies have shown that the application of graduated compression garments can significantly decrease the symptoms of venous insufficiency, including leg swelling and the sensation of heaviness, thereby improving the quality of life for affected individuals. Furthermore, in the context of lipedema, compression therapy has been instrumental in managing chronic pain, a prevalent symptom that profoundly impacts patients' daily functioning and well-being. Mobility improvements have also been documented, with patients reporting enhanced ability to perform daily activities and increased exercise tolerance. Case studies further substantiate these findings, providing detailed accounts of individual patient experiences that underscore the personalized nature of compression therapy and its adaptability to meet specific patient needs. These narratives, combined with quantitative data from clinical trials, offer a comprehensive understanding of the multifaceted role of compression therapy in treatment regimens, reinforcing its status as a cornerstone of effective management for conditions characterized by compromised lymphatic and venous circulation.

Compression therapy, while effective, presents several challenges that can impact patient compliance and overall treatment success. Common issues faced by patients include discomfort, difficulty in donning and doffing compression garments, skin irritation, and the aesthetic concerns associated with wearing these garments daily. Addressing comfort and compliance is crucial to ensuring patients continue with their prescribed therapy. Solutions to these challenges have evolved through clinical innovation and patient feedback.

For instance, the development of donning aids and garments with more user-friendly materials has significantly eased the application process, enhancing patient autonomy and reducing dependence on caregivers. Manufacturers have also focused on creating compression garments that balance efficacy with aesthetics, offering a variety of colors and styles to meet patient preferences and reduce self-consciousness associated with garment use. Additionally, education plays a role in improving compliance; healthcare providers offering clear instructions and demonstrations on garment use, as well as regular follow-up to adjust therapy as needed, can greatly enhance patient comfort and adherence to treatment. Integrating patient education with the use of improved garment technology and support systems addresses the common challenges in compression therapy, leading to better outcomes and patient satisfaction.

The landscape of compression therapy is continually evolving, with advancements in technology leading to more effective and user-friendly treatment options. Among these innovations, pneumatic compression devices stand out for their ability to provide dynamic, adjustable compression. These devices use air-filled chambers that sequentially inflate and deflate, mimicking natural lymphatic flow and venous return, thus offering an alternative to traditional static compression garments. Additionally, the development of innovative materials and garment designs has significantly improved patient compliance and comfort. Materials that offer greater breathability, moisture-wicking properties, and enhanced elasticity ensure that compression garments can be worn comfortably for extended periods. Garment designs now also incorporate user feedback, leading to features such as easier donning mechanisms and aesthetically pleasing options that cater to patient preferences. Looking to the future, trends in compression therapy suggest a move toward personalized medicine, with wearable technology providing real-time adjustments to compression levels based on individual patient needs and activity levels. Furthermore, integration with digital health platforms may allow for remote monitoring of therapy adherence and effectiveness, offering healthcare providers valuable insights to tailor treatment plans. These advancements promise to enhance the efficacy of compression therapy, making it a more adaptable, comfortable, and effective treatment modality for patients with venous and lymphatic disorders.

The psychosocial considerations associated with compression therapy, especially in the context of lipedema, are profound, influencing both body image and lifestyle. The chronic nature of lipedema, coupled with the visible symptoms and the necessity for ongoing use of compression garments, can significantly impact patients' perception of their bodies and their social interactions. Addressing patient concerns and expectations is crucial; healthcare providers must engage in open, empathetic conversations about the goals of compression therapy, realistically setting what can be achieved while acknowledging the emotional and psychological challenges patients may face. In summarizing the role of compression therapy in lipedema, it is essential to highlight its efficacy in managing symptoms and improving quality of life but also to recognize that it is part of a broader, holistic treatment approach. This approach should encompass not only physical interventions but also support for the psychological well-being of patients, through counseling, support groups, or therapy, to address body image issues, self-esteem, and coping strategies. By emphasizing the importance of a holistic treatment approach, healthcare providers can help patients navigate the complexities of lipedema management, ensuring a more compassionate and comprehensive care pathway that acknowledges the interplay between physical symptoms and psychosocial health.

Suggested Reading

Wold L.E., Hines JR E.A., Allen E.V. Lipedema of the legs: A syndrome characterized by fat legs and edema. *Ann. Intern. Med.* 1951;**34**:1243–1250.

Forner-Cordero I., Szolnoky G., Forner-Cordero A., Keméy L. Lipedema: An overview of its clinical manifestations, diagnosis and treatment of the disproportional fatty deposition syndrome–systematic review. *Clin. Obes.* 2012;**2**:86–95. doi: https://doi.org/10.1111/j.1758-8111.2012.00045.x.

Herbst K., Chava Y., Te C.H.T., Mirkovskaya L., Bharhagava A. Lipedema Fat and Signs and Symptoms of Illness, Increase with Advancing Stage. *Arch. Med.* 2015;**7**:1–8..

Bertsch T., Erbacher G., Elwell R. Lipoedema: A paradigm shift and consensus. *J. Wound Care.* 2020;**29**:1–51. doi: https://doi.org/10.12968/jowc.2020.29.Sup11b.1.

Bosman J. Lipoedema: Poor knowledge, neglect or disinterest? *J. Lymphoedema.* 2011;**6**:109–111.

Buso G., Depairon M., Tomson D., Raffoul W., Vettor R., Mazzolai L. Lipedema: A Call to Action! *Obesity.* 2019;**27**:1567–1576. doi: https://doi.org/10.1002/oby.22597.

Herbst K.L., Kahn L.A., Iker E., Ehrlich C., Wright T., McHutchison L., Schwartz J., Sleigh M., Donahue P.M.C., Lisson K.H. Standard of care for lipedema in the United States. *Phlebology.* 2021;**36**:779–796. doi: https://doi.org/10.1177/02683555211015887.
Erbacher G., Bertsch T. Lipoedema and Pain: What is the role of the psyche?–Results of a pilot study with 150 patients with Lipoedema. *Phlebologie.* 2020;**49**:305–316. doi: https://doi.org/10.1055/a-1238-6657.
Peled A.W., Kappos E.A. Lipedema: Diagnostic and management challenges. *Int. J. Womens Health.* 2016;**8**:389. doi: https://doi.org/10.2147/IJWH.S106227.
Child A.H., Sharpe P., Gordon K.D., Brice G., Ostergaard P., Jeffery S., Mortimer P.S. Lipedema: An inherited condition. *Am. J. Med. Genet. Part A.* 2010;**152**:970–976. doi: https://doi.org/10.1002/ajmg.a.33313.
Herpertz U. Lipedema—Pathogenesis, Diagnosis and Treatment Options. *Dtsch. Aerzteblatt Int.* 2021;**118**:39.
Langendoen S.I., Habbema L., Nijsten T.E.C., Neumann H.A.M. Lipoedema: From clinical presentation to therapy. A review of the literature. *Br. J. Dermatol.* 2009;**161**:980–986. doi: https://doi.org/10.1111/j.1365-2133.2009.09413.x.
Bauer A.-T., von Lukowicz D., Lossagk K., Aitzetmueller M., Moog P., Cerny M., Erne H., Schmauss D., Duscher D., Machens H.-G. New Insights on Lipedema: The Enigmatic Disease of the Peripheral Fat. *Plast. Reconstr. Surg.* 2019;**144**:1475–1484. doi: https://doi.org/10.1097/PRS.0000000000006280.
Romeijn J.R.M., de Rooij M.J.M., Janssen L., Martens H. Exploration of Patient Characteristics and Quality of Life in Patients with Lipoedema Using a Survey. *Dermatol. Ther.* 2018;**8**:303–311. doi: https://doi.org/10.1007/s13555-018-0241-6.
Crescenzi R., Mahany H.B., Lants S.K., Wang P., Donahue M.J., Marton A., Titze J., Donahue P.M.C., Beckman J.A. Tissue Sodium Content is Elevated in the Skin and Subcutaneous Adipose Tissue in Women with Lipedema. *Obesity.* 2018;**26**:310–317. doi: https://doi.org/10.1002/oby.22090.
Aksoy H., Karadag A.S., Wollina U. Cause and management of lipedema-associated pain. *Dermatol. Ther.* 2020;**34**:e14364. doi: https://doi.org/10.1111/dth.14364.
Sucker C., Schmidt-Lucke J.-A., Litmathe J. Hämatomneigung bei Lipödem: Kutane Genese oder Gerinnungsdefekt? *Wien. Med. Wochenschr.* 2021;**171**:48–52. doi: https://doi.org/10.1007/s10354-020-00792-9.
Melander C., Juuso P., Olsson M. Women's experiences of living with lipedema. *Health Care Women Int.* 2021;**43**:54–69. doi: https://doi.org/10.1080/07399332.2021.1932894.
Czerwińska M., Ostrowska P., Hansdorfer-Korzon R. Lipoedema as a Social Problem. A Scoping Review. *Int. J. Environ. Res. Public Health.* 2021;**18**:10223. doi: https://doi.org/10.3390/ijerph181910223.
Dudek J.E., Białaszek W., Gabriel M. Quality of life, its factors, and sociodemographic characteristics of Polish women with lipedema. *BMC Womens Health.* 2021;**21**:1–9. doi: https://doi.org/10.1186/s12905-021-01174-y.
Dudek J.E., Białaszek W., Ostaszewski P., Smidt T. Depression and appearance-related distress in functioning with lipedema. *Psychol. Health Med.* 2018;**23**:846–853. doi: https://doi.org/10.1080/13548506.2018.1459750.
Williams A. Understanding the challenges of lipoedema. *J. Community Nurs.* 2018;**32**:34–41.
Fetzer A. Specialist approaches to managing lipoedema. *Br. J. Community Nurs.* 2016;**21**:30–35. doi: https://doi.org/10.12968/bjcn.2016.21.Sup4.S30.
Bertsch T. Compression garments for pain management, comfort and freedom of movement in lipoedema patients: Clinical benefits of JOBST® Confidence. *Br. J. Community Nurs.* 2022;**27**:S22. doi: https://doi.org/10.12968/bjcn.2022.27.Sup9.S22.
Paling I., Macintyre L. Survey of lipoedema symptoms and experience with compression garments. *Br. J. Community Nurs.* 2020;**25**:S17–S22. doi: https://doi.org/10.12968/bjcn.2020.25.Sup4.S17.

Czerwińska M., Teodorczyk J., Hansdorfer-Korzon R. A Scoping Review of Available Tools in Measurement of the Effectiveness of Conservative Treatment in Lipoedema. *Int. J. Environ. Res. Public Health.* 2022;**19**:7124. doi: https://doi.org/10.3390/ijerph19127124.

Szél E., Kemény L., Groma G., Szolnoky G. Pathophysiological dilemmas of lipedema. *Med. Hypotheses.* 2014;**83**:599–606. doi: https://doi.org/10.1016/j.mehy.2014.08.011.

Yuan Y., Gao J., Ogawa R. Mechanobiology and mechanotherapy of adipose tissue-effect of mechanical force on fat tissue engineering. *Plast. Reconstr. Surg. Glob. Open.* 2015;**3**:e578. doi: https://doi.org/10.1097/GOX.0000000000000564.

Lipoedema UK Big Survey 2014 Research Report. 2016. [(accessed on 22 December 2022)]. Available online: https://www.lipoedema.co.uk/wp-content/uploads/

Atan T., Bahar-Özdemir Y. The Effects of Complete Decongestive Therapy or Intermittent Pneumatic Compression Therapy or Exercise Only in the Treatment of Severe Lipedema: A Randomized Controlled Trial. *Lymphat. Res. Biol.* 2021;**19**:86–95. doi: https://doi.org/10.1089/lrb.2020.0019.

Herbst K.L., Ussery C., Eekema A. Pilot study: Whole body manual subcutaneous adipose tissue (SAT) therapy improved pain and SAT structure in women with lipedema. *Horm. Mol. Biol. Clin. Investig.* 2017;**33** doi: https://doi.org/10.1515/hmbci-2017-0035.

Ibarra M., Eekema A., Ussery C., Neuhardt D., Garby K., Herbst K.L. Subcutaneous adipose tissue therapy reduces fat by dual X-ray absorptiometry scan and improves tissue structure by ultrasound in women with lipoedema and Dercum disease. *Clin. Obes.* 2018;**8**:398–406. doi: https://doi.org/10.1111/cob.12281.

Amato A.C.M., Saucedo D.Z., Santos K.D.S., Benitti D.A. Ultrasound criteria for lipedema diagnosis. *Phlebology.* 2021;**36**:651–658. doi: https://doi.org/10.1177/02683555211002340.

Hirsch T., Schleinitz J., Marshall M., Faerber G. Is the differential diagnosis of lipoedema by means of high-resolution ultrasonography possible. *Phlebologie.* 2018;**47**:182–187.

MLD

Manual lymphatic drainage (MLD) (Fig. 1) is a therapeutic technique distinct from traditional massage, aimed at enhancing the natural flow of lymph fluid within the body to aid in the removal of waste products from tissues. The lymphatic system, reliant on the peristalsis of smooth muscle cells in lymph vessels and the movement of skeletal muscles, propels lymph toward the heart, integrating it with the cardiovascular system. MLD employs light pressure and rhythmic circular motions, a method developed in the 1930s by Danish doctors Emil Vodder and Estrid Vodder, initially as a treatment for chronic sinusitis and immune disorders. Noticing swollen lymph nodes in patients with chronic colds, the Vodders experimented with gentle hand movements to stimulate lymph flow, later formalizing their technique and disseminating it post–World War II.

The traditional Vodder method involves semicircular hand movements, which have been foundational in lymphedema treatment for decades. However, in 1999, Godoy and Godoy introduced a novel approach to MLD, advocating for linear motions that follow the lymphatic vessels toward the lymph nodes, using hand pressure instead of rollers. This method emphasizes maintaining consistent pressure along the vessels' path. The efficacy of these techniques, including the changes in limb volume they induce, has been substantiated through various assessments such as lymphoscintigraphy, volumetry, and bioimpedance, marking a significant evolution in lymphedema management and various aesthetic procedures.

Manual lymphatic drainage (MLD) therapy is a specialized massage technique that is used to stimulate the lymphatic system and promote the natural drainage of lymph fluid from the body. The lymphatic system is a network of vessels and nodes that help to remove waste products and excess fluids from the body. When the lymphatic system is not functioning properly, it can lead to swelling, fluid retention, and other symptoms.

During MLD therapy, a certified therapist uses gentle, rhythmic strokes and light pressure to stimulate lymphatic flow and encourage the natural drainage of lymph

G. Laur, *Lipoedema*, https://doi.org/10.1007/978-981-96-8939-2_20

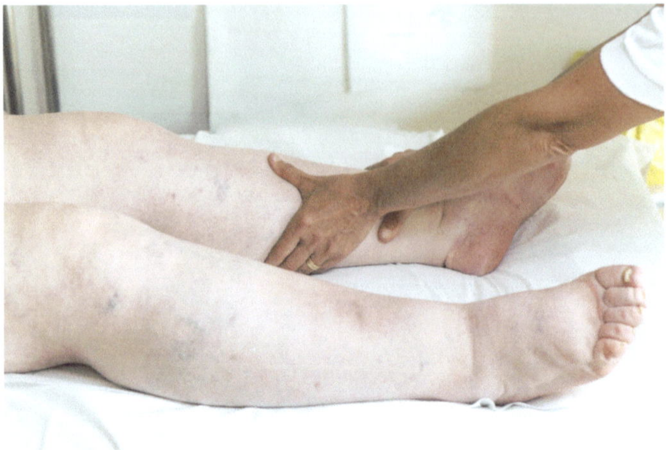

Fig. 1 Manual lymphatic drainage massage for a patient with swelling effect

fluid from the body. The therapist will use their hands to move the skin in specific directions, working to stimulate lymphatic vessels and nodes in the affected area.

MLD therapy is often used as a noninvasive treatment option for conditions such as lymphedema, which is a condition characterized by swelling and fluid retention in the limbs. MLD therapy can also be used to help manage other conditions that are related to poor lymphatic function, such as lipedema.

Manual lymphatic drainage (MLD) is an essential therapeutic intervention in the management of lipedema, a condition marked by irregular fat distribution and associated with lymphatic dysfunction. As a specialized form of massage, MLD aims to enhance the function of the lymphatic system, facilitating the removal of excess lymphatic fluid and thus reducing the painful swelling commonly experienced in lipedema. This gentle, rhythmic technique is designed to stimulate the natural circulation of lymph through the body, which can be particularly beneficial in the early stages of lipedema to prevent progression to secondary lymphedema. The effectiveness of MLD in lipedema management is supported by its ability to improve lymph flow, ameliorate symptoms, and potentially slow disease progression. While MLD does not reduce fat deposits directly, it contributes to a decrease in discomfort and an improvement in limb mobility and quality of life for patients. For optimal outcomes, MLD should be integrated into a comprehensive treatment plan that includes compression therapy, exercise, and nutrition counseling. Moreover, the regular application of MLD by trained therapists, alongside self-massage techniques for ongoing self-care, represents a proactive approach to managing the chronic symptoms of lipedema, underscoring the significant role of MLD within the multidisciplinary care of this condition.

The lymphatic system is a critical component of the body's immune and circulatory systems, functioning primarily to transport lymph, a fluid containing white blood cells, throughout the body. It plays a central role in fluid homeostasis, immune response, and the absorption of dietary fats. The mechanism of action of manual lymphatic drainage (MLD) is intricately tied to the enhancement of this system's functions.

MLD employs a gentle, systematic massage technique that encourages the natural movement of lymph fluids around the body, particularly from congested areas to more centrally located lymph vessels that drain into the venous system. Through specific hand movements and sequences, MLD stimulates the lymphangions to contract more frequently, increasing the rate of lymph flow and facilitating the clearance of excess interstitial fluid.

In the context of lipedema treatment, the goals of MLD are multifold. Primarily, it aims to alleviate the often painful edema associated with lipedema by improving lymph flow, thereby reducing swelling and discomfort. Additionally, MLD seeks to prevent the development of secondary lymphedema, a common complication of lipedema, by maintaining lymphatic efficiency. MLD also aims to enhance the overall functional status of the affected limbs, thereby improving mobility and quality of life for patients with lipedema. Importantly, while MLD does not directly impact fat deposition, it can serve as a supportive therapy in comprehensive lipedema management plans, which may include compression therapy, exercise, dietary changes, and, in some cases, surgical interventions. The application of MLD in lipedema care is thus a cornerstone in the conservative management of the condition, addressing both the physiological and symptomatic aspects to provide a holistic treatment approach.

The efficacy of manual lymphatic drainage (MLD) therapy in the management of lipedema is substantiated by a body of research and clinical evidence. Studies have consistently demonstrated that MLD, a specialized form of gentle skin manipulation designed to enhance the flow of lymph, offers symptomatic relief for lipedema, particularly in the early stages of the disease. Clinical trials and patient reports have provided evidence supporting the role of MLD in reducing the hallmark symptoms of lipedema, such as pain, swelling, and restricted mobility. Pain relief is often reported by patients receiving MLD, attributed to the reduction in excess interstitial fluid and the gentle, soothing nature of the therapy. Swelling, or edema, is also significantly impacted by MLD; the therapy's ability to promote lymph flow can help diminish fluid accumulation in the affected tissues, thereby alleviating the physical discomfort and tightness associated with this symptom. Furthermore, by decreasing pain and swelling, MLD indirectly contributes to improved mobility, allowing patients to engage more actively in daily activities and exercise, which are essential components of comprehensive lipedema management. The effectiveness of MLD in enhancing quality of life for patients with lipedema, while not a curative approach, affirms its value as an integral part of the multidisciplinary treatment paradigm for this condition.

Manual lymphatic drainage (MLD) therapy, while beneficial for lipedema, is not without its challenges. A primary issue is the varying levels of patient compliance and motivation, which are crucial for the success of MLD as it often requires regular and sometimes lengthy sessions to achieve optimal results. Educating patients on the benefits and potential for improved quality of life can enhance adherence to therapy schedules. Tailoring treatment plans to individual needs and schedules and setting realistic goals can also improve compliance. Additionally, the physical discomfort of lipedema can make MLD a sensitive procedure for patients, particularly in areas with significant pain or tenderness. To address this, therapists are trained to apply gentle techniques and to adjust pressure accordingly to ensure patient comfort while still effectively stimulating lymphatic flow. This may involve starting with very light touches and gradually increasing pressure as tolerated, as well as using supportive measures such as cushions or foam padding to alleviate discomfort during treatment.

Moreover, incorporating patient feedback actively into the session can empower patients and make them active participants in their treatment, thereby enhancing the therapeutic experience. Implementing these strategies can help in overcoming the challenges associated with MLD in lipedema management, ultimately leading to improved patient outcomes and adherence to therapy.

The integration of manual lymphatic drainage (MLD) with compression therapy represents a synergistic approach in the management of lipedema, aiming to optimize treatment outcomes. MLD is designed to manually stimulate the lymphatic flow, reducing fluid congestion within the tissues. When combined with the use of compression garments, the effectiveness of MLD is enhanced; the garments help maintain the reduced limb volume achieved by MLD by providing continuous external pressure, which supports the lymphatic and venous systems and prevents the re-accumulation of fluid. This combination therapy is widely advocated in clinical practice, and its efficacy is reflected in numerous case studies. For example, patients presenting with lipedema-related lymphedema have shown significant and sustained reductions in limb girth and improvements in pain and mobility when treated with both MLD and subsequent compression therapy. The sequential use of MLD followed by the application of compression garments is a standard protocol, as MLD can initially reduce swelling, making the limbs more amenable to fitting into compression garments. Such combined treatment approaches are evidenced in the case of a patient who, after receiving a series of MLD sessions, was fitted with custom-made compression stockings and reported not only a reduction in limb volume but also an increased ability to participate in daily activities and an improved overall quality of life. These anecdotal outcomes underscore the need for further structured research to solidify the combined use of MLD and compression therapy as a cornerstone in the multidisciplinary approach to lipedema management.

In conclusion, manual lymphatic drainage (MLD) is an indispensable component of a comprehensive lipedema treatment plan, playing a significant role in the management of the condition's symptoms and patient well-being. The therapeutic technique of MLD, with its unique mechanism of encouraging lymph flow, has been consistently validated as a means of alleviating the pain, swelling, and mobility issues associated with lipedema. When integrated with other treatment modalities, such as compression therapy, physical activity, and nutritional guidance, MLD contributes to a holistic approach that addresses the multifactorial nature of lipedema.

The consistent application of MLD has shown to improve lymphatic system function, reduce edema, and enhance the quality of life for individuals with lipedema. It serves not only to manage the physical symptoms but also to empower patients to take an active role in the management of their condition. The success of MLD, however, hinges on patient compliance and the skillful adaptation of the therapy to each patient's needs, especially when treating sensitive or painful areas.

Furthermore, the role of MLD within the broader spectrum of lipedema management strategies underscores the importance of patient education, motivation, and the establishment of supportive healthcare relationships. The case examples of combined treatment approaches provide a promising outlook on the potential for improved patient outcomes when MLD is effectively incorporated into the treatment regimen.

Therefore, MLD should be recognized as a cornerstone of lipedema management, emphasizing the need for continued research, education, and refinement of techniques to enhance its efficacy. The healthcare community's commitment to integrating MLD into lipedema care will continue to be a critical factor in advancing the standard of treatment and support for individuals affected by this challenging condition.

Suggested Reading

Chikly BJ. Manual techniques addressing the lymphatic system: Origins and development. *J Am Osteopath Assoc.* 2005;105:457–474.

Eisenhart AW, Gaeta TJ, Yens DP. Osteopathic manipulative treatment in the emergency department for patients with acute ankle sprains. *J Am Osteopath Assoc.* 2003;103:417–421.

Lesho EP. An overview of osteopathic medicine. *Arch Fam Med.* 1999;8:477–484.

Weiss JM. Treatment of leg edema and wound = s in a patient with severe musculoskeletal injuries. *Phys fler.* 1998;78:1104–1113.

Korosec BJ. Manual lymphatic drainage therapy. *Home Health Care Mang Pract.* 2004;17:499–511

Patterson MM. Mechanisms of change: Animal models in osteopathic research. *J Am Osteopath Assoc.* 2007;107:593–597

Kasseroller RG. The Vodder school: The Vodder method. *Cancer.* 1998;83:2840–2842

Birrer RB, Fani-Salek MH, Totten VY, Herman LM, Polti V. Managing ankle injuries in the emergency department. *J Emerg Med.* 1999;17:751–770.

McKeon PO, Medina JM, Hertel J. Hierarchy of evidence–based clinical research in sports medicine. *Athletic fler Today.* 2006;11:42–45.

Medina JM, McKeon PO, Hertel J. Rating the levels of evidence in sports medicine research. *Athletic fler Today.* 2006;11:38–41

Schillinger A, Koening D, Haefele C, et al. Effect of manual lymph drainage on the course of serum levels of muscle enzymes after treadmill exercise. *Am J Phys Med Rehabil.* 2006;85:516–520.

Härén K, Backman C, Wiberg M. Effect of manual lymph drainage as described by Vodder on œdema of the hand after fracture of the distal radius: A prospective clinical study. *Scand J Plast Reconstr Surg Hand Surg.* 2000;34:367–372.

Asplund R. Manual lymph drainage therapy using light massage for fibromyalgia sufferers: A pilot study. *Phys fler.* 2003;7:192–196.

Lancaster DG, Crow WT. Osteopathic manipulative treatment of a 26-year-old woman with Bell's palsy. *J Am Osteopath Assoc.* 2006;106:285–289.

Déry MA, Yonuschot G, Winterson BJ. The effects of manually applied intermittent pulsation pressure to a rat ventral thorax on lymph transport. *Lymphology.* 2000;33:58–61.

Knott EM, Tune JD, Stoll ST, Downey HF. Increased lymphatic flow in the thoracic duct during manipulative intervention. *J Am Osteopath Assoc.* 2005;105:447–456.

Hodge LM, King HH, Williams AG, et al. Abdominal lymphatic pump treatment increases leukocyte count flux in thoracic duct lymph. *Lymph Res Biol.* 2007;5:127–134.

Ernst E. The safety of massage therapy. *Rheumatology.* 2003;42:1101–1106.

Fritz JM, Cleland J. Effectiveness versus efficacy: More than a debate over language. *J Orthop Sports Phys fler.* 2003;33:163–165.

Exercise

Exercise can be an important component of the management of lipedema. Regular exercise can help improve overall fitness, reduce inflammation, increase lymphatic and blood flow, and improve muscle tone, all of which can help alleviate some of the symptoms associated with lipedema.

When developing an exercise program for lipedema, it is important to take into account the individual needs and limitations of the patient. Low-impact exercises that do not put excessive stress on the joints and tissues, such as swimming, cycling, and walking, are often recommended. Strength training exercises that target the affected areas can also help improve muscle tone and support lymphatic drainage.

It is important to start slowly and gradually increase the duration and intensity of the exercise program. Overexertion and high-impact activities can worsen lipedema symptoms and should be avoided. Patients with lipedema should also wear compression garments while exercising to help support lymphatic flow and prevent fluid buildup.

In addition to formal exercise programs, incorporating more physical activity into daily life can also be beneficial for managing lipedema. Simple activities such as taking the stairs instead of the elevator, walking instead of driving short distances, and taking regular breaks to stretch and move during prolonged sitting can all help improve lymphatic and blood flow and reduce inflammation.

Understanding the role of physical activity in the management of lipedema is crucial for both mitigating the progression of the condition and enhancing the overall well-being of affected individuals. Physical activity, particularly low-impact exercises such as swimming, cycling, and walking, plays a role in managing lipedema by promoting lymphatic drainage, improving cardiovascular health, and aiding in weight management. These activities help in reducing the excessive accumulation of lipedematous fat, alleviating pain, and decreasing the risk of secondary complications such as lymphedema and joint issues. Furthermore, regular exercise contributes to the improvement of mobility and flexibility, enabling patients to maintain an active lifestyle despite the challenges posed by lipedema. Beyond the physical benefits, engaging in physical activity has been shown to have positive

G. Laur, *Lipoedema*, https://doi.org/10.1007/978-981-96-8939-2_21

effects on mental health, including reducing symptoms of depression and anxiety and improving self-esteem and body image. It is essential for patients with lipedema to incorporate a tailored exercise regimen, developed in consultation with healthcare professionals, into their comprehensive treatment plan. This approach ensures that the exercise program is both effective and safe, taking into consideration the individual's symptoms, stage of lipedema, and overall health status. Through a balanced integration of physical activity into lipedema management, patients can achieve significant improvements in their condition, leading to a better quality of life.

Understanding safe exercise practices is paramount in the management of lipedema, as it ensures the effectiveness of physical activity while minimizing the risk of exacerbating the condition. The primary goals of exercise in lipedema management include promoting lymphatic drainage to reduce fluid accumulation, enhancing cardiovascular fitness to support overall health, and maintaining or improving range of motion and muscle strength to counteract the physical limitations imposed by lipedema. Additionally, exercise aims to support weight management, which can mitigate the progression of lipedema symptoms and reduce the risk of comorbid conditions. Adapting exercise to individual needs and abilities is critical; what is beneficial for one patient may not be suitable for another, given the variability in lipedema stages, the presence of coexisting conditions, and differing physical capabilities. A personalized exercise program, ideally developed in collaboration with healthcare professionals specialized in lipedema, might include a combination of low-impact aerobic activities, strength training, and flexibility exercises. Careful consideration of the patient's pain levels, fatigue, and potential mobility issues is essential in tailoring the exercise regimen, ensuring that it not only addresses the specific needs of the individual but also fosters long-term engagement and adherence. By prioritizing safe exercise practices and adapting programs to meet the unique needs of each patient, individuals with lipedema can maximize the health benefits of physical activity while navigating the challenges of their condition.

In the management of lipedema, a condition characterized by the pathological accumulation of fat in the lower extremities, incorporating a variety of beneficial exercises is paramount for alleviating symptoms and enhancing overall well-being. Low-impact cardiovascular exercises, such as walking, cycling, and using an elliptical trainer, are highly recommended for promoting lymphatic drainage and improving cardiovascular health without placing excessive stress on the joints. Strength training and muscle toning exercises, when performed with careful consideration to avoid overexertion, can help in building lean muscle mass, boosting metabolism, and supporting the structural integrity of the limbs. Flexibility and stretching exercises are crucial for maintaining joint mobility and preventing the stiffness and reduced range of motion often associated with lipedema. Aquatic therapy and water-based exercises emerge as particularly advantageous due to the buoyancy of water, which reduces the gravitational pull on the body, thereby minimizing pain and pressure on the limbs while enhancing lymphatic flow. The resistance offered by water also aids in strengthening muscles and improving endurance. Tailoring these exercise modalities to individual needs and abilities, while ensuring they are performed under the guidance of professionals experienced in lipedema management, can significantly contribute to the effective control of lipedema symptoms, promote physical and mental health, and improve patients' quality of life.

Tailoring exercise to accommodate the varying stages of lipedema is essential for ensuring both the efficacy and safety of physical activity for individuals affected by this condition. In the early stages of patients with lipedema typically have fewer physical limitations, allowing for a broader range of exercise options. During this phase, a combination of low-impact cardiovascular exercises, strength training, and flexibility routines can be highly beneficial. These activities help in maintaining a healthy weight, improving blood flow, and enhancing lymphatic drainage, potentially slowing the progression of lipedema. As the condition advances to more severe stages, exercise adjustments become necessary to accommodate increased sensitivity, pain, and mobility restrictions. The focus may shift more toward gentle, low-impact exercises such as swimming or water aerobics, which reduce stress on the joints and provide natural compression through water resistance. Aquatic therapy is particularly advantageous for individuals with advanced lipedema, offering a means to exercise effectively while minimizing discomfort.

For those with severe lipedema, special considerations include closely monitoring intensity levels and incorporating rest periods to prevent overexertion. Exercises may need to be performed under the guidance of a physical therapist specialized in lymphatic disorders, ensuring that movements are performed correctly and safely. The goal remains to enhance mobility, reduce symptoms, and improve overall well-being, but with a heightened awareness of the patient's limitations and potential risks. This personalized approach to exercise, adapted to the individual's stage of lipedema and unique needs, underscores the importance of a careful, informed strategy in managing this complex condition, emphasizing that physical activity remains a cornerstone of effective lipedema management across all stages.

Integrating exercise with compression therapy represents a synergistic approach in the management of lipedema, leveraging the combined benefits of both strategies to optimize patient outcomes. The application of compression garments during exercise enhances the effectiveness of physical activity by improving venous return and lymphatic flow, reducing the risk of swelling, and potentially mitigating the accumulation of lipedematous fat. This combination not only aids in alleviating the symptoms associated with lipedema but also contributes to increased exercise efficiency, enabling patients to engage in physical activities with reduced discomfort and improved mobility.

Guidelines for wearing compression during exercise recommend the use of well-fitted garments that provide adequate pressure without restricting movement or blood flow. The selection of appropriate compression levels should be individualized, taking into account the severity of lipedema, the specific type of exercise being performed, and the patient's comfort and tolerance. Practical examples and case studies have underscored the value of this integrated approach. For instance, patients who participated in regular low-impact cardiovascular exercises while wearing compression garments reported not only a decrease in limb volume and pain but also an enhanced sense of well-being and increased ability to perform daily activities.

This evidence highlights the importance of a comprehensive treatment plan that includes both exercise and compression therapy. By combining these modalities, patients with lipedema can achieve greater symptom relief and a higher quality of life, underscoring the need for healthcare providers to advocate for and guide the implementation of these combined strategies in the management of lipedema.

Pain management is a critical aspect of facilitating physical activity in individuals experiencing pain, particularly in conditions such as lipedema where pain and sensitivity are prevalent. Developing strategies for managing pain during exercise involves a multifaceted approach, including modifying exercises to ensure they are low-impact and do not exacerbate pain or sensitivity. For instance, aquatic exercises can be particularly beneficial as the buoyancy of water reduces stress on painful joints and tissues while still providing resistance for strength and cardiovascular fitness. Additionally, the incorporation of gradual warm-ups and cool-downs can help prepare the body for physical activity and reduce postexercise discomfort.

The importance of ongoing pain assessment and monitoring cannot be overstated. Individuals are encouraged to maintain an open dialogue with healthcare providers about their pain levels and any discomfort experienced during or after physical activity. This continuous feedback loop allows for the adjustment of exercise regimens in real time, ensuring that activities remain within a therapeutic range that promotes health benefits without causing harm. Furthermore, understanding personal pain thresholds and employing pain relief techniques such as controlled breathing, mindfulness, and the use of compression garments during exercise can enhance pain management. These strategies not only facilitate participation in physical activity despite the presence of pain but also empower individuals to take an active role in managing their condition and improving their quality of life.

Lymphatic considerations play a crucial role in tailoring exercise programs for individuals with conditions affecting lymphatic flow, such as lipedema. Exercises that enhance lymphatic drainage are pivotal, as they can significantly impact the management and progression of such conditions. Low-impact cardiovascular exercises, including walking, swimming, and cycling, are particularly beneficial as they encourage the movement of lymph fluid without overburdening the lymphatic system. The rhythmic contraction of muscles during these activities acts as a pump, facilitating lymphatic flow and reducing the risk of lymph accumulation and subsequent swelling. Understanding the impact of physical activity on the lymphatic system is essential; it requires a delicate balance to ensure that exercise intensity does not exacerbate lymphatic overload, which could worsen symptoms. Balancing exercise intensity with lymphatic health involves starting with low-impact activities and gradually increasing intensity based on individual tolerance, ensuring regular intervals of rest and recovery. Incorporating manual lymphatic drainage (MLD) techniques before or after exercise can also support lymphatic function, optimizing the benefits of physical activity while minimizing potential adverse effects. This comprehensive approach underscores the importance of a well-considered exercise regimen that acknowledges the specific needs and limitations imposed by lymphatic health considerations, thereby ensuring that exercise serves as an effective adjunct therapy in the management of lymphatic-related conditions.

Overcoming barriers to exercise, particularly in the context of chronic conditions like lipedema, requires a multifaceted approach that addresses both psychological and physical challenges. Common psychological barriers include lack of motivation, fear of injury, and self-consciousness about exercising in public spaces. Addressing these concerns involves providing education on the benefits of exercise, setting realistic goals, and fostering a supportive community or finding a workout buddy to enhance accountability and encouragement. For individuals facing physical and mobility challenges, solutions may involve adapting exercises to meet their specific needs, such as incorporating seated or water-based exercises that reduce strain on the joints while still promoting lymphatic flow and cardiovascular health. Accessibility to tailored exercise programs can be improved through the guidance of physical therapists or fitness professionals experienced in working with patients with lipedema. Building a sustainable exercise routine is crucial; this includes identifying activities that the individual enjoys, gradually increasing the intensity and duration of workouts to prevent burnout, and incorporating variety to maintain engagement. Establishing a routine that is flexible, enjoyable, and adapted to the individual's capabilities can significantly reduce the barriers to regular physical activity, facilitating long-term adherence and contributing positively to the management of lipedema and overall well-being.

Developing an individualized exercise plan necessitates a holistic approach that begins with an assessment of fitness levels and the setting of realistic, attainable goals. This initial evaluation should consider the individual's current physical condition, medical history, and specific challenges or limitations, providing a foundation upon which a tailored exercise regimen can be built. Collaboration with healthcare professionals, including physicians, physical therapists, and exercise physiologists, is essential in ensuring the exercise plan is not only effective but also safe, especially for individuals with conditions such as lipedema. These professionals can offer expert guidance on the types of exercises that will best support the individual's health goals while minimizing the risk of injury or exacerbation of symptoms. Monitoring progress is a critical component of the individualized exercise plan, involving regular assessments to track improvements in fitness, adjustments to the intensity and type of exercises as the individual progresses, and the integration of new goals to keep the regimen challenging and engaging. Adjusting the plan based on feedback and ongoing assessments ensures that the exercise program remains aligned with the individual's evolving needs and preferences, thereby maximizing adherence and facilitating long-term health benefits. This dynamic, personalized approach underscores the importance of a thoughtful and informed strategy in developing an exercise plan, ensuring it supports the individual's health journey in a meaningful and sustainable way.

Nutrition and hydration play roles in optimizing exercise performance for individuals with lipedema, necessitating tailored dietary considerations to support physical activity and overall health. A balanced diet rich in anti-inflammatory foods, such as fruits, vegetables, whole grains, and lean proteins, can help manage inflammation associated with lipedema and provide the necessary nutrients for muscle recovery and energy during exercise. Carbohydrates are particularly important for fueling exercise, while adequate protein intake supports muscle repair and growth. Given the propensity for water retention in lipedema, managing sodium intake is also crucial to prevent exacerbating swelling.

Hydration is another critical aspect, as adequate fluid intake is essential for maintaining optimal lymphatic function and preventing dehydration, which can thicken the lymph fluid and hinder its flow. Individuals should ensure they are well-hydrated before starting exercise, consume water or electrolyte-replenishing fluids during physical activity to replace fluids lost through sweat, and continue hydrating after exercise to aid in recovery and lymphatic drainage. Monitoring urine color can be a practical guide for hydration status, aiming for a pale straw color as an indicator of proper hydration. By integrating these nutritional and hydration strategies, individuals with lipedema can enhance their exercise performance, support their body's lymphatic and circulatory systems, and contribute positively to their overall management of lipedema.

The role of exercise in the management of lipedema is pivotal, providing long-term benefits that significantly contribute to the overall health and quality of life for those affected by this condition. Regular physical activity, tailored to the individual's capabilities and stages of lipedema, offers a multitude of advantages, including improved lymphatic drainage, enhanced cardiovascular health, and increased muscle strength and flexibility. These benefits facilitate the reduction of lipedema symptoms such as pain, swelling, and mobility issues. Moreover, exercise plays a critical role in weight management, helping to prevent additional stress on the lymphatic system and potentially slowing the progression of lipedema. Beyond the physical improvements, engaging in regular exercise promotes psychological well-being, reducing the risk of depression and anxiety, and improving self-esteem and body image.

The integration of exercise into lipedema management requires a thoughtful approach, beginning with an assessment of fitness levels, setting realistic goals, and potentially collaborating with healthcare professionals to ensure the safety and effectiveness of the exercise regimen. By emphasizing the long-term benefits of physical activity, individuals with lipedema can empower themselves to manage their condition proactively, enhancing their ability to lead active, fulfilling lives.

Suggested Reading

Földi M, Foldi E, Strossenreuther RHK, Kubik S. *Földi's Textbook of Lymphology for Physicians and Lymphedema Therapists*, 2nd ed. Trento, Italy: Urban & Fischer; 2006

Torre YS, Wadeea R, Rosas V, Herbst KL. Lipedema: Friend and foe. *Horm Mol Biol Clin Investig* 2018; 33(1). https://doi.org/10.1515/hmbci-2017-0076

Herbst KL, Kahn LA, Iker E, et al. Standard of care for lipedema in the United States. Phlebology 2021

Wold LE, Hines EA Jr., Allen EV. Lipedema of the legs; a syndrome characterized by fat legs and edema. *Ann Intern Med* 1951; 34:1243–1250

Crescenzi R, Donahue PMC, Petersen KJ, et al.. Upper and lower extremity measurement of tissue sodium and fat content in patients with lipedema. *Obesity (Silver Spring)* 2020; 28:907–915
Petersen KJ, Garza M, Donahue PMC, et al.. Neuroimaging of cerebral blood flow and sodium in women with lipedema. *Obesity (Silver Spring)* 2020; 28:1292–1300
Buck DW, 2nd, Herbst KL. Lipedema: A relatively common disease with extremely common misconceptions. *Plast Reconstr Surg Glob Open* 2016; 4:e1043
Kruglikov IL, Joffin N, Scherer PE. The MMP14-caveolin axis and its potential relevance for lipoedema. *Nat Rev Endocrinol* 2020; 16:669–674
Dudek JE, Bialaszek W, Ostaszewski P. Quality of life in women with lipoedema: A contextual behavioral approach. *Qual Life Res* 2016; 25:401–408
Buso G, Depairon M, Tomson D, Raffoul W, Vettor R, Mazzolai L. Lipedema: A call to action! Obesity (Silver Spring) 2019; 27:1567–1576
Fetzer A, Fetzer S. Lipoedema UK Big Survey 2014 Research Report. Lipoedema UK, 2016
Reich-Schupke S, Schmeller W, Brauer WJ, et al.. S1 guidelines: Lipedema. *J Dtsch Dermatol Ges* 2017; 15:758–767
Warren Peled A, Kappos EA. Lipedema: Diagnostic and management challenges. *Int J Womens Health* 2016; 8:389–395
Szolnoky G, Varga E, Varga M, Tuczai M, Dosa-Racz E, Kemeny L. Lymphedema treatment decreases pain intensity in lipedema. *Lymphology* 2011; 44:178–182
Szolnoky G, Ifeoluwa A, Tuczai M, et al.. Measurement of capillary fragility: A useful tool to differentiate lipedema from obesity? *Lymphology* 2017; 50:203–209
Allen EV, Hines EA. Lipedema of the legs: A syndrome characterized by fat legs and orthostatic edema. *Proc Staff Mayo Clinic* 1940; 15:184–187
Beltran K, Herbst KL. Differentiating lipedema and Dercum's disease. *Int J Obes (Lond)* 2017; 41:240–245
van Esch-Smeenge J, Damstra, RJ, Hendrickx, AS. Muscle strength and functional exercise capacity in patients with lipoedema and obesity: A comparative study. *J Lymphoedema* 2017; 12:27–31
Kruppa P, Georgiou I, Biermann N, Prantl L, Klein-Weigel P, Ghods M. Lipedema-pathogenesis, diagnosis, and treatment options. *Dtsch Arztebl Int* 2020; 117:396–403
Langendoen SI, Habbema L, Nijsten TE, Neumann HA. Lipoedema: From clinical presentation to therapy. A review of the literature. *Br J Dermatol* 2009; 161:980–986
Tzani I, Tsichlaki M, Zerva E, Papathanasiou G, Dimakakos E. Physiotherapeutic rehabilitation of lymphedema: State-of-the-art. *Lymphology* 2018; 51:1–12
Cho Y, Do J, Jung S, Kwon O, Jeon JY. Effects of a physical therapy program combined with manual lymphatic drainage on shoulder function, quality of life, lymphedema incidence, and pain in breast cancer patients with axillary web syndrome following axillary dissection. *Support Care Cancer* 2016; 24:2047–2057
Shah C, Arthur DW, Wazer D, Khan A, Ridner S, Vicini F. The impact of early detection and intervention of breast cancer-related lymphedema: A systematic review. *Cancer Med* 2016; 5:1154–1162
Bertsch T, Erbacher G, Elwell R. Lipoedema: A paradigm shift and consensus. *J Wound Care* 2020; 29:1–51
Esmer M, Schingale FJ, Unal D, Yazıcı MV, Güzel NA. Physiotherapy and rehabilitation applications in lipedema management: A literature review. *Lymphology* 2020; 53:88–95
Crescenzi R, Marton A, Donahue PMC, et al.. Tissue sodium content is elevated in the skin and subcutaneous adipose tissue in women with lipedema. *Obesity (Silver Spring)* 2018; 26:310–317
Executive Committee. The diagnosis and treatment of peripheral lymphedema: 2016 Consensus document of the International Society of Lymphology. *Lymphology* 2016; 49:170–184
Executive Committee of the International Society of Lymphology. The diagnosis and treatment of peripheral lymphedema: 2020 Consensus Document of the International Society of Lymphology. *Lymphology* 2020; 53:3–19

Stratford P, Gill C, Westaway M, Binkley J. Assessing disability and change on individual patients: A report of a patient specific measure. *Physiotherapy Canada* 1995; 47:258–263
Abbott JH, Schmitt J. Minimum important differences for the patient-specific functional scale, 4 region-specific outcome measures, and the numeric pain rating scale. *J Orthop Sports Phys Ther* 2014; 44:560–564
Hays RD, Morales LS. The RAND-36 measure of health-related quality of life. *Ann Med* 2001; 33:350–357
Kopp C, Linz P, Wachsmuth L, et al.. (23)Na magnetic resonance imaging of tissue sodium. *Hypertension* 2012; 59:167–172
Cohen J. A power primer. *Psychol Bull* 1992; 112:155–159
Ahmed E. Endermologie technique versus decongestive lymphatic therapy on post-mastectomy related lymphedema. *J Nov Physiother* 2013; 3:155
Herbst KL, Ussery C, Eekema A. Pilot study: Whole body manual subcutaneous adipose tissue (SAT) therapy improved pain and SAT structure in women with lipedema. *Horm Mol Biol Clin Investig* 2017; 33
Volkan-Yazıcı M, Yazici G, Esmer M. The effects of complex decongestive physiotherapy applications on lower extremity circumference and volume in patients with lipedema. *Lymphat Res Biol* 2021; 19:111–114
Schneider R. Low-frequency vibrotherapy considerably improves the effectiveness of manual lymphatic drainage (MLD) in patients with lipedema: A two-armed, randomized, controlled pragmatic trial *Physiother Theory Pract* 2020; 36:63–70
Machnik A, Dahlmann A, Kopp C, et al.. Mononuclear phagocyte system depletion blocks interstitial tonicity-responsive enhancer binding protein/vascular endothelial growth factor C expression and induces salt-sensitive hypertension in rats. *Hypertension* 2010; 55:755–761
Machnik A, Neuhofer W, Jantsch J, et al.. Macrophages regulate salt-dependent volume and blood pressure by a vascular endothelial growth factor-C-dependent buffering mechanism. *Nat Med* 2009; 15:545–552
Gould DJ, El-Sabawi B, Goel P, Badash I, Colletti P, Patel KM. Uncovering lymphatic transport abnormalities in patients with primary lipedema. *J Reconstr Microsurg* 2020; 36:136–141
Bilancini S, Lucchi M, Tucci S, Eleuteri P. Functional lymphatic alterations in patients suffering from lipedema. *Angiology* 1995; 46:333–339
Lohrmann C, Foeldi E, Langer M. MR imaging of the lymphatic system in patients with lipedema and lipo-lymphedema. *Microvasc Res* 2009; 77:335–339
Farrow W. Phlebolymphedema—A common underdiagnosed and undertreated problem in the wound care clinic. *J Am Col Certif Wound Spec* 2010; 2:14–23
Rasmussen JC, Zhu B, Morrow JR, et al.. Degradation of lymphatic anatomy and function in early venous insufficiency. *J Vasc Surg Venous Lymphat Disord* 2021; 9:720 730

Mental Health

The mental health impact of lipedema extends beyond the physical symptoms of the condition, deeply affecting patients' emotional and psychological well-being. Patients with lipedema are at an increased risk of developing psychological disorders such as anxiety and depression, a vulnerability that can be exacerbated by underlying difficulties in emotion regulation (ER). For instance, Al-Wardat et al. (2022) found in their international survey of 1358 patients with lipedema that 28% reported emotional lability, indicating a significant prevalence of rapid and exaggerated mood changes among those afflicted. This emotional instability suggests that a considerable number of individuals with lipedema struggle with ER, which involves controlling emotional experiences and expressions, as well as the ability to process a full spectrum of emotions adaptively. The challenges faced by patients with lipedema, including accessing adequate healthcare, coping with unmanageable changes in body appearance, and dealing with weight stigma and social isolation, can lead to or exacerbate these ER difficulties.

As ER is crucial for modulating the intensity of emotions and preventing the escalation of negative emotional states, the high incidence of emotional lability among patients with lipedema highlights the need for targeted interventions focusing on enhancing ER skills to mitigate the mental health burden associated with the condition.

Patients with lipedema endure considerable psychological strain, which varies according to the condition's progression. Around 40% of patients have reported feelings of depression, and 16% have identified struggles with eating disorders. These figures align with studies employing validated measures that have identified a depression prevalence rate of 31–59% among patients with lipedema and an 18% incidence of eating disorders. Notably, those in the more advanced stages of lipedema, stages 3 and 4, are more prone to suffer from depression and eating disorders compared to individuals in the initial stages, 1 and 2. This corroborates findings that the exacerbation of lipedema symptoms correlates with an increase in depression severity and a greater frequency of depression and eating disorders among individuals with a body mass index (BMI) of 40 or above. The research

G. Laur, *Lipoedema*, https://doi.org/10.1007/978-981-96-8939-2_22

further revealed that patients with lipedema often deal with emotional disturbances such as hypersensitivity, persistent thoughts about their condition, feelings of worthlessness, solitude, self-imposed isolation, emotional outbursts, irritability, and anxiety, which they attribute to their condition. Such emotional turmoil suggests a heightened self-focus and a sense of inferiority among lipedema sufferers, potentially stemming from shame and the fear of societal judgment, leading to withdrawal and a sense of isolation.

Moreover, individuals in the latter stages of lipedema, specifically stages 3 and 4, reported more significant social difficulties, including increased feelings of anxiety, loneliness, and a tendency to isolate themselves more than those in earlier stages, supporting existing research on lipedema's impact on social engagement. This enhanced social difficulty in later stages may be attributed to a greater likelihood of encountering weight stigma. For instance, qualitative studies involving women with stage 3 lipedema revealed frequent encounters with weight stigma and discrimination, which adversely affected their self-esteem and social interactions, promoting a withdrawal from social and professional settings. These findings underscore the profound impact of social disconnection on mental health, emphasizing the critical need for holistic support that addresses the physical, social, and emotional challenges faced by individuals with lipedema, alongside encouraging proactive support-seeking behavior.

The body image of patients with lipedema is significantly impacted by the condition, reflecting a complex interplay between physical manifestations and psychological responses. Lipedema, characterized by an abnormal accumulation of fat in the lower body, often leads to a disproportionate body shape that diverges from societal norms of attractiveness and health. This divergence can profoundly affect self-perception and self-esteem, leading to body dissatisfaction and negative body image. Research indicates that the visible and palpable aspects of lipedema—such as limb size asymmetry, pain, and tenderness—not only contribute to physical discomfort but also to psychological distress, manifesting as shame, embarrassment, and a decreased sense of personal worth. The stigma associated with obesity, often erroneously applied to lipedema due to its appearance, exacerbates these feelings, further entrenching negative body image. Furthermore, the progressive nature of lipedema and its resistance to conventional weight loss strategies can lead to feelings of helplessness and frustration, undermining efforts toward positive body image.

Studies suggest that these challenges are pervasive among patients with lipedema, necessitating a holistic approach to treatment that addresses both physical symptoms and the psychological need for body image rehabilitation. The establishment of support networks, psychoeducation, and counseling is critical in helping patients navigate the complexities of body image associated with lipedema, promoting a healthier self-image and overall well-being.

The prevalence of eating disorders among patients with lipedema underscores a critical aspect of the condition's psychological impact, meriting thorough investigation within the medical and psychological fields. Lipedema, a chronic condition characterized by abnormal fat accumulation primarily in the lower extremities, not only presents significant physical challenges but also contributes to complex psychosocial stressors, including issues related to body image and self-esteem. This intricate relationship can predispose individuals to disordered eating behaviors as patients may resort to restrictive diets or other unhealthy eating patterns in an often futile attempt to manage or mitigate the progression of their condition. The misunderstanding and misattribution of lipedema symptoms to obesity-related issues further compound the risk, as patients experience increased pressure to conform to societal standards of body size and shape, despite the ineffectiveness of conventional weight loss methods on lipedema fat. Research indicates a notable incidence of eating disorders in this patient population, suggesting a bidirectional link where the psychological burden of living with lipedema can lead to the development of eating disorders, while the presence of such disorders can exacerbate the emotional distress caused by lipedema. Addressing eating disorders in patients with lipedema requires a multidisciplinary approach that encompasses not only medical management of lipedema but also psychological support and interventions aimed at treating the eating disorder and improving body image and self-acceptance. This holistic approach is vital for the effective care and support of patients with lipedema, highlighting the need for increased awareness and understanding of the unique challenges faced by this population.

Diagnosing and treating mental health conditions in the context of lipedema involves navigating a complex interplay of physiological, psychological, and social factors, requiring a nuanced and multidisciplinary approach. Lipedema, characterized by the pathological accumulation of fat in the lower extremities and often accompanied by pain and mobility issues, presents unique challenges in mental health management. The condition's physical manifestations can significantly impact patients' quality of life, leading to psychological distress, body image disturbances, and social isolation. These factors contribute to a heightened risk of developing mental health conditions, including depression, anxiety, and eating disorders. However, the overlapping symptoms of psychological distress and lipedema, such as fatigue and decreased activity levels, may complicate the diagnostic process, potentially leading to misdiagnosis or underdiagnosis of mental health issues. Furthermore, the stigma associated with both lipedema and mental health conditions can deter individuals from seeking help, exacerbating their psychological and physical suffering. Treatment approaches must therefore be comprehensive, integrating physical management strategies for lipedema with psychological support. This includes educating healthcare providers about the psychological aspects of lipedema to ensure accurate diagnosis and treatment, as well as offering patients access to mental health professionals skilled in addressing the unique challenges posed by chronic physical health conditions. Additionally, fostering a supportive community and advocating for increased awareness can mitigate stigma and encourage engagement with both physical and mental health services.

Ultimately, recognizing the interconnectedness of physical and psychological health is paramount in the effective care of individuals with lipedema, underscoring the importance of a holistic, patient-centered approach in treatment planning.

Effective management of mental health in individuals with lipedema necessitates a comprehensive and empathetic approach, incorporating a range of therapy options and support systems tailored to address the multifaceted nature of the condition. Cognitive-behavioral therapy (CBT) stands out as an intervention, offering strategies to modify negative thought patterns and behaviors associated with body image distress, depression, and anxiety, thereby improving coping mechanisms and enhancing quality of life. Furthermore, mindfulness-based stress reduction (MBSR) and acceptance and commitment therapy (ACT) can be instrumental in fostering a more compassionate self-relationship and acceptance, crucial for individuals grappling with the chronic and visible symptoms of lipedema. Beyond individual therapy, group therapy and support groups provide invaluable platforms for sharing experiences and strategies, reducing feelings of isolation by connecting with others facing similar challenges. These settings not only facilitate emotional support but also promote the exchange of practical advice on navigating the healthcare system, advocating for oneself, and managing lipedema's physical aspects. Additionally, integrating physical health management with psychological support, such as physiotherapy and nutritional counseling, in a multidisciplinary team approach ensures that treatment plans are holistic and patient-centered. The role of online communities and resources should also be acknowledged, offering accessible avenues for support and information. Ultimately, effective management of mental health in patients with lipedema requires a personalized, multifaceted strategy that addresses both the psychological and physical dimensions of the condition, underscoring the importance of integrated care pathways and the empowerment of individuals through education and community support.

The role of healthcare professionals in addressing mental health issues in patients with lipedema is pivotal, demanding a holistic and informed approach that transcends the traditional focus on physical symptoms alone. Given the significant psychological impact of lipedema, including body image disturbances, depression, anxiety, and social isolation, healthcare providers must adopt a multifaceted strategy that incorporates mental health screening, referral, and management as integral components of lipedema care. Early identification of mental health conditions through routine screening can facilitate timely interventions, enhancing patient outcomes. Primary care physicians, dermatologists, and specialists in lymphatic disorders play critical roles in recognizing the psychological burdens of lipedema and should be prepared to refer patients to mental health professionals, including psychologists and psychiatrists, for specialized care. Additionally, the incorporation of interdisciplinary teams, comprising physical therapists, dietitians, and occupational therapists, can offer comprehensive support, addressing both the physical and emotional aspects of the condition. Education and ongoing communication between healthcare professionals and patients about the nature of lipedema, its treatment options, and its impact on mental health are essential for reducing stigma and empowering patients. Furthermore, healthcare professionals should advocate for and facilitate access to support groups and community resources, fostering a network of support that encourages patients to share experiences and coping strategies.

Ultimately, the role of healthcare professionals in managing lipedema extends beyond physical treatment to include advocating for holistic care that recognizes and addresses the complex mental health needs of this patient population.

In conclusion, the comprehensive management of lipedema necessitates a holistic care approach that equally prioritizes the physical and mental health needs of individuals afflicted by this complex condition. Lipedema, characterized by the disproportionate accumulation of fat in the lower extremities and often accompanied by pain, mobility issues, and a distinct set of psychological challenges, requires a multifaceted treatment strategy. This strategy should encompass not only medical interventions aimed at alleviating the physical symptoms but also psychological support mechanisms to address the mental health concerns that frequently co-occur. The integration of cognitive-behavioral therapy, mindfulness practices, and support groups into the treatment plan has been underscored as essential for managing the psychological impact, including body image disturbances, depression, anxiety, and social isolation, experienced by many individuals with lipedema.

Healthcare professionals play a crucial role in the delivery of holistic care, necessitating an informed, empathetic, and coordinated approach to both diagnose and treat lipedema effectively. The early screening for mental health issues, interdisciplinary collaboration, and patient education about lipedema are critical components of comprehensive care. Furthermore, fostering a supportive community, both online and in-person, can significantly mitigate the feelings of isolation and stigma that often accompany this condition.

The importance of holistic care in the management of lipedema cannot be overstated. It not only addresses the immediate physical and psychological symptoms but also contributes to the long-term well-being and quality of life of individuals living with lipedema. This approach underscores the need for ongoing research, increased awareness, and improved healthcare practices to support the multifaceted needs of this population. In embracing holistic care, healthcare providers, patients, and the wider community can work together toward a more understanding, effective, and compassionate approach to lipedema management, ensuring that individuals receive the comprehensive support they require to navigate the complexities of this condition.

Suggested Reading

Kruppa P, Georgiou I, Biermann N, Prantl L, Klein-Weigel P, Ghods M. Lipedema-pathogenesis, diagnosis, and treatment options. *Deutsches Arzteblatt International.* 2020;117(22–23):396–403. https://doi.org/10.3238/arztebl.2020.0396

Herbst KL, Kahn LA, Iker E, Ehrlich C, Wright T, McHutchison L, Schwartz J, Sleigh M, Donahue PM, Lisson KH, Faris T, Miller J, Lontok E, Schwartz MS, Dean SM, Bartholomew JR, Armur P, Correa-Perez M, Pennings N, Wallace EL, Larson E. Standard of care for lipedema in the United States. *Phlebology.* 2021 https://doi.org/10.1177/02683555211015887

Forner-Cordero I, Szolnoky G, Forner-Cordero A, Kemény L. Lipedema: An overview of its clinical manifestations, diagnosis and treatment of the disproportional fatty deposition syndrome – systematic review. *Clinical Obesity.* 2012;2(3–4):86–95. https://doi.org/10.1111/j.1758-8111.2012.00045.x

Herbst, K. L., Mirkovskaya, L., Bharhagava, A., Chava, Y., & Te, C. H. T. (2015). Lipedema fat and signs and symptoms of illness, increasing with advancing stage. *Archives of Medicine*, 7(4):

10. https://www.archivesofmedicine.com/medicine/lipedema-fat-and-signs-and-symptoms-of-illness-increase-with-advancing-stage.php?aid=6744

Wounds UK. *Best Practice Guidelines: The Management of Lipoedema.* London: Wounds UK; 2017

Fetzer, A., & Fetzer, S. (2016). *Lipoedema UK big survey 2014 research report.* Lipoedema UK. Retrieved August 14, 2022, from https://www.lipoedema.co.uk/wp-content/uploads/2016/04/UK-Big-Surey-version-web.pdf.

Kinavey H, Cool C. The broken lens: How anti-fat bias in psychotherapy is harming our clients and what to do about it. *Women & Therapy.* 2019;42(1–2):116–130. https://doi.org/10.1080/02703149.2018.1524070

Romejin JRM, de Rooij MJM, Janssen L, Martens H. Exploration of patient characteristics and quality of life in patients with lipoedema using a survey. *Dermatology and Therapy.* 2018;8:303–311. https://doi.org/10.1007/s13555-018-0241-6

Fetzer A, Wise C. Living with lipoedema: Reviewing different self-management techniques. *British Journal of Community Nursing.* 2015;20(Sup10):S14–S19. https://doi.org/10.12968/bjcn.2015.20.Sup10.S14

Macdonald JM, Sims N, Mayrovitz HN. Lymphoedema, lipoedema and the open wound: The role of compression therapy. *Surgical Clinics of North America.* 2003;83:639–658. https://doi.org/10.1016/S0039-6109(02)00201-3

Fetzer A. Women in dire need: The far-reaching impact of lipoedema on women's lives. *British Journal of Community Nursing.* 2020;25(Sup4):S6–S9. https://doi.org/10.12968/bjcn.2020.25

Fetzer, S., & Warrilow, M. (2021). Living with lipoedema: Liposuction and other treatments [Poster]. British Lymphology Society Conference 2021 (BLS2021), Online.

Frambach Y, Baumgartner A, Schmeller W, Hanse-Klinik L. Lipödem und Lebensqualität. *Vasomed.* 2015;27(5):248–249

Alwardat N, Di Renzo L, Alwardat M, Romano L, De Santis G, Gualtieri P, Carrano E, Nocerino P, De Lorenzo A. The effect of lipedema on health-related quality of life and psychological status: A narrative review of the literature. *Eating and Weight Disorders.* 2020;25(4):851–856

Dudek, J., (2017) *Quality of life and psychological functioning of patients 13* [Conference session]. Fat Disorders Research Society, Lipedema & Dercum's Disease: Goals for the Future and Tools for Today, Salt Lake City, UT, Retrieved August 14, 2022, from https://www.youtube.com/watch?v=xV-IVc0eVQM

Dudek J, Białaszek W, Gabriel M. Quality of life, its factors, and sociodemographic characteristics of Polish women with lipedema. *BMC Women's Health.* 2021;21(1):27. https://doi.org/10.1186/s12905-021-01174-y

Erbacher G, Bertsch T. Lipoedema and pain: What is the role of the psyche?—Results of a pilot study with 150 patients with lipoedema. *Phlébologie.* 2020;49:305–316. https://doi.org/10.1055/a-1238-6657

Stutz, J. (2015). *Lipedema can be life-threatening: Increased rates of suicide attempts, depression, and eating disorders among women with lipedema.* [Conference session]. 25th World Congress of Lymphology, San Francisco, California, Retrieved August 14, 2022, from https://www.lymfologi.se/anvandarbilder/221/files/Program%20book%20Final%20Sent%20for%20publication%2026Aug15.pdf

Reich-Schupke S, Schmeller W, Justus Brauer W, Cornely ME, Faerber G, Ludwig M, Lulay G, Miller A, Rapprich S, Richter DF, Schacht V, Schrader K, Stücker M, Ure C. S1 guidelines: Lipedema. *Journal of the German Society for Dermatology.* 2015;15(7):758–767. https://doi.org/10.1111/ddg.13036

Baumgartner A, Hueppe M, Schmeller W. Long-term benefit of liposuction in patients with lipoedema: A follow-up study after an average of 4 and 8 years. *British Journal of Dermatology.* 2016;174(5):1061–1067. https://doi.org/10.1111/bjd.14289

Dadras M, Mallinger P, Corterier C, Theodosiadi S, Ghods M. Liposuction in the treatment of lipedema: A longitudinal study. *Archives of Plastic Surgery.* 2017;44(4):324–331. https://doi.org/10.5999/aps.2017.44.4.324

Rapprich S, Baum S, Kaak I, Kottmann T, Podda M. Treatment of lipoedema using liposuction. *Results of our own surveys. Phlebologie.* 2015;44(3):121–132. https://doi.org/10.12687/phleb2265-3-2015

Lawrence B, Kerr D, Pollard C, Theophilus M, Alexander E, Haywood D, O'Connor M. Weight bias among health professionals: A systematic review and meta-analysis. *Obesity.* 2021;29:1082–1812. https://doi.org/10.1002/oby.23266

Phelan S, Burgess D, Yeazel M, Hellerstedt W, Griffin J, Van Ryn M. Impact of weight bias and stigma on quality of care and outcomes for patients with obesity. *Obesity Reviews.* 2015;16(4):319–326. https://doi.org/10.1111/obr.12266

World Health Organization. Regional Office for Europe. (2017). *Weight bias and obesity stigma: Considerations for the WHO European region.* World Health Organization. Regional Office for Europe. Retrieved August 14, 2022, from https://apps.who.int/iris/handle/10665/353613

Bidstrup H, Brennan L, de la Kaufmann L, Piedad Garcia X. Internalised weight stigma as a mediator of the relationship between experienced/perceived weight stigma and biopsychosocial outcomes: A systematic review. *International Journal of Obesity.* 2021 https://doi.org/10.1038/s41366-021-00982-4

Carter A, Gilbert P, Kirby J. Compassion-focused therapy for body weight shame: A mixed methods pilot trial. *Clinical Psychology and Psychotherapy.* 2021;28(1):93–108. https://doi.org/10.1002/cpp.2488

Fetzer, S., & Fetzer, A. (2019). *Women in dire need denied surgery and treatments: Preview results of 2019 Lipoedema UK survey report.* Lipoedema UK. Retrieved August 14, 2022, from https://www.lipoedema.co.uk/wp-content/uploads/2019/02/lipoedema-A4-2019-surgery.pdf

Al-Wardat, M.; Clarke, C.; Alwardat, N.; Kassab, M.; Salimei, C.; Gualtieri, P.; Marchetti, M.; Best, T.; Di Renzo, L. The Difficulties in Emotional Regulation among a Cohort of Females with Lipedema. Int. J. Environ. Res. Public Health 2022, 19, 13679. https://doi.org/10.3390/ijerph192013679

Shockwave and Cavitation Ultrasound

Cavitation ultrasound treatment is a noninvasive cosmetic procedure that is sometimes promoted as a way to reduce the appearance of lipedema. However, there is limited scientific evidence to support its effectiveness for treating lipedema.

Cavitation ultrasound uses high-frequency sound waves to break down fat cells. The procedure is typically performed by a licensed professional using a handheld device that emits the sound waves. The sound waves create pressure changes in the fat cells, causing them to break apart and be eliminated from the body.

While cavitation ultrasound may temporarily reduce the appearance of lipedema, it does not address the underlying cause of the condition. In fact, some experts caution against using any type of liposuction or fat-reducing procedure for lipedema, as it can worsen the condition and cause additional swelling and discomfort.

Instead, conservative management strategies such as compression therapy, exercise, and manual lymphatic drainage are typically recommended as the first line of treatment for lipedema. These treatments can help to reduce swelling, improve lymphatic flow, and increase mobility and quality of life for people with lipedema. It is important to consult with a healthcare provider before trying any new treatments or procedures for lipedema.

Shockwave therapy, also known as extracorporeal shockwave therapy (ESWT), is a noninvasive treatment that uses high-energy sound waves to promote tissue healing and reduce pain. While there have been some studies investigating the use of shockwave therapy for conditions such as cellulite and other forms of localized adiposity, there is currently limited research on the use of shockwave therapy for lipedema.

While some practitioners may promote shockwave therapy as a potential treatment for lipedema, there is currently no scientific evidence to support its effectiveness for this condition. In fact, some experts caution against using shockwave therapy or any other invasive procedures for lipedema, as it can worsen the condition and cause additional swelling and discomfort.

Instead, conservative management strategies such as compression therapy, exercise, and manual lymphatic drainage are typically recommended as the first line of

G. Laur, *Lipoedema*, https://doi.org/10.1007/978-981-96-8939-2_23

treatment for lipedema. These treatments can help to reduce swelling, improve lymphatic flow, and increase mobility and quality of life for people with lipedema. It is important to consult with a healthcare provider before trying any new treatments or procedures for lipedema.

Shockwave therapy, a noninvasive treatment modality, employs high-energy acoustic waves that interact with tissue, leading to a cascade of biological effects. Its mechanism of action is believed to be multifaceted: the acoustic waves induce microtrauma to the affected tissue, which stimulates the body's intrinsic repair mechanisms, promoting neovascularization and enhancing blood flow to regenerate damaged tissue. Additionally, shockwave therapy has been shown to have analgesic effects, possibly due to the disruption of pain mediators and the stimulation of nerve fibers that modulate pain perception.

Shockwave therapy (SWT) exerts a range of biological effects on tissue, which are fundamental to its therapeutic applications. At the cellular level, SWT is known to induce microtrauma that triggers a cascade of biological responses leading to tissue regeneration and healing. The mechanical stress and strain applied by the shockwaves result in increased cell permeability, which enhances the flow of ions and signaling molecules into the cell, prompting the release of growth factors such as vascular endothelial growth factor (VEGF) and fibroblast growth factor (FGF).

These growth factors are instrumental in initiating neovascularization, thereby improving blood supply and oxygenation to the treated area.

Moreover, SWT has been shown to stimulate the production of nitric oxide (NO), a molecule that promotes vasodilation and angiogenesis, contributing to the restoration of blood flow and the reduction of ischemia. The mechanical stimulus provided by shockwaves also appears to facilitate the breakdown of calcified deposits within soft tissues, a process beneficial in conditions such as calcific tendinitis. Additionally, there is evidence to suggest that SWT can modulate inflammatory processes, reducing the concentration of pro-inflammatory cytokines and enhancing the anti-inflammatory response, which can alleviate pain and swelling in various musculoskeletal conditions.

In the context of connective tissue, the application of SWT can disrupt fibrous tissue structures, thereby decreasing tissue stiffness and improving elasticity and mobility. This is particularly relevant in the treatment of fibrotic conditions and scars. The induced biological effects of shockwave therapy—ranging from cellular to systemic—make it a versatile treatment modality with the potential to address a spectrum of pathological tissue alterations.

The historical development of shockwave therapy dates back to its initial medical applications in the dissolution of kidney stones, a process known as lithotripsy, first performed in the early 1980s. Since then, its utility has expanded to treat a variety of musculoskeletal disorders, including tendinopathies, plantar fasciitis, and delayed bone healing. The therapeutic benefits, such as promoting inflammation for healing, breaking down calcifications, and restoring normal tissue function, have led to its exploration in other medical applications.

Shockwave therapy (SWT) is a medical treatment that utilizes high-energy acoustic waves to deliver targeted energy to affected tissues within the body. This modality is based on the principles of sound wave propagation and employs either focused or radial shockwaves that invoke a series of biological responses within the tissue, including neovascularization, anti-inflammatory effects, and direct cellular effects that stimulate healing and regeneration. SWT has a long-standing history of application in the fragmentation of kidney stones, known as lithotripsy and has since expanded into orthopedics, physiotherapy, and wound healing due to its restorative properties.

Cavitation ultrasound, on the other hand, involves the use of ultrasonic waves, typically at frequencies above 20 kHz, which create oscillating pressure waves in a liquid medium. This process generates microbubbles that grow and implode, a phenomenon known as cavitation. The implosion of these microbubbles releases significant energy, which can disrupt adjacent structures. In a therapeutic context, cavitation ultrasound is utilized for its ability to break down adipose tissue, enhance the delivery of topical medications through increased cell membrane permeability, and promote tissue repair and healing through mechanical and thermal mechanisms.

While both SWT and cavitation ultrasound are rooted in the application of acoustic energy for therapeutic purposes, their mechanisms of action, operational frequencies, and clinical indications differ.

Specifically, in the context of lipedema treatment, SWT is emerging as a therapeutic option to address the fibrosis and impaired vascular function inherent to the condition, while cavitation ultrasound may be explored for its potential in adipose tissue modulation. Both modalities offer noninvasive alternatives that expand the arsenal of available treatments for conditions traditionally managed by more invasive procedures.

In the context of lipedema treatment, shockwave therapy has specific relevance. The condition's pathological basis in the fibrotic deposition and dysfunctional adipose tissue suggests that the regenerative and reparative effects of shockwave therapy may be beneficial. Preliminary studies have indicated that shockwave therapy can alleviate fibrosis, improve lymphatic drainage, and reduce the volume of pathological adipose deposits in lipedema. This leads to potential reductions in pain and swelling and improvements in limb function and mobility for patients with lipedema. While more extensive clinical trials are necessary to establish definitive protocols, the current evidence positions shockwave therapy as a promising adjunct to the multidisciplinary management of lipedema, offering a novel approach to addressing the complex pathophysiology of this condition.

Ultrasound cavitation is a noninvasive technology used primarily for reducing localized fat deposits and cellulite, leveraging the principles of low-frequency ultrasound waves. This technique induces the formation of microbubbles within the interstitial fluid of adipose tissue, which expand and implode due to the pressure variations caused by the ultrasound waves. The process of cavitation creates shock waves that selectively disrupt the membranes of adipocytes (fat cells), leading to the release of their lipid contents without harming surrounding tissues, such as blood vessels, nerves, and connective tissues. The liquefied fat is then metabolized by the body and expelled through the lymphatic and vascular systems, ultimately processed by the liver.

The underlying mechanism of ultrasound cavitation is grounded in the physics of acoustic waves and their interaction with biological tissues, highlighting the specificity of the method for targeting adipose tissue with minimal invasiveness. This specificity is attributed to the choice of ultrasound frequency, which is crucial for ensuring that the cavitation effect occurs within the fat layer without causing damage to other tissue types. Clinical and aesthetic applications of ultrasound cavitation have demonstrated its efficacy in body contouring, emphasizing its role as a safe and effective alternative to surgical liposuction for patients seeking fat reduction and cellulite improvement.

Despite its benefits, the effectiveness of ultrasound cavitation depends on various factors, including the treated area's size and the individual's physiological response to the treatment. It often requires multiple sessions to achieve desired results, and its effectiveness can be enhanced by combining it with other treatments such as lymphatic drainage massages to aid in the elimination of the released fatty acids. Understanding ultrasound cavitation involves recognizing both its potential as a cosmetic treatment and its limitations, requiring a comprehensive approach to patient selection, treatment planning, and post-treatment care to optimize outcomes.

Cavitation ultrasound operates through a sophisticated mechanism at the cellular level that exploits the physical properties of acoustic waves to induce targeted effects within adipose tissue.

When low-frequency ultrasound waves penetrate the skin and reach the adipose layer, they generate rapid pressure changes in the fluid surrounding the fat cells. This leads to the formation of microbubbles in a process known as cavitation. These microbubbles oscillate due to the acoustic pressure waves, growing in size until they reach a point where they can no longer absorb energy and implode. The implosion of these microbubbles generates localized shock waves and produces strong shear forces. These forces exert mechanical stress on the adipocytes, causing disruption of their cell membranes and leading to the release of triglycerides and other lipid contents into the interstitial space.

The lipid molecules released from the adipocytes are then transported through the lymphatic system to be metabolized and eliminated by the body's natural metabolic processes. This cellular-level mechanism allows for the selective reduction of fat without damaging surrounding tissues, such as blood vessels, nerves, and connective tissue, which are less susceptible to the mechanical effects induced by cavitation. Furthermore, the process stimulates the production of collagen and can enhance skin elasticity and firmness as the body responds to the ultrasonic and mechanical stimuli by initiating tissue repair processes. The efficacy of cavitation ultrasound in body contouring and fat reduction is thus deeply rooted in its ability to precisely target adipose cells and stimulate physiological responses that facilitate the removal and breakdown of fat, underscoring the importance of understanding and leveraging these cellular mechanisms for therapeutic and aesthetic applications.

Cavitation ultrasound has emerged as a significant advancement in adipose tissue management, offering a nonsurgical approach to fat reduction and body contouring. This technology specifically targets adipose cells by employing low-frequency ultrasound waves that create cavitation effects—microscopic bubbles that expand

and implode within the fatty tissue. This process leads to the disruption of fat cell membranes, causing the release of their lipid contents into the interstitial fluid. Subsequently, these lipids are metabolized by the body's natural processes, primarily through the liver and lymphatic system, leading to a reduction in the volume of the treated adipose tissue areas.

The applications of cavitation ultrasound in adipose tissue management include targeted fat reduction in areas resistant to diet and exercise, such as the abdomen, thighs, and buttocks, offering a contouring effect that enhances body shape. Additionally, it has been utilized in the treatment of cellulite, where the mechanical action of the ultrasound waves can help break down the fibrous tissue bands causing skin dimpling, improving skin texture and appearance. Beyond aesthetic enhancements, the technique's noninvasiveness and specificity for adipose tissue make it an attractive option for patients seeking alternatives to liposuction and other more invasive procedures.

The effectiveness of cavitation ultrasound in adipose tissue management is dependent on various factors, including the treated area's size, the treatment protocol's consistency, and the patient's overall health and lifestyle. It often requires multiple sessions to achieve optimal results, emphasizing the need for a comprehensive approach that may include diet, exercise, and hydration to support fat metabolism and removal. As research and clinical practice continue to refine the applications and outcomes of cavitation ultrasound, its role in adipose tissue management represents a promising area of noninvasive cosmetic and therapeutic interventions.

The efficacy and clinical outcomes of treatments targeting lipedema symptoms, notably pain reduction and improved lymphatic function, have been the focus of numerous research studies and clinical trials. A systematic review of these studies reveals a consensus on the positive impact of interventions such as manual lymphatic drainage (MLD), compression therapy, and low-level laser therapy (LLLT) on alleviating the symptoms associated with lipedema. Specifically, MLD has been shown to enhance lymphatic drainage, thereby reducing edema and associated pain, a critical concern for patients with lipedema. Compression therapy, both through garments and pneumatic pumps, has similarly demonstrated effectiveness in managing lipedema by improving lymphatic flow and reducing limb volume, which contributes to pain alleviation.

Clinical trials exploring the efficacy of LLLT have reported promising results in terms of pain reduction and tissue softening, suggesting improvements in lymphatic function and a potential reduction in fibrotic tissue typical of advanced lipedema. These interventions directly address the pathophysiological mechanisms underlying lipedema, offering symptomatic relief and improving patients' quality of life. However, the literature also indicates variability in individual responses to these treatments, underscoring the need for personalized treatment plans and further research into identifying predictors of treatment success. Overall, the accumulation of clinical evidence supports the use of these therapies in comprehensive lipedema management plans, highlighting their role in reducing pain, enhancing lymphatic drainage, and ultimately improving clinical outcomes for individuals with lipedema.

In conclusion, shockwave therapy and cavitation ultrasound have emerged as innovative and noninvasive modalities in the management of lipedema, offering new avenues for addressing the complex symptomatology of this condition. Shockwave therapy, with its ability to induce neovascularization, improve lymphatic drainage, and alleviate fibrosis, presents a promising option for patients with lipedema, particularly those with painful symptoms and limited mobility. Its mechanical stimulation has shown potential in reducing the fibrotic components of lipedema, thereby improving tissue elasticity and function. On the other hand, cavitation ultrasound targets adipose tissue directly, utilizing acoustic waves to disrupt fat cells and facilitate their removal through the body's natural metabolic processes. This technique offers a targeted approach to reducing fat deposits characteristic of lipedema, potentially improving body contour and reducing the burden of excess adipose tissue.

The integration of shockwave therapy and cavitation ultrasound into lipedema management underscores the importance of a comprehensive and multidisciplinary treatment plan. Such plans should not only focus on symptom alleviation but also on addressing the underlying pathophysiological mechanisms of lipedema. This requires a holistic approach that combines these innovative therapies with established treatments such as manual lymphatic drainage, compression therapy, and lifestyle modifications to achieve optimal outcomes.

Furthermore, the necessity for personalized treatment planning cannot be overstated. Given the heterogeneity in lipedema presentations and responses to treatment, individual assessment and tailored therapy plans are paramount. This individualized approach, combined with ongoing research and clinical trials, will enhance our understanding of the efficacy and mechanisms of action of shockwave and cavitation ultrasound in lipedema treatment. Ultimately, the goal is to improve the quality of life for individuals with lipedema by providing effective, evidence-based, and patient-centered care options.

Suggested Reading

Akbari, A.H., Sagheb, H.M. and Rashidi, H.J.: "Effects of vacuum-compression therapy on healing of diabetic foot ulcers: Randomized controlled trail." JRRD; 44(5): 631–636, 2007.

Alstead, S.A. and Girdwood, R.H.: "Textbook of medical treatment‘. 22th edition. Edinburgh: Churchill Livingstone, 2005.

Amman, B.R., Fanzeck, U.K. and Bollinger, A.K.: Microlymphatic aneurysms in patients with lipoedema. Lymphology; 34: 170–175,2001.

Barker, A.T., Jaffe, I.F. and Vance, J.W.: "Obesity and lower limb lipoedema". Am J Physiol. 22: R38-R44, 2010.

Benison, J.D.: Lipoedema and the non-lymphatic masquerader. Angiology; 15: 66–72, 2004.

Berlin, C.B., Erlandsen, S.L. and Butcher, E.C.: "Lymphocyte attachment and rolling under physiologic flow". Cell 10: 44–52, 2008.

Biiancini, S.S., Lucchi, M.R. and Tucci, S.T.: Functional lymphatic alterations in patients suffering from lipoedema. Angiology; 16: 22–28, 2009.

Brauer, W.J., Veissleder, H.M. and Ergebnis, B.C.: Erfahrungen bei·924 Patienten. Phlebologie; 31: 118–125, 2009.

Breu, F.X., Marshal, M.N. and Ergebnis, B.C.: Diagnostik des Lip- und. Lymphödems:Kompressi onssonographie mit einer neuen 13-M Hz-Linearsonde. Phlebologie; 22: 14–22,2008.

Chen, A.H., Frangos, S.G. and Sumpio, B.E. Intermittent compression devices physioiogic mechanisms of action Eur J Vase Endovasc Surg; 21: 383–392, 2009.
Chen, A.H., Hsu, S.D. and Chen, T.M.: Painful fat syndrome in a male patient. Br J Plast Surg; 57: 282·286, 2004.
Curd, S.B.: Fibrosclsrotica (Llposklerose) Ein nosoloqisches Problem. In: Ges. ML Vodder, ed. Schriftenreihe Manuelle Lymphdrainagenach Dr. Vedder, K.F. Haug, Heidelberg: 10–22, 2008.
DeFrantz, A.J., Hall, J.H. and Herring, S.M.: Adiposis dolorosa (Dercums disease):Liposuction is an effective form of treatment. Plast Reconstr Surg; 15: 89–96, 2009.
Derry, G.A., Veissleder, H.J. and Vergleichende, V.C.: prä- undposttherapeutische Volurnenmessungen in Beinsegmenten beim Lipodem. Lymphf-orsch; 10 (3): 55–61, 2009.
Dirnakakos, P.B., Stefanopoulos, T.P. and Antoniou, A.R. MRI and ultrasonographicfindings in the investigation' of lymphedema and lipeclema: Int Surg; 10: 44–52, 2007.
Fahlman, A.S. and Lambert, H.G.: "Effects of vacuum-cavitation on lipoedema in elderly women". Gerontology; 10: 17–24, 2010.
Fasshauer, M.J., Bluher, M.D. and Paschke, R.H.: Adipokine: Mogliches Bindeglied zwischen lnsullnresistenz und Adipositas. Dtsch Arzteblatt; 101 3491–3495, 2005.
Fasshauer, M.J., Bluher, M.D. and Paschke, R.H.: Adipokine: Moqliches Bindegiiedzwischen Insulinresistenz und Adipositas.Dtsch Arzteblatt; 101 3491–3495, 2006.
Fearon, A.S. and Locksley, E.S.: "Role of vacuum-cavitation on lipoedema". Science. 22:30, 2006.
Feddar, E.W., Klotz, G.F. and Gentzkow, A.W.: "vacuum-cavitation and lipoedema".Phys Ther. 11: 69–77, 2010.
Pipkin, F.B.: Medical statistics made easy. Edinburgh. London, Melbourne and New York,1984.

Surgical Management

Lipectomy

Understanding the role and scope of lipectomy in the management of lipedema is crucial for both patients and healthcare providers navigating treatment options for this complex condition. Lipedema is a chronic disorder characterized by the abnormal accumulation of fat in the lower extremities, leading to pain, tenderness, and, in many cases, mobility issues. Despite being a predominantly nonsurgical condition, surgical interventions such as lipectomy have emerged as significant options for managing advanced cases where conservative treatments have not yielded sufficient relief.

Lipectomy, specifically liposuction, for lipedema involves the removal of pathological adipose tissue to alleviate the symptoms associated with the condition. Unlike cosmetic liposuction, lipectomy for lipedema targets the fibrotic fat that is resistant to diet and exercise, aiming to reduce limb volume, improve mobility, and decrease pain. The procedure has shown promising outcomes in reducing the burden of lipedema, with many patients reporting improved quality of life post-surgery. Additionally, it can help in mitigating the progression of lipedema to more severe stages, potentially reducing the risk of developing secondary lymphedema, a condition characterized by excessive lymph fluid retention and swelling.

The decision to pursue lipectomy as a treatment option should be made within the context of a comprehensive care plan, considering the individual patient's symptoms, stage of lipedema, and overall health status. Preoperative evaluation by a multidisciplinary team, including vascular specialists, plastic surgeons, and physical therapists, is essential to assess the suitability for surgery and to optimize postoperative outcomes. Furthermore, lipectomy should be viewed as part of an integrated treatment approach, complemented by conservative measures such as compression therapy, manual lymphatic drainage, and lifestyle modifications to manage lipedema effectively.

Lipectomy procedures (Fig. 1) for the treatment of lipedema have evolved, incorporating both traditional techniques and more recent innovations such as tumescent liposuction, to effectively target the condition's pathological adipose tissue. Traditional lipectomy techniques, typically involving direct excision of fat tissue,

G. Laur, *Lipoedema*, https://doi.org/10.1007/978-981-96-8939-2_24

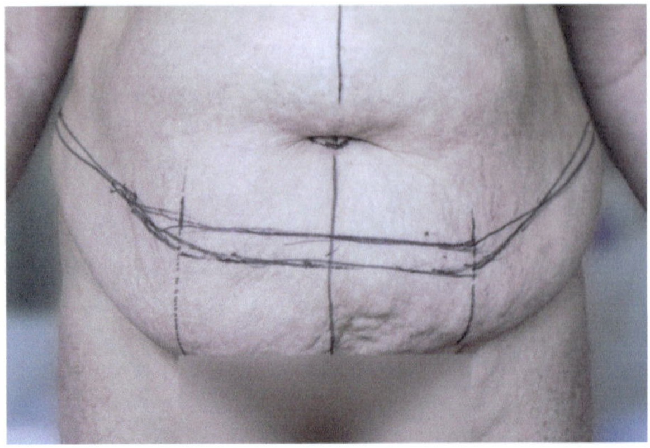

Fig. 1 Selective focus of a mature woman and markings for beltectomy, panniculectomy or apron removal, and liposuction on inner thighs. A tummy tuck extending to the spine. Mummy tummy, sagging loose skin

have been largely supplanted in the context of lipedema by liposuction methods due to the need for precise removal of abnormal fat while minimizing damage to the lymphatic system. Tumescent liposuction, a significant advancement in this field, involves the infusion of a large volume of a dilute solution of local anesthesia and epinephrine into the fatty tissue before liposuction. This technique reduces blood loss, minimizes postoperative bruising and swelling, and facilitates the easier removal of fat. Adaptations of tumescent liposuction for lipedema, such as water-assisted liposuction (WAL) and power-assisted liposuction (PAL), further refine the approach to specifically address the fibrotic adipose tissue characteristic of lipedema.

These adaptations allow for a gentler and more controlled removal of lipedemic fat, significantly improving patient outcomes in terms of pain reduction, mobility enhancement, and aesthetic results. The evolution of lipectomy procedures, particularly the introduction and adaptation of tumescent liposuction techniques, marks an advancement in the surgical management of lipedema, offering hope for effective symptom management and improved quality of life for patients suffering from this challenging condition.

The lipectomy procedure, particularly when adapted for the treatment of lipedema, involves meticulous planning and execution, with specific emphasis on anesthesia considerations and intraoperative management to ensure patient safety and optimal outcomes. Initially, anesthesia considerations are paramount, with the choice between general anesthesia and tumescent local anesthesia being dictated by the extent of the procedure and patient-specific factors. Tumescent local anesthesia, favored for its reduced systemic effects and enhanced recovery, involves the infusion of a dilute solution of lidocaine and epinephrine into the subcutaneous tissue, providing localized numbness and vasoconstriction to minimize bleeding. Once anesthesia is established, the intraoperative phase begins with the careful mapping of the lipedemic areas to be addressed. Surgeons employ techniques such as tumescent liposuction, which requires the strategic infusion of the tumescent solution followed by the insertion of small cannulas through tiny incisions to aspirate the pathological adipose tissue. This phase is critical for preserving the integrity of the lymphatic and vascular structures while effectively removing lipedemic fat.

Intraoperative monitoring of fluid balance and vital signs is essential to manage the large volume of tumescent fluid and to ensure the patient's stability throughout the procedure.

Advances in technology, such as ultrasound-assisted and power-assisted liposuction, offer additional precision in targeting fibrotic adipose tissue, facilitating a more effective removal while reducing trauma to surrounding tissues. The comprehensive approach to the lipectomy procedure, from anesthesia to intraoperative management, underscores the importance of tailored surgical strategies to address the unique challenges presented by lipedema, aiming for significant symptom relief and improvement in patients' quality of life.

The efficacy and outcomes of lipectomy for the treatment of lipedema have been increasingly documented, showcasing both short-term and long-term benefits for patients suffering from this chronic condition. In the short term, patients often experience significant reductions in limb volume, alleviation of pain, and improvements in mobility and quality of life. These immediate effects arc largely attributed to the removal of fibrotic adipose tissue that characterizes lipedema, which is resistant to diet and exercise. Long-term outcomes further validate the procedure's efficacy, with sustained improvements in limb size, continued pain relief, and enhanced physical function being reported. Additionally, lipectomy can have a psychological impact, improving patients' self-esteem and mental health, which are often adversely affected by lipedema.

Case studies and patient outcomes further underscore the procedure's effectiveness. For instance, a retrospective study may highlight a series of patients with lipedema who underwent lipectomy, demonstrating not only reductions in the volume of the affected limbs but also marked improvements in symptoms such as tenderness, bruising, and fluid retention. Moreover, these studies often reveal a significant decrease in the need for conservative treatments, such as compression therapy and manual lymphatic drainage, post-surgery.

Despite these positive outcomes, it is crucial to note that lipectomy is not a cure for lipedema and is most effective when integrated into a comprehensive treatment plan that includes lifestyle modifications, physical therapy, and ongoing management of the condition. The variability in patient outcomes also highlights the need for individualized treatment plans and realistic expectations regarding the results of the surgery. Overall, lipectomy for lipedema offers a promising option for symptom management, with a significant potential to improve patients' quality of life.

The undertaking of lipectomy, like any surgical intervention, carries inherent risks and potential complications, both in the immediate postoperative period and over the long term. Common surgical risks include infection, bleeding, and adverse reactions to anesthesia, alongside procedure-specific concerns such as damage to the lymphatic vessels, which could exacerbate lymphedema in patients with lipedema. Effective strategies to minimize these risks involve meticulous surgical technique, stringent aseptic protocols, and careful selection and management of anesthesia, tailored to individual patient needs and health status. Postoperative complications such as seroma formation, contour irregularities, and temporary sensory changes in the treated areas require vigilant management, including the use of compression garments, close monitoring of wound sites, and physical therapy to ensure optimal lymphatic drainage and healing.

Long-term risks and considerations for patients undergoing lipectomy for lipedema include the potential for regrowth of adipose tissue if the underlying hormonal and genetic contributors to lipedema are not managed, underscoring the necessity of continued lifestyle interventions and support. Additionally, patients must be counseled on the realistic expectations of surgical outcomes, emphasizing that lipectomy is a symptomatic treatment rather than a cure for lipedema. Integrating surgical treatment with comprehensive care plans that address the multifactorial nature of lipedema can mitigate long-term risks and enhance overall patient well-being. Thus, a multidisciplinary approach involving surgeons, primary care providers, physical therapists, and nutritionists is essential for managing the complexities of lipedema, optimizing surgical outcomes, and ensuring the long-term health and satisfaction of patients.

Postoperative care and recovery following a lipectomy procedure, especially for patients with lipedema, are critical components of the treatment pathway, demanding meticulous attention to ensure optimal outcomes. Guidelines for postoperative care typically emphasize the importance of compression therapy to manage swelling and support the healing tissues, as well as the initiation of gentle manual lymphatic drainage (MLD) to facilitate lymphatic function and prevent fluid accumulation. Pain management, infection prevention strategies, and wound care are also central to postoperative protocols, with patients receiving detailed instructions on medication management, signs of infection to watch for, and techniques for caring for incision sites. The recovery timeline can vary, with initial improvements in symptoms and mobility often observed within weeks, although the full benefits of the surgery and the complete resolution of swelling may take several months to manifest.

The importance of follow-up and monitoring cannot be overstressed, as these allow for the timely identification and management of any complications, such as infections or lymphatic damage. Regular follow-up appointments provide opportunities to assess healing progress, adjust compression garment fittings, and update rehabilitation exercises to enhance recovery. Long-term monitoring is equally important, as it aids in evaluating the sustainability of the surgical outcomes and addressing any emerging issues related to lipedema progression or the development of secondary conditions. This continuous care and interaction with the healthcare team reinforce the patient's understanding of the chronic nature of lipedema, underlining the necessity for ongoing management and lifestyle adjustments even after surgical intervention, to maintain the gains achieved and support overall well-being.

The integration of lipectomy with other therapeutic modalities such as compression therapy, manual lymphatic drainage (MLD), and physical therapy represents a comprehensive, multidisciplinary approach to the management of lipedema, aiming for optimal outcomes. This holistic strategy acknowledges the multifaceted nature of lipedema, addressing not only the excessive adipose tissue but also the associated symptoms and complications, such as lymphatic dysfunction and mobility restrictions. Compression therapy, applied postoperatively, is essential for reducing swelling, improving lymphatic flow, and shaping the limbs. MLD further complements this by gently stimulating the lymphatic system to remove excess fluids and reduce the risk of lymphedema. Physical therapy plays a critical role in enhancing mobility, strength, and overall function, facilitating a quicker return to daily activities and improving quality of life.

Case examples of combined treatment plans underscore the effectiveness of this integrative approach. For instance, a patient undergoing lipectomy for lipedema may begin with preoperative MLD and physical therapy to maximize lymphatic function and physical conditioning, followed by surgery, and then transition into a postoperative regimen that includes compression garments and continued MLD and physical therapy. This coordinated care plan not only addresses the immediate surgical recovery but also focuses on long-term management of lipedema, preventing complications and supporting the patient's overall well-being.

A multidisciplinary team, including surgeons, physiotherapists, lymphedema therapists, and other specialists, is crucial for designing and implementing such comprehensive treatment plans. This team approach ensures that all aspects of the patient's condition are considered, enabling personalized care that maximizes the benefits of lipectomy while minimizing risks and complications. Through this collaborative strategy, patients with lipedema can achieve significant improvements in symptoms, functionality, and quality of life, demonstrating the value of integrating surgical and nonsurgical therapies in the management of this complex condition.

The emotional and psychological impact of surgery for conditions such as lipedema cannot be understated, necessitating comprehensive counseling and support both before and after the procedure. Undergoing surgery, especially lipectomy, can be a significant emotional journey for patients, many of whom may have struggled with the symptoms and aesthetic concerns of lipedema for years. Preoperative counseling plays a crucial role in setting realistic expectations, preparing patients for the physical outcomes, and addressing any anxieties or fears regarding the surgery. Postoperatively, continued psychological support is essential to navigate the recovery process, which may involve adjustments to changes in body image, coping with post-surgical pain, and managing expectations regarding the final outcomes.

The improvements in body image and quality of life post-lipectomy can be profound, with many patients reporting increased self-esteem and decreased psychological distress as they observe reductions in limb size and symmetry. These changes often translate to enhanced mobility and engagement in social and physical activities that were previously hindered by lipedema, further contributing to an overall improvement in quality of life. However, it is important to acknowledge that the journey does not end with surgery; ongoing support, including psychotherapy or participation in support groups, can be invaluable in helping patients fully integrate these changes into their self-concept and life narrative.

The intersection of physical and psychological care underscores the importance of a holistic approach to the treatment of lipedema, where surgical interventions are integrated with emotional and psychological support. Such an approach not only addresses the physical manifestations of the condition but also fosters a supportive environment for emotional healing and psychological resilience, ensuring that patients receive comprehensive care that truly meets their needs as individuals navigating the complexities of lipedema.

In conclusion, lipectomy emerges as a significant intervention within the multifaceted landscape of lipedema treatment, offering a targeted approach to reducing the burden of pathologically accumulated adipose tissue characteristic of this condition. By addressing one of the core physical manifestations of lipedema, lipectomy can significantly alleviate symptoms, improve mobility, and enhance the quality of life for patients.

However, the decision to pursue lipectomy must be carefully balanced against potential risks and complications, underscoring the necessity of a thorough preoperative evaluation and a personalized treatment plan that aligns with the individual patient's health status, goals, and concerns.

The efficacy of lipectomy in managing lipedema highlights not only the potential for significant physical improvement but also underscores the importance of comprehensive care in the treatment of lipedema. Integrating surgical options with conservative therapies such as compression garments, manual lymphatic drainage, and physical therapy, alongside psychological support, creates a holistic care framework essential for addressing the wide-ranging impacts of lipedema. This comprehensive approach ensures that both the physical and emotional health of the patient are prioritized, fostering a supportive environment for recovery and long-term management.

Ultimately, the journey of managing lipedema is highly individual, with treatment plans needing to be as dynamic and multifaceted as the condition itself. Lipectomy stands as a valuable tool within the broader therapeutic arsenal against lipedema, offering hope and improved outcomes for many patients. Yet, its optimal utilization hinges on the recognition of lipedema as a complex, systemic condition that necessitates a coordinated, patient-centered approach to care. Through such comprehensive management strategies, patients with lipedema can achieve meaningful improvements in their symptoms and overall quality of life, marking significant strides in the ongoing battle against this challenging condition.

Suggested Reading

Schook CC, Mulliken JB, Fishman SJ, et al.. Differential diagnosis of lower extremity enlargement in pediatric patients referred with a diagnosis of lymphedema. *Plast Reconstr Surg.* 2011;127:1571–1581

Herpertz U. Krankheitsspektrum des Lipödems an einer Lymphologischen Fachklinik—Erscheinungsformen, Mischbilder und Behandlungsmöglichkeiten. *Vasomed.* 1997;5:301–307

Forner-Cordero I, Szolnoky G, Forner-Cordero A, et al.. An overview of its clinical manifestations, diagnosis and treatment of the disproportional fatty deposition syndrome – systematic review. *Clinical Obesity.* 2012;2:86–95

Angst F, Lehmann S, Aeschlimann A, et al.. Cross-sectional validity and specificity of comprehensive measurement in lymphedema and lipedema of the lower extremity: a comparison of five outcome instruments. *Health Qual Life Outcomes.* 2020;18:245

Felson DT, Niu J, Gross KD, et al.. Valgus malalignment is a risk factor for lateral knee osteoarthritis incidence and progression: findings from the Multicenter Osteoarthritis Study and the Osteoarthritis Initiative. *Arthritis Rheum*. 2013;65:355–362

Rowe PJ, Myles CM, Walker C, et al.. Knee joint kinematics in gait and other functional activities measured using flexible electrogoniometry: how much knee motion is sufficient for normal daily life? *Gait Posture*. 2000;12:143–155

Kikkert LHJ, de Groot MH, van Campen JP, et al.. Gait dynamics to optimize fall risk assessment in geriatric patients admitted to an outpatient diagnostic clinic. *PLoS One*. 2017;12:e0178615

Crescenzi R, Donahue PMC, Hartley KG, et al.. Lymphedema evaluation using noninvasive 3 T MR lymphangiography. *J Magn Reson Imaging*. 2017;46:1349–1360

Gould DJ, El-Sabawi B, Goel P, et al.. Uncovering lymphatic transport abnormalities in patients with primary lipedema. *J Reconstr Microsurg*. 2019;36:136–141

van de Pas CB, Boonen RS, Stevens S, et al.. Does tumescent liposuction damage the lymph vessels in lipoedema patients? *Phlebology*. 2020;35:231–236

Reich-Schupke S, Schmeller W, Brauer WJ, et al.. S1 guidelines: lipedema. *J Dtsch Dermatol Ges*. 2017;15:758–768

Gensior M, Cornely M. Complications and their management in the surgical treatment of lipohyperplasia dolorosa. *Dermatologie (Heidelb)*. 2023;74:114–120

Baumgartner A, Hueppe M, Schmeller W. Long-term benefit of liposuction in patients with lipoedema: a follow-up study after an average of 4 and 8 years. *Br J Dermatol*. 2015;174:1061–1067

Peled AW, Slavin SA, Brorson H. Long-term outcome after surgical treatment of lipedema. *Ann Plast Surg*. 2012;68:303–307

Rasmussen JC, Aldrich MB, Fife CE, et al.. Lymphatic function and anatomy in early stages of lipedema. *Obesity (Silver Spring, Md)*. 2022;30:1391–1400

van Heumen S, Riksen JJM, Bramer WM, et al.. Imaging of the lymphatic vessels for surgical planning: a systematic review. *Ann Surg Oncol*. 2023;30:462–479

van Heumen S, Riksen JJM, Bramer WM, et al.. Imaging of the lymphatic vessels for surgical planning: a systematic review. *Ann Surg Oncol*. 2022;29:628

Herbst K, Mirkovskaya L, Bharhagava A, et al.. Lipedema fat and signs and symptoms of illness, increase with advancing stage. *Archives of Medicine*. 2015;7:1–8

Frick A, Hoffmann JN, Baumeister RG, et al.. Liposuction technique and lymphatic lesions in lower legs: anatomic study to reduce risks. *Plast Reconstr Surg*. 1999;103:1868–73; discussion 1874

Hoffmann JN, Fertmann JP, Baumeister RG, et al.. Tumescent and dry liposuction of lower extremities: differences in lymph vessel injury. *Plast Reconstr Surg*. 2004;113:718–24; discussion 725

Wright TF, Herbst KL. A case series of lymphatic injuries after suction lipectomy in women with lipedema. *Am J Case Rep*. 2022;23:e935016

Dean SM, Valenti E, Hock K, et al.. The clinical characteristics of lower extremity lymphedema in 440 patients. *J Vasc Surg Venous Lymphat Disord*. 2020;8:851–859

Child AH, Gordon KD, Sharpe P, et al.. Lipedema: an inherited condition. *Am J Med Genet A*. 2010;152A:970–976

Wold LE, Hines EA, Jr, Allen EV. Lipedema of the legs: a syndrome characterized by fat legs and edema. *Ann Intern Med*. 1951;34:1243–1250

Wu S, Coombs DM, Gurunian RL. Liposuction: concepts, safety, and techniques in body-contouring surgery. *Cleve Clin J Med*. 2020;87:367–375

Wright T, Scarfino CD, O'Malley EM. Effect of pneumatic compression device and stocking use on symptoms and quality of life in women with lipedema: a proof-in-principle randomized trial. *Phlebology*. 2023;38:51–61

Campisi CC, Ryan M, Boccardo F, et al.. Fibro-lipo-lymph-aspiration with a lymph vessel sparing procedure to treat advanced lymphedema after multiple lymphatic-venous anastomoses: the complete treatment protocol. *Ann Plast Surg*. 2017;78:184–190

Klein JA. *Tumescent Technique. Tumescent Anesthesia and Microcannular Liposuction.*: Mosby; 2000

Cronin M, Dengler N, Krauss ES, et al.. Completion of the Updated Caprini Risk Assessment Model (2013 version). *Clin Appl Thromb Hemost.* 2019;25:1076029619838052
Golemi I, Salazar Adum JP, Tafur A, et al.. Venous thromboembolism prophylaxis using the Caprini score. *Dis Mon.* 2019;65:249–298
PROMIS physical function scoring manual. Available at https://www.healthmeasures.net/administrator/components/com_instruments/uploads/PROMIS%20Physical%20Function%20Scoring%20Manual.pdf Published 2019. Accessed November 8, 2022.
Ware JE, Jr, Sherbourne CD. The MOS 36-item short-form health survey (SF-36) I Conceptual framework and item selection. *Med Care.* 1992;30:473–483
Rapprich S, Dingler A, Podda M. Liposuction is an effective treatment for lipedema-results of a study with 25 patients. *J Dtsch Dermatol Ges.* 2011;9:33–40
Baumgartner A, Hueppe M, Meier-Vollrath I, et al.. Improvements in patients with lipedema 4, 8 and 12 years after liposuction. *Phlebology.* 2021;36:152–159
Alcolea JM, Alonso Alvarez B, Arroyo Bielsa A, et al.., ed. *Documento de Consenso Lipedema 2018.* In: 33rd National Congress of the Spanish Society of Aesthetic Medicine (SEME); 22–24 February 2018; Malaga/Barcelona, Spain. Barcelona, Spain: LITOGAMA S.L.; 2018
Coppel T, Cunneen J, Fetzer S, et al.. Best practice guidelines: the management of lipoedema. *Wounds UK.* 2017;13:1–36
Nichols CI, Vose JG. Clinical outcomes and costs within 90 days of primary or revision total joint arthroplasty. *J Arthroplasty.* 2016;31:1400–1406.e3
Hua Y, Salcedo J. Cost-effectiveness analysis of robotic-arm assisted total knee arthroplasty. *PLoS One.* 2022;17:e0277980
Ramkumar PN, Chu CT, Harris JD, et al.. Causes and rates of unplanned readmissions after elective primary total joint arthroplasty: a systematic review and meta-analysis. *Am J Orthop (Belle Mead NJ).* 2015;44:397–405
Clair AJ, Evangelista PJ, Lajam CM, et al.. Cost analysis of total joint arthroplasty readmissions in a bundled payment care improvement initiative. *J Arthroplasty.* 2016;31:1862–1865
Park KK, Chang CB, Kang YG, et al.. Correlation of maximum flexion with clinical outcome after total knee replacement in Asian patients. *J Bone Joint Surg Br.* 2007;89:604–608
Maradit Kremers H, Larson DR, Crowson CS, et al.. Prevalence of Total Hip and Knee Replacement in the United States. *J Bone Joint Surg Am.* 2015;97:1386–1397
Weinstein AM, Rome BN, Reichmann WM, et al.. Estimating the burden of total knee replacement in the United States. *J Bone Joint Surg Am.* 2013;95:385–392
Houck J, Jacobson R, Bass M, et al.. Improving interpretation of the patient-reported outcomes measurement information system (PROMIS) physical function scale for specific tasks in community-dwelling older adults. *J Geriatr Phys Ther.* 2020;43:142–152
Oh-Park M, Wang C, Verghese J. Stair negotiation time in community-dwelling older adults: normative values and association with functional decline. *Arch Phys Med Rehabil.* 2011;92:2006–2011
Khalil LS, Darrith B, Franovic S, et al.. Patient-reported outcomes measurement information system (PROMIS) global health short forms demonstrate responsiveness in patients undergoing knee arthroplasty. *J Arthroplasty.* 2020;35:1540–1544
Klemt C, Tirumala V, Oganesyan R, et al.. Single-stage revision of the infected total knee arthroplasty is associated with improved functional outcomes: a propensity score-matched cohort study. *J Arthroplasty.* 2021;36:298–304
Shim J, Hamilton DF. Comparative responsiveness of the PROMIS-10 Global Health and EQ-5D questionnaires in patients undergoing total knee arthroplasty. *Bone Joint J.* 2019;101-B:832–837
Amitkumar M, Singh PK, Singh KJ, et al.. Surgical outcome in spinal operation in patients aged 70 years and above. *Neurol India.* 2020;68:45–51
Herbst KL, Hansen EA, Cobos Salinas LM, et al.. Survey outcomes of lipedema reduction surgery in the United States. *PRS Global Open.* 2021;9:e3553

Cárdenas-Camarena L, Tobar-Losada A, Lacouture AM. Large-volume circumferential liposuction with tumescent technique: a sure and viable procedure. *Plast Reconstr Surg*. 1999;104:1887–1899

Chow I, Alghoul MS, Khavanin N, et al.. Reply: is there a safe lipoaspirate volume? A risk assessment model of liposuction volume as a function of body mass index. *Plast Reconstr Surg*. 2016;137:756e–758e

Yeh RW, Valsdottir LR, Yeh MW, et al.; PARACHUTE Investigators. Parachute use to prevent death and major trauma when jumping from aircraft: randomized controlled trial. *BMJ*. 2018;363:k5094

Bariatric Surgery

Bariatric surgery is a type of surgery that aims to help obese individuals lose weight by altering the digestive system. The procedure has been used for many years to treat severe obesity, and its benefits for improving overall health have been well documented. However, it is important to note that bariatric surgery is not a cure for obesity, and it requires significant lifestyle changes and ongoing support to achieve long-term success.

In recent years, there has been growing interest in the use of bariatric surgery as a treatment for lipedema. This is because many individuals with lipedema struggle with their weight, despite efforts to diet and exercise. Bariatric surgery has been shown to be effective in helping individuals with severe obesity lose weight and improve their overall health, and it is possible that it could be similarly effective for patients with lipedema.

History of Bariatric Surgery

The history of bariatric surgery (Fig. 1) dates back to the 1950s when the jejunoileal bypass procedure was developed. This procedure involved rerouting a portion of the small intestine to bypass the duodenum and jejunum, resulting in malabsorption of food and weight loss. However, this procedure had many complications, and it fell out of favor in the 1970s when safer and more effective procedures were developed.

In the 1980s and 1990s, the gastric band and gastric bypass procedures were developed. These procedures involved reducing the size of the stomach or rerouting the digestive tract to limit the amount of food that could be consumed and absorbed. These procedures were found to be more effective and had fewer complications than earlier procedures, and they quickly became the most commonly performed bariatric surgeries.

G. Laur, *Lipoedema*, https://doi.org/10.1007/978-981-96-8939-2_25

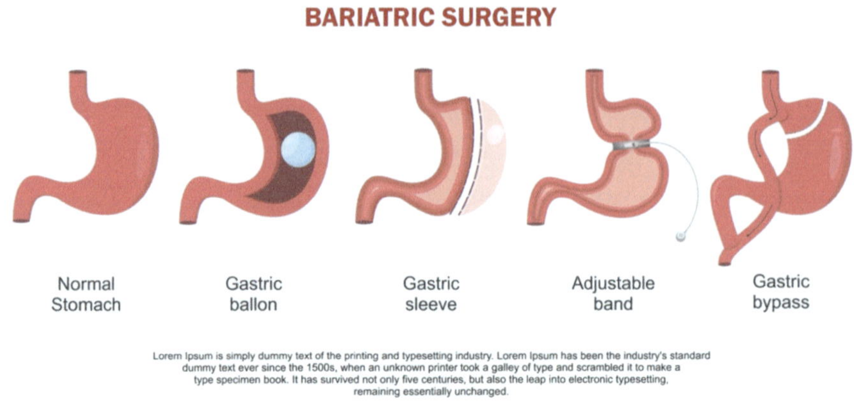

Fig. 1 Diagram showing the different techniques of bariatric surgery

In recent years, new procedures have been developed, including the sleeve gastrectomy and the duodenal switch. These procedures have been found to be effective in helping individuals lose weight and improve their overall health.

This detailed study reveals significant insights into the use of bariatric surgery for patients with lipedema, particularly in relation to thigh volume reduction, challenging previous assumptions about the condition's resistance to weight loss.

The study reveals a significant decrease of 33.4% in thigh volume among patients with lipedema after undergoing bariatric surgery, specifically either sleeve gastrectomy or bypass surgery. This discovery is significant as it challenges prior assumptions and research indicating that thigh volume in patients with lipedema is impervious to weight reduction. The decrease in thigh volume among patients with lipedema was determined to be statistically comparable to that observed in control groups. This suggests that bariatric surgery can be equally successful for patients with lipedema as it is for persons who do not have the disorder. The study concluded that both the type of bariatric surgery and the obesity category of the patient had no significant impact on the decrease in thigh volume. Previous studies have attributed the persistence of reduced leg volume in people with lipedema to initial research. Nevertheless, this study proposes that the resistance shown may not be an inherent characteristic of lipedema. Liposuction is advised in lipedema recommendations as a means to reduce leg volume and alleviate pain. Nevertheless, the efficacy of liposuction has been called into question as a result of insufficient evidence. By comparison, the leg volume decrease observed in this study after bariatric surgery (33.7%) significantly surpasses the typical reduction achieved by liposuction (about 7%). The study revealed that weight loss in patients with lipedema was comparable to that of the control group, contradicting previous findings that indicated compromised total weight reduction in these individuals. The study's retrospective approach may have generated selection bias. The diagnosis of lipedema was solely reliant on the clinical presentation, hence increasing the potential for misdiagnosis. The study primarily examined the loss in thigh volume, without considering other symptoms associated with lipedema. The study finds that bariatric surgery is a viable and efficient choice for decreasing leg volume in patients suffering from obesity and lipedema, warranting additional research.

This finding opens new avenues for treatment options and suggests that bariatric surgery could play a significant role in managing lipedema, especially in cases where traditional methods like diet, exercise, and liposuction are less effective or not viable.

In summary, bariatric surgery emerges from this study as a promising intervention for patients with lipedema and obesity, offering substantial benefits in terms of thigh volume reduction. This contradicts earlier beliefs about the condition's resistance to weight loss and underscores the importance of ongoing research and reassessment of treatment strategies in the field of lipedema management.

Risks and Benefits of Bariatric Surgery

Bariatric surgery is a major surgical procedure, and it carries risks like any other surgery. The risks of bariatric surgery include bleeding, infection, blood clots, and complications related to anesthesia. In addition, there are specific risks associated with each type of bariatric surgery, and patients should carefully consider these risks before deciding to undergo surgery.

Despite the risks, bariatric surgery has been shown to be an effective treatment for severe obesity, and it can lead to significant improvements in overall health. Bariatric surgery has been found to reduce the risk of obesity-related health conditions, such as type 2 diabetes, high blood pressure, and sleep apnea. In addition, bariatric surgery has been shown to improve quality of life and increase lifespan.

Complications of Bariatric Surgery

While bariatric surgery can be an effective treatment for severe obesity and lipedema, there are potential complications that can occur. These complications can be mild or severe and can include.

1. Nausea and vomiting
2. Abdominal pain
3. Dumping syndrome (a condition where food moves too quickly through the digestive system)
4. Malnutrition
5. Infection
6. Blood clots
7. Hernias
8. Gallstones
9. Bowel obstruction

It is important for patients to carefully consider the risks and benefits of bariatric surgery and to discuss any concerns they may have with their healthcare provider.

In conclusion, bariatric surgery is a significant surgical intervention that may serve as an effective treatment option for individuals with severe obesity and, in selected cases, lipedema. Nonetheless, it is essential for patients to thoroughly evaluate the potential risks and benefits in consultation with their healthcare providers. When undertaken with appropriate preoperative assessment, postoperative care, and long-term multidisciplinary support, bariatric surgery can be a valuable component of a comprehensive management strategy aimed at improving health outcomes and quality of life.

Suggested Reading

Fink JM, Schreiner L, Marjanovic G, Erbacher G, Seifert GJ, Foeldi M, Bertsch T. Leg Volume in Patients with Lipoedema following Bariatric Surgery. Visc Med. 2021 Jun;37(3):206–211. https://doi.org/10.1159/000511044

Aksoy H, Karadag AS, Wollina U. Cause and management of lipedema-associated pain. Dermatol Ther. 2021;34(1):e14364

Child AH, Gordon KD, Sharpe P, Brice G, Ostergaard P, Jeffery S, Mortimer PS. Lipedema: an inherited condition. Am J Med Genet A. 2010 Apr;152A(4):970–6

Kruppa P, Georgiou I, Biermann N, Prantl L, Klein-Weigel P, Ghods M. Lipedema-Pathogenesis, Diagnosis, and Treatment Options. Dtsch Arztebl Int. 2020 Jun 01;117(22–23):396–403

Paolacci S, Precone V, Acquaviva F, Chiurazzi P, Fulcheri E, Pinelli M, Buffelli F, Michelini S, Herbst KL, Unfer V, Bertelli M., GeneOb Project. Genetics of lipedema: new perspectives on genetic research and molecular diagnoses. Eur Rev. Med Pharmacol Sci. 2019 Jul;23(13):5581–5594

Herbst KL. Subcutaneous Adipose Tissue Diseases: Dercum Disease, Lipedema, Familial Multiple Lipomatosis, and Madelung Disease. In: Feingold KR, Anawalt B, Blackman MR, Boyce A, Chrousos G, Corpas E, de Herder WW, Dhatariya K, Dungan K, Hofland J, Kalra S, Kaltsas G, Kapoor N, Koch C, Kopp P, Korbonits M, Kovacs CS, Kuohung W, Laferrère B, Levy M, McGee EA, McLachlan R, New M, Purnell J, Sahay R, Shah AS, Singer F, Sperling MA, Stratakis CA, Trence DL, Wilson DP, editors. Endotext [Internet]. MDText.com, Inc.; South Dartmouth (MA): Dec 14, 2019

Katzer K, Hill JL, McIver KB, Foster MT. Lipedema and the Potential Role of Estrogen in Excessive Adipose Tissue Accumulation. Int J Mol Sci. 2021 Oct 29;22(21)

Szél E, Kemény L, Groma G, Szolnoky G. Pathophysiological dilemmas of lipedema. Med Hypotheses. 2014 Nov;83(5):599–606

Nemes A, Kovács Z, Kormányos Á, Domsik P, Kalapos A, Piros GÁ, Kemény L, Forster T, Szolnoky G. The mitral annulus in lipedema: Insights from the three-dimensional speckle-tracking echocardiographic MAGYAR-Path Study. Echocardiography. 2019 Aug;36(8):1482–1491

Herbst KL. Rare adipose disorders (RADs) masquerading as obesity. Acta Pharmacol Sin. 2012 Feb;33(2):155–72

Crescenzi R, Donahue PMC, Weakley S, Garza M, Donahue MJ, Herbst KL. Lipedema and Dercum's Disease: A New Application of Bioimpedance. Lymphat Res Biol. 2019 Dec;17(6):671–679

Buso G, Depairon M, Tomson D, Raffoul W, Vettor R, Mazzolai L. Lipedema: A Call to Action! Obesity (Silver Spring). 2019 Oct;27(10):1567–1576

Buck DW, Herbst KL. Lipedema: A Relatively Common Disease with Extremely Common Misconceptions. Plast Reconstr Surg Glob Open. 2016 Sep;4(9):e1043

Keith L, Seo CA, Rowsemitt C, Pfeffer M, Wahi M, Staggs M, Dudek J, Gower B, Carmody M. Ketogenic diet as a potential intervention for lipedema. Med Hypotheses. 2021 Jan;146:110435

Warren Peled A, Kappos EA. Lipedema: diagnostic and management challenges. Int J Womens Health. 2016;8:389–95

Shin BW, Sim YJ, Jeong HJ, Kim GC. Lipedema, a rare disease. Ann Rehabil Med. 2011 Dec;35(6):922–7

Reich-Schupke S, Altmeyer P, Stücker M. Thick legs – not always lipedema. J Dtsch Dermatol Ges. 2013 Mar;11(3):225–33

Herbst KL, Hansen EA, Cobos Salinas LM, Wright TF, Larson EE, Schwartz JS. Survey Outcomes of Lipedema Reduction Surgery in the United States. Plast Reconstr Surg Glob Open. 2021 Apr;9(4):e3553

Peprah K, MacDougall D. Liposuction for the Treatment of Lipedema: A Review of Clinical Effectiveness and Guidelines [Internet]. Canadian Agency for Drugs and Technologies in Health; Ottawa (ON): Jun 07, 2019

Dadras M, Mallinger PJ, Corterier CC, Theodosiadi S, Ghods M. Liposuction in the Treatment of Lipedema: A Longitudinal Study. Arch Plast Surg. 2017 Jul;44(4):324–331

Torre YS, Wadeea R, Rosas V, Herbst KL. Lipedema: friend and foe. Horm Mol Biol Clin Investig. 2018 Mar 09;33(1)

Halk AB, Damstra RJ. First Dutch guidelines on lipedema using the international classification of functioning, disability and health. Phlebology. 2017 Apr;32(3):152–159

Schneider R. Low-frequency vibrotherapy considerably improves the effectiveness of manual lymphatic drainage (MLD) in patients with lipedema: A two-armed, randomized, controlled pragmatic trial. Physiother Theory Pract. 2020 Jan;36(1):63–70

Pfister C, Dawczynski H, Schingale FJ. Selenium Deficiency in Lymphedema and Lipedema-A Retrospective Cross-Sectional Study from a Specialized Clinic. Nutrients. 2020 Apr 25;12(5)

Reich-Schupke S, Schmeller W, Brauer WJ, Cornely ME, Faerber G, Ludwig M, Lulay G, Miller A, Rapprich S, Richter DF, Schacht V, Schrader K, Stücker M, Ure C. S1 guidelines: Lipedema. J Dtsch Dermatol Ges. 2017 Jul;15(7):758–767

Hansson E, Svensson H, Brorson H. Review of Dercum's disease and proposal of diagnostic criteria, diagnostic methods, classification and management. Orphanet J Rare Dis. 2012 Apr 30;7:23.

Liposuction

Surgical excision is another approach for the management of lipedema. The technique involves the removal of the subcutaneous fat and lymphatic tissue from the affected areas. This procedure is also known as "liposuction" or "lipectomy" and has been used for the treatment of lipedema for several decades. However, there are limited studies that focus on the long-term outcomes of this procedure.

The history of surgical excision in lipedema dates back to the 1920s when Charles Dercum, a prominent American neurologist, first described the condition. At that time, surgical interventions were limited, and conservative treatments such as compression stockings and diuretics were the only options available. However, as surgical techniques developed, the use of liposuction became more common.

The first liposuction procedure was performed in 1974 by a French surgeon named Dr. Yves-Gerard Illouz. Since then, the technique has been refined, and different methods have been developed. One of the most common techniques used today is tumescent liposuction. This method involves the injection of a solution containing local anesthetic and epinephrine into the fatty tissue. This solution helps to numb the area and reduce bleeding during the procedure.

During the surgery, small incisions are made in the skin, and a thin, hollow tube called a cannula is inserted into the fatty tissue (Fig. 1). The cannula is attached to a vacuum device, which is used to suction out the fat cells. The goal of the surgery is to remove as much of the diseased tissue as possible while preserving the surrounding healthy tissue.

While liposuction can be an effective treatment for lipedema, there are risks and complications associated with the procedure. These include bleeding, infection, fluid accumulation, and changes in sensation or skin texture. In rare cases, more serious complications such as blood clots or damage to surrounding tissues may occur.

In addition, liposuction is not a cure for lipedema, and there is a risk of recurrence. It is important that patients maintain a healthy lifestyle and continue with conservative treatments such as compression therapy and exercise to minimize the risk of recurrence.

G. Laur, *Lipoedema*, https://doi.org/10.1007/978-981-96-8939-2_26

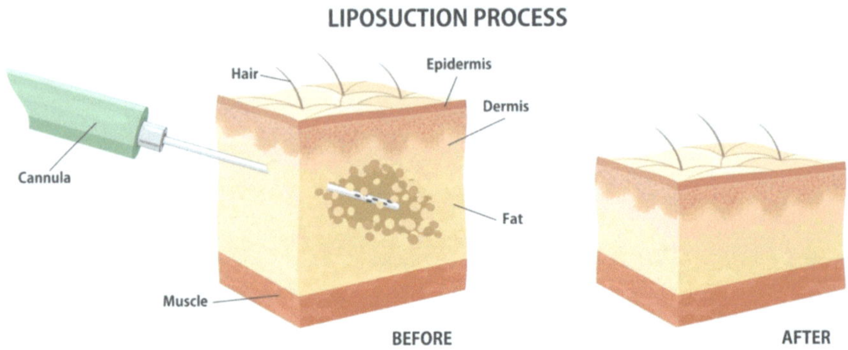

Fig. 1 Diagram of liposuction

Overall, surgical excision is a viable treatment option for patients with lipedema who have not responded to conservative measures. However, it is important that patients discuss the risks and benefits of the procedure with their healthcare provider and choose a qualified and experienced surgeon.

Lipedema is a chronic condition characterized by the symmetrical buildup of adipose tissue in the legs and arms, often leading to pain, mobility issues, and psychological distress. Traditional management strategies have focused on conservative measures such as compression therapy, manual lymphatic drainage, and lifestyle modifications, with varying degrees of success.

However, the introduction of liposuction as a treatment option has marked a significant advancement in the management of lipedema. This surgical approach aims to remove the pathologic fat cells, thereby reducing limb volume, alleviating pain, and improving mobility and quality of life for patients. The role of liposuction in lipedema management has been increasingly recognized, supported by a growing body of evidence that highlights its effectiveness in reducing the symptoms and progression of the disease. Unlike traditional liposuction, which targets cosmetic fat removal, liposuction for lipedema focuses on the removal of fibrotic, diseased fat tissues, necessitating specialized techniques and an understanding of the disease's pathophysiology. This chapter delves into the integration of liposuction into lipedema management, exploring its mechanisms, outcomes, and the evolving understanding of its role as a transformative treatment option for those suffering from this underdiagnosed and often debilitating condition.

Liposuction has emerged as a treatment option in the management of lipedema, a chronic condition characterized by the abnormal accumulation of fat in the lower body, leading to pain, swelling, and mobility issues. The decision to employ liposuction in lipedema management is contingent upon a set of rigorous criteria aimed at ensuring the suitability and safety of the procedure for the patient. These criteria include a definitive diagnosis of lipedema, typically distinguished from similar conditions such as lymphedema and obesity through clinical examination and patient history. Additionally, candidates for liposuction should have a stable weight, as significant weight fluctuations post-surgery can undermine the outcomes of the procedure. Conservative treatments, such as compression therapy, diet, exercise, and manual lymphatic drainage, should have been trialed and found insufficient in managing the symptoms effectively. Furthermore, the patient's overall health and ability to tolerate surgery and anesthesia are critical considerations, alongside a realistic expectation of the surgery's outcomes. It is essential that patients understand that while liposuction can significantly reduce the burden of lipedema fat and alleviate symptoms, it is not a cure for the condition and may require adjunctive therapies for comprehensive management.

Assessing suitability for liposuction treatment in individuals with lipedema involves a multifaceted approach that encompasses clinical evaluation, patient history, and a thorough understanding of the patient's goals and expectations. The initial step involves confirming the diagnosis of lipedema, which is often misdiagnosed as obesity or lymphedema. This distinction is crucial as it informs the treatment strategy and expected outcomes. Clinicians assess the stage of lipedema, the distribution of lipedematous fat, and the presence of symptoms such as pain, tenderness, and mobility limitations. Suitability also hinges on the patient's overall health status, including the absence of contraindications to surgery such as significant cardiovascular or coagulation disorders. Psychological assessment is equally important, ensuring that the patient has realistic expectations regarding the results of the surgery and is prepared for the postoperative care regimen. Moreover, it is vital that the patient has attempted conservative management strategies, such as compression therapy and lifestyle modifications, without satisfactory improvement in symptoms. Through this comprehensive evaluation, healthcare providers can identify candidates for whom liposuction could offer substantial relief from the physical and psychological burdens of lipedema, paving the way for improved quality of life.

The preoperative evaluation and patient selection process for lipedema treatment through liposuction is a critical step to ensure optimal outcomes and patient safety. This process begins with a thorough medical history and physical examination to confirm the diagnosis of lipedema, differentiate it from other conditions, such as lymphedema or obesity, and determine the severity and distribution of lipedematous tissue. Important aspects of the evaluation include documenting the patient's symptomatology, such as pain, bruising, and mobility issues, as well as previous interventions attempted, including diet, exercise, compression therapy, and manual lymphatic drainage. Imaging studies, such as lymphoscintigraphy or MRI, may be utilized to further assess the extent of fat deposition and rule out secondary causes of lymphedema. The patient's overall health, including any comorbid conditions that could affect surgical risk or recovery, is carefully considered. Psychological assessment is also integral to ensure that the patient has realistic expectations of the surgical outcomes and is psychologically prepared for the procedure and its aftermath. Additionally, the patient's commitment to postoperative care, including continued use of compression garments and engagement in a healthy lifestyle, is assessed as part of the selection process. This comprehensive approach ensures that liposuction is offered to those who are most likely to benefit from it, with a clear understanding of the procedure's limitations and potential for significant improvement in quality of life.

The realm of liposuction has evolved significantly, encompassing both traditional and advanced techniques tailored to address various clinical needs, including the management of conditions like lipedema. Traditional liposuction, often referred to as tumescent liposuction, involves the infiltration of a large volume of dilute local anesthesia into subcutaneous fat, followed by the removal of fat using small cannulas through suction. This technique has been lauded for its effectiveness in fat removal and its minimally invasive nature, allowing for outpatient procedures with reduced recovery times. On the other hand, advanced liposuction techniques have expanded the arsenal of options for more specific or challenging cases. Techniques such as ultrasound-assisted liposuction (UAL), power-assisted liposuction (PAL), and laser-assisted liposuction (LAL) leverage technology to enhance fat breakdown and removal. UAL uses ultrasonic energy to liquefy fat cells, making them easier to remove, while PAL employs a mechanically vibrating cannula to break up fat cells with less force, potentially reducing tissue trauma. LAL utilizes laser energy to dissolve fat cells and coagulate small blood vessels, aiming to reduce bleeding and bruising. Each of these techniques offers distinct advantages, including improved precision, reduced recovery times, and enhanced skin tightening effects. The choice of technique is influenced by the patient's specific condition, the volume of fat to be removed, and the surgeon's expertise, ensuring a tailored approach to each patient's needs.

For patients with lipedema considering liposuction, specific considerations are paramount to ensure the effectiveness of the treatment and minimize potential complications. Unlike traditional fat removal, liposuction for lipedema requires a nuanced understanding of the condition's pathology, focusing on removing fibrotic lipedematous tissue while preserving lymphatic structures to prevent exacerbating lymphatic dysfunction. Preoperatively, a detailed mapping of the affected areas is essential to plan the removal of diseased fat deposits strategically. Surgeons specialized in lipedema must employ gentle techniques, such as tumescent liposuction or water-assisted liposuction, to reduce trauma to the tissue and minimize postoperative pain and swelling. The volume of fat removed during a single session may be limited to reduce the risk of fluid shifts and hemodynamic instability. Postoperative care is critical, with an emphasis on early mobilization, lymphatic drainage massage, and the use of compression garments to support recovery and lymphatic flow.

Patients should be informed about the potential need for multiple procedures to achieve optimal results and the importance of maintaining a healthy lifestyle to prevent the progression of lipedema. Tailoring the liposuction approach to address the unique challenges posed by lipedema can significantly improve symptoms, enhance mobility, and positively impact the patient's quality of life.

The customization of liposuction techniques to the individual needs of patients with lipedema is a critical component of achieving optimal outcomes and enhancing patient satisfaction. Lipedema, characterized by its heterogeneity in fat distribution, severity, and symptomatology, necessitates a tailored approach to surgical intervention. This personalized strategy begins with a comprehensive assessment of the patient, including the staging of lipedema, the specific areas affected, the density of fibrotic tissue, and the patient's overall health status and aesthetic goals. Advanced liposuction techniques, such as tumescent, water-assisted, or ultrasound-assisted liposuction, are selected and adapted based on these factors to effectively target and remove the abnormal adipose tissue while minimizing damage to surrounding structures. The volume of fat removed, the choice of anesthesia, and the number of sessions planned are also customized to accommodate the patient's medical history, tolerance for surgery, and recovery capacity. Importantly, postoperative care plans, including compression therapy, manual lymphatic drainage, and physical therapy, are individualized to support healing, promote lymphatic function, and optimize functional outcomes. This patient-centric approach underscores the importance of understanding the unique aspects of lipedema and the need for surgeons to possess specialized skills and knowledge to adapt surgical techniques to the nuanced demands of treating this complex condition.

The rationale for employing liposuction in the treatment of lipedema lies in its targeted approach to reducing the pathologically accumulated fat deposits that are resistant to conventional weight loss methods. Lipedema fat, characterized by its fibrotic nature and abnormal distribution, primarily affects the legs, arms, and in some cases, other areas of the body, leading to pain, mobility issues, and psychosocial distress. Liposuction, specifically techniques such as tumescent or water-assisted liposuction, enables the precise removal of these lipedematous fat cells while minimizing damage to the surrounding tissues, including the lymphatic vessels. This specificity is crucial, as preserving lymphatic integrity prevents worsening of lymphatic dysfunction, a potential complication of lipedema.

The expected benefits and outcomes of liposuction for patients with lipedema extend beyond mere aesthetic improvements. Clinically, patients often report significant reductions in pain and tenderness, improvement in limb mobility, and a decrease in the frequency of bruising episodes. Psychologically, the removal of lipedema fat deposits can lead to improved body image and self-esteem, contributing to overall quality of life enhancements. Furthermore, by alleviating the physical burden of lipedema, liposuction can facilitate patients' engagement in physical activities and exercise, promoting healthier lifestyles and potentially slowing the progression of the disease. Although liposuction is not a cure for lipedema, it represents a critical component of a comprehensive treatment strategy, offering patients symptomatic relief and a path toward a more active and fulfilling life.

Water-assisted tumescent liposuction (WATL) is a refined, minimally invasive procedure designed to extract lipedematous fat with precision, minimizing tissue trauma and promoting a faster recovery. The procedure commences with the infusion of a tumescent solution—comprising saline, lidocaine, and epinephrine—into the subcutaneous tissue.

This solution facilitates the swelling and firming of the fat, reducing bleeding by causing vasoconstriction and providing local anesthesia. Following tumescence, a water-jet-assisted device is used to simultaneously infuse saline solution and aspirate the fat cells with gentle force. This technique allows for the selective removal of fat while preserving the integrity of surrounding tissues, including blood vessels and lymphatic channels.

Anesthesia considerations in WATL are significant, as the tumescent technique typically reduces the need for general anesthesia, thereby mitigating associated risks and promoting quicker postoperative recovery. Patients may undergo the procedure under local anesthesia, supplemented by sedation as needed, which contributes to the safety profile of WATL, especially important for individuals with lipedema who may have an increased sensitivity to pain or a predisposition to lymphatic complications.

The minimally invasive nature of WATL, characterized by small incisions and the gentle removal of fat, plays a role in its effectiveness and safety. This approach reduces the risk of postoperative complications, such as infections and lymphedema exacerbation, and facilitates a quicker return to daily activities. The precision of water-assisted liposuction, coupled with the benefits of the tumescent technique, makes it an ideal choice for managing lipedema, offering patients symptomatic relief and an enhanced quality of life with reduced surgical risks.

Liposuction has been increasingly recognized for its efficacy in managing lipedema, with both short-term and long-term results, highlighting its potential to significantly improve patient outcomes. In the short term, patients often experience a notable reduction in the volume of the affected limbs, leading to immediate improvements in contour and a decrease in physical discomfort. The reduction in excess fatty tissue can alleviate the constant pressure on joints and lymphatic vessels, resulting in diminished pain and enhanced mobility. This immediate relief is frequently accompanied by a psychological boost, as patients observe visible changes in their body shape and experience fewer limitations in physical activities.

Long-term outcomes of liposuction for lipedema are particularly promising, with sustained reductions in limb volume and improvements in symptoms. Over time, patients report a lasting decrease in the frequency and intensity of pain, which can be attributed to the removal of fibrotic fatty tissues that contribute to discomfort and inflammation. Improved mobility and physical function are sustained benefits, enabling patients to engage more actively in daily activities and exercise, which further supports lymphatic health and overall well-being. Additionally, the aesthetic improvements achieved through liposuction can have profound effects on self-esteem and mental health, contributing to a better quality of life.

The impact of liposuction on lipedema symptoms extends beyond physical relief, fostering a cycle of positive outcomes. As pain is reduced and mobility is enhanced, patients are more likely to maintain an active lifestyle, which can help in managing the progression of lipedema. However, it is important to note that liposuction is not a cure for lipedema; it is a treatment that addresses the symptoms and can significantly improve the patient's quality of life. Continuous management through compression therapy, diet, exercise, and possibly additional liposuction sessions may be necessary to maintain the outcomes and manage the chronic aspects of lipedema.

Liposuction, while highly effective for the treatment of lipedema, carries inherent surgical risks, including infection, bleeding, and adverse reactions to anesthesia. Unique to patients with lipedema is the potential exacerbation of lymphatic dysfunction, leading to lymphedema, and uneven contours or asymmetry due to the uneven removal of fatty tissues. To minimize these risks, meticulous surgical planning, technique, and postoperative management are essential. Surgeons must employ gentle liposuction techniques, such as tumescent or water-assisted liposuction, which are less traumatic to the lymphatic vessels and surrounding tissues. Postoperative care is important in managing complications; this includes the use of compression garments to reduce swelling and support the lymphatic system, as well as engaging in manual lymphatic drainage therapy to enhance lymphatic function and prevent fluid accumulation. Monitoring for signs of infection and managing pain effectively are also critical components of postoperative care. For patients with lipedema, a thorough preoperative assessment to identify any underlying conditions that may affect healing is crucial. Tailoring the liposuction procedure to the individual's specific needs, coupled with a comprehensive approach to postoperative care, significantly reduces the risk of complications and maximizes the safety and efficacy of liposuction for lipedema management.

The recovery timeline and expectations following liposuction for lipedema vary, reflecting the individualized nature of the procedure and the patient's condition. Generally, initial recovery is observed within the first few weeks, during which significant swelling and bruising may occur, gradually subsiding over time. Most patients can resume light daily activities within a few days post-surgery, with a return to a full range of activities typically advised after 4–6 weeks, contingent upon the extent of the liposuction and individual healing processes. The critical role of compression garments cannot be overstated in this period; they are essential for reducing swelling, facilitating lymphatic drainage, and shaping the contours of the treated areas. These garments should be worn continuously for a specified duration, often several weeks to months, as advised by the surgeon.

Follow-up care is paramount to monitor the healing progress, manage any complications promptly, and assess the efficacy of the treatment in alleviating lipedema symptoms. During these visits, adjustments to compression garment use and guidance on lymphatic drainage exercises or massage may be provided to enhance recovery outcomes. Long-term expectations include a gradual improvement in symptoms such as pain reduction and enhanced mobility, with the full impact of the liposuction becoming evident as the body adapts and stabilizes, typically within 6–12 months post-surgery. It is crucial for patients to have realistic expectations and understand that while liposuction significantly reduces the burden of lipedematous fat and improves quality of life, ongoing management may be necessary to address the chronic nature of lipedema. Through adherence to postoperative guidelines, including the use of compression garments and active participation in follow-up care, patients can optimize their recovery and outcomes from liposuction in the management of lipedema.

The recovery timeline and expectations following liposuction for lipedema vary, reflecting the individualized nature of the procedure and the patient's condition. Generally, initial recovery is observed within the first few weeks, during which significant swelling and bruising may occur, gradually subsiding over time. Most patients can resume light daily activities within a few days post-surgery, with a return to a full range of activities typically advised after 4–6 weeks, contingent upon the extent of the liposuction and individual healing processes.

The critical role of compression garments cannot be overstated in this period; they are essential for reducing swelling, facilitating lymphatic drainage, and shaping the contours of the treated areas. These garments should be worn continuously for a specified duration, often several weeks to months, as advised by the surgeon.

Follow-up care is paramount to monitor the healing progress, manage any complications promptly, and assess the efficacy of the treatment in alleviating lipedema symptoms. During these visits, adjustments to compression garment use and guidance on lymphatic drainage exercises or massage may be provided to enhance recovery outcomes. Long-term expectations include a gradual improvement in symptoms such as pain reduction and enhanced mobility, with the full impact of the liposuction becoming evident as the body adapts and stabilizes, typically within 6–12 months post-surgery. It is crucial for patients to have realistic expectations and understand that while liposuction significantly reduces the burden of lipedematous fat and improves quality of life, ongoing management may be necessary to address the chronic nature of lipedema. Through adherence to postoperative guidelines, including the use of compression garments and active participation in follow-up care, patients can optimize their recovery and outcomes from liposuction in the management of lipedema.

Integrating liposuction with compression therapy, manual lymphatic drainage (MLD), and exercise forms a comprehensive treatment approach for lipedema, enhancing outcomes and addressing the multifaceted nature of the condition. Post-liposuction, compression therapy plays a crucial role in reducing swelling, improving lymphatic drainage, and aiding in the reshaping of the treated areas, thereby facilitating recovery and optimizing the surgical results. Manual lymphatic drainage, a specialized form of massage that encourages the natural circulation of the lymph fluid, is essential for managing lipedema both pre- and post-surgery. MLD can significantly reduce postoperative swelling, accelerate healing, and prevent fibrosis, making it a vital component of the post-liposuction care regimen. Exercise, tailored to the patient's capabilities and recovery stage, is fundamental in maintaining the functionality of the lymphatic system, improving overall vascular health, and promoting weight management. Engaging in low-impact activities such as swimming, walking, or cycling can enhance lymphatic flow, reduce the risk of lipedema progression, and improve joint mobility and pain. This integrated approach not only addresses the immediate surgical recovery needs but also contributes to the long-term management of lipedema, supporting patient well-being and quality of life. By combining liposuction with compression therapy, MLD, and exercise, patients can achieve more significant, sustainable improvements, mitigating the symptoms of lipedema and fostering a proactive stance toward managing this chronic condition.

Post-liposuction improvements in body image and quality of life for patients with lipedema are profound and multifaceted, underscoring the psychological and social benefits of this surgical intervention. Liposuction, by significantly reducing the diseased fat deposits characteristic of lipedema, directly impacts patients' perceptions of their bodies, leading to enhanced body image and self-esteem. This transformation is not merely physical; the reduction in limb volume and improvement in body contours can alleviate the social stigma and emotional distress associated with the condition, fostering a more positive self-image and confidence. Moreover, the alleviation of lipedema symptoms such as pain, heaviness, and mobility restrictions through liposuction contributes significantly to improving quality of life.

Patients often report increased physical activity levels, participation in social activities, and overall life satisfaction post-surgery, highlighting the interconnection between physical improvements and psychological well-being. The enhanced ability to engage in everyday activities without the previous physical and emotional burdens of lipedema can lead to a renewed sense of normalcy and autonomy. However, it is crucial to recognize the importance of ongoing support and counseling for some patients to address long-standing body image issues and adjust to their new physical selves. Thus, liposuction for lipedema offers not just a physical remedy but also a pathway to psychological recovery and a better quality of life, emphasizing the holistic benefits of addressing both the physical and emotional aspects of the condition.

Long-term follow-up care is essential in the comprehensive management of lipedema, especially after liposuction, to ensure sustained management of the condition and the longevity of treatment outcomes. Regular follow-up visits allow healthcare providers to monitor the progression of lipedema and assess the need for potential revisions or additional interventions. These sessions are critical for evaluating the effectiveness of liposuction in reducing lipedema symptoms, such as pain and mobility issues, and in detecting any changes in the condition that may require further treatment. Follow-up care also offers an opportunity to reinforce and adjust individualized management plans, including ongoing compression therapy, manual lymphatic drainage (MLD), and exercise programs, which are pivotal in maintaining the results achieved through liposuction. Strategies for maintaining outcomes over time include patient education on lifestyle modifications, such as nutrition and weight management, to prevent further accumulation of lipedematous fat and to support overall health. Moreover, psychological support may be provided as part of long-term care to address body image issues and enhance the patient's quality of life. By emphasizing the importance of long-term follow-up care, healthcare providers can support patients in navigating the chronic nature of lipedema, ensuring that they continue to benefit from the initial treatment and maintain an improved quality of life.

Liposuction plays a transformative role in the management of lipedema, offering patients a potential reduction in the chronic symptoms and physical limitations associated with this condition. By selectively targeting and removing the pathologically accumulated fat that is unresponsive to diet and exercise, liposuction provides significant relief from pain, improves mobility, and enhances body contour, thereby improving overall quality of life. However, the decision to proceed with liposuction requires a careful balancing of benefits and risks, tailored to the individual patient's health status, stage of lipedema, and personal goals. This necessitates a thorough preoperative evaluation to assess suitability for surgery, consider potential complications, and ensure realistic expectations of the outcomes.

The importance of comprehensive care in the treatment of lipedema with liposuction cannot be overstated. A multidisciplinary approach, incorporating postoperative care such as compression therapy, manual lymphatic drainage (MLD), and personalized exercise programs, is critical for optimizing surgical outcomes, minimizing the risk of complications, and managing the chronic aspects of lipedema. Additionally, long-term follow-up care is essential for monitoring the patient's progress, addressing any emerging needs, and providing ongoing support. This holistic approach underscores the necessity of viewing liposuction not merely as a standalone intervention but as a component of a broader, integrated treatment strategy aimed at addressing the multifaceted challenges of lipedema.

Through this comprehensive framework, liposuction emerges as a valuable tool in the armamentarium against lipedema, offering patients a path toward improved physical and psychological well-being.

Suggested Reading

Dadras M, Mallinger PJ, Corterier CC, Theodosiadi S, Ghods M. Liposuction in the treatment of lipedema: a longitudinal study. *Arch Plast Surg*. 2017;44(4):324–331

Halk AB, Damstra RJ. First Dutch guidelines on lipedema using the international classification of functioning, disability and health. *Phlebology*. 2017;32(3):152–159

Buck DW, 2nd, Herbst KL. Lipedema: a relatively common disease with extremely common misconceptions. *Plast Reconstr Surg Glob Open*. 2016;4(9):e1043

Wollina U, Heinig B. Treatment of lipedema by low-volume micro-cannular liposuction in tumescent anesthesia: Results in 111 patients. *Dermatol Ther*. 2019;32(2):e12820

Reich-Schupke S, Schmeller W, Brauer WJ, et al. S1 guidelines: lipedema. *J Dtsch Dermatol Ges*. 2017;15(7):758–767

Warren Peled A, Kappos EA. Lipedema: diagnostic and management challenges *Int J Women Health*. 2016;8:389–395

Felson S. Lipedema. *WebMD* 2017; https://www.webmd.com/women/guide/lipedema-symptoms-treatment-causes#1.

Wounds UK. Best practice guidelines: the management of lipoedema. London (UK): Wounds UK; 2017: https://www.lipoedema.co.uk/wp-content/uploads/2017/05/WUK_Lipoedema-BPS_Web.pdf. Accessed 2019 May 28.

Schmeller W, Hueppe M, Meier-Vollrath I. Tumescent liposuction in lipoedema yields good long-term results. *Br J Dermatol*. 2012;166(1):161–168

Basic overview of liposuction for lipedema. *Lipedma* https://www.lipedema.net/overview-liposuction-lipedema.html.

Rapprich S, Dingler A, Podda M. Liposuction is an effective treatment for lipedema-results of a study with 25 patients. *J Dtsch Dermatol Ges*. 2011;9(1):33–40

Baumgartner A, Hueppe M, Schmeller W. Long-term benefit of liposuction in patients with lipoedema: a follow-up study after an average of 4 and 8 years. *Br J Dermatol*. 2016;174(5):1061–1067

Fetzer A. Specialist approaches to managing lipoedema. *Br J Community Nurs*. 2016;Suppl:S30–35

Rapprich S, Baum S, Kaak I, Kottmann T, Podda M. Treatment of lipoedema using liposuction: results of our own surveys. *Phlebologie*. 2015;44(3):121–132.

Downs SH, Black N. The feasibility of creating a checklist for the assessment of the methodological quality both of randomised and non-randomised studies of health care interventions.

J Epidemiol Community Health. 1998;52(6):377–384. http://www.ncbi.nlm.nih.gov/pmc/articles/PMC1756728/pdf/v052p00377.pdf. Accessed 2019 Jun 07

Agree Next Steps Consortium. The AGREE II Instrument. Hamilton (ON): AGREE Enterprise; 2017: https://www.agreetrust.org/wp-content/uploads/2017/12/AGREE-II-Users-Manual-and-23-item-Instrument-2009-Update-2017.pdf. Accessed 2019 Jun 07.

Liberati A, Altman DG, Tetzlaff J, et al. The PRISMA statement for reporting systematic reviews and meta-analyses of studies that evaluate health care interventions: explanation and elaboration. *J Clin Epidemiol*. 2009;62(10):e1–e34

Wollina U. Lipedema-an update. *Dermatol Ther*. 2019;32(2):e12805

Holistic Management

Associated Cardiovascular Comorbidities

Lipedema is a chronic and often underdiagnosed condition characterized by the pathological accumulation of adipose tissue, primarily in the lower extremities, leading to pain, tenderness, and swelling. Unlike typical fat distribution, lipedema fat is symmetrically distributed and does not improve with weight loss efforts. While the exact etiology remains unclear, hormonal changes and genetic predispositions are thought to play significant roles in its development. The condition predominantly affects women and often begins or worsens at puberty, pregnancy, or menopause. Beyond the physical manifestations, lipedema may have a potential connection with cardiovascular disorders. The excessive fat accumulation can lead to venous insufficiency, a condition where the flow of blood through the veins is inadequate, causing blood to pool in the legs. This can increase the risk of varicose veins and, in more severe cases, chronic venous insufficiency, which is a risk factor for cardiovascular disease. Additionally, the chronic inflammation associated with lipedema can contribute to endothelial dysfunction, a key factor in the development of atherosclerosis. The impaired lymphatic drainage seen in lipedema can further exacerbate cardiovascular strain by contributing to fluid retention and increased leg volume, potentially elevating blood pressure. Recognizing and addressing lipedema through a multidisciplinary approach is crucial not only for alleviating its direct symptoms but also for mitigating its potential impact on cardiovascular health. This underscores the importance of early diagnosis and comprehensive management strategies that encompass lifestyle modifications, compression therapy, and, in some cases, pharmacological or surgical interventions.

Cardiovascular comorbidities that might be seen with increased prevalence among individuals with lipedema include venous insufficiency, varicose veins, and, potentially, an elevated risk of developing conditions related to systemic inflammation and obesity, such as hypertension, atherosclerosis, and coronary artery disease. The relationship between lipedema and these cardiovascular conditions could be attributed to several factors:

G. Laur, *Lipoedema*, https://doi.org/10.1007/978-981-96-8939-2_27

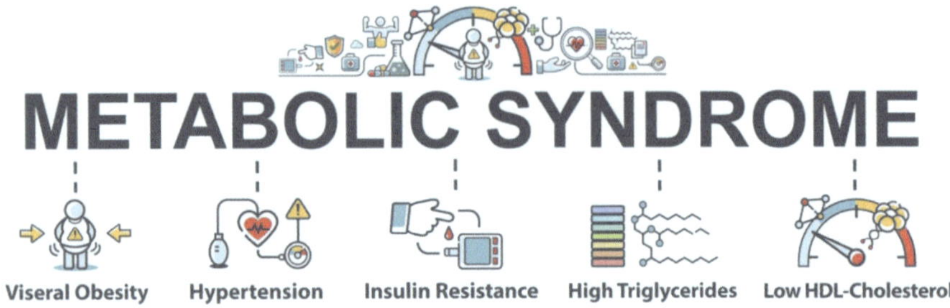

Fig. 1 Key features of metabolic syndrome

1. Venous Insufficiency and Varicose Veins: The excessive accumulation of fat in the legs can exert pressure on the venous system, impairing venous return and leading to venous insufficiency and varicose veins.
2. This venous dysfunction can exacerbate swelling and pain, further limiting mobility and physical activity, which are key for cardiovascular health.
3. Inflammation: Lipedema tissue may be associated with chronic inflammation, which is a known risk factor for various cardiovascular diseases, including atherosclerosis, which can lead to coronary artery disease and stroke.
4. Obesity and Metabolic Syndrome (Fig. 1): While lipedema is distinct from obesity, many individuals with lipedema are also overweight or obese, potentially due to decreased mobility and the psychological impact of the disease, such as depression and anxiety, leading to increased food intake for emotional comfort. The presence of obesity and metabolic syndrome, which includes a cluster of conditions such as high blood pressure, high blood sugar, excess body fat around the waist, and abnormal cholesterol levels, significantly increases the risk for cardiovascular disease.

Despite these associations, it is crucial to note that lipedema and its connection to cardiovascular comorbidities is an area still in need of further research. Studies focusing on the cardiovascular risks specific to lipedema are necessary to understand fully the extent of these comorbidities and to develop targeted interventions to reduce cardiovascular risk in this population. Clinicians managing patients with lipedema should be vigilant for signs of cardiovascular issues and consider comprehensive, multidisciplinary approaches that address both lipedema symptoms and associated comorbidities to optimize health outcomes.

Hypertension, or high blood pressure, is a common comorbidity in patients with lipedema. The relationship between high blood pressure (hypertension) and lipedema is an area of increasing interest within medical research, due to the potential implications for the management and treatment of individuals suffering from lipedema. Lipedema is characterized by the pathological accumulation of fat in the lower extremities, leading to pain, swelling, and mobility issues. This condition predominantly affects women and can often be mistaken for simple obesity or lymphedema.

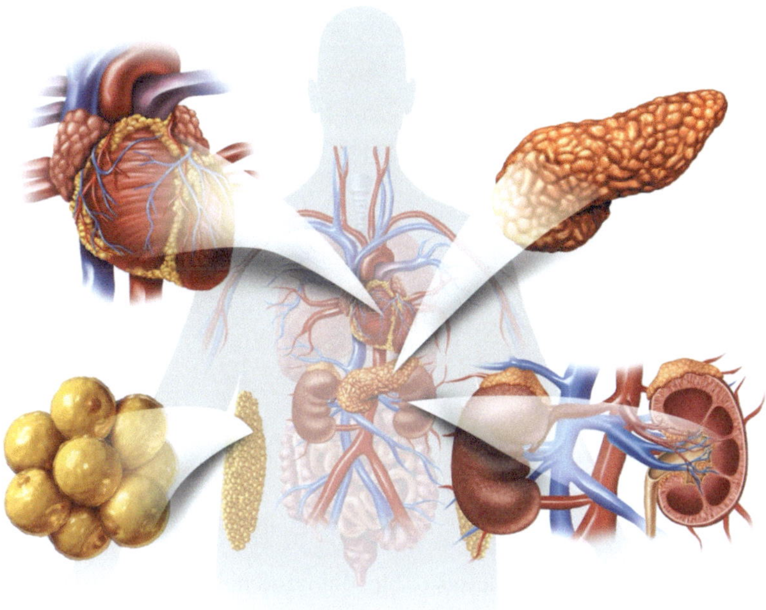

Fig. 2 The main area of impact by metabolic syndrome

Hypertension as a comorbidity in patients with lipedema may not be directly caused by lipedema itself but can result from several interconnected factors common in patients with lipedema. First, the chronic pain and reduced mobility associated with lipedema can lead to a sedentary lifestyle, contributing to weight gain and obesity, which are well-established risk factors for high blood pressure. Furthermore, the excessive adipose tissue characteristic of lipedema can contribute to systemic inflammation and increased oxidative stress, conditions that have been linked to endothelial dysfunction and, subsequently, elevated blood pressure.

Moreover, the psychological stress of living with a chronic, often misdiagnosed, and visually stigmatizing condition like lipedema can exacerbate risk factors for hypertension. Stress is known to contribute to high blood pressure through mechanisms involving the nervous and endocrine systems.

While specific studies focusing on the prevalence of hypertension within the lipedema population are limited, it is clear that the condition's indirect effects on lifestyle, mental health, and systemic inflammation could contribute to an increased risk of developing high blood pressure. Therefore, managing lipedema with a holistic approach that includes weight management, stress reduction techniques, and regular physical activity is crucial not only for addressing the direct symptoms of lipedema but also for mitigating the risk of developing comorbid conditions such as hypertension. Collaborative care involving vascular specialists, physiotherapists, dietitians, and mental health professionals can offer a comprehensive strategy to manage both lipedema and its associated risks (Fig. 2).

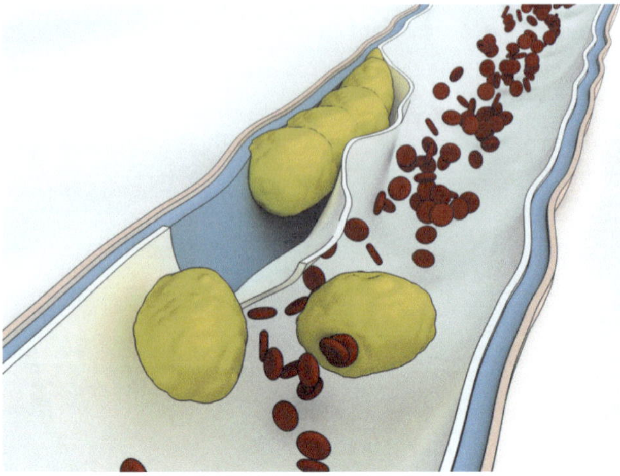

Fig. 3 Lobule of fat reaching the systemic system

Dyslipidemia, or abnormal levels of blood lipids (cholesterol and triglycerides), is also sometimes associated with lipedema. The connection between dyslipidemia and lipedema highlights the intricate interplay between adipose tissue dysfunction and lipid metabolism, raising important considerations for the management and treatment of individuals with lipedema. Dyslipidemia, characterized by abnormal lipid levels in the blood, including elevated total cholesterol, low-density lipoprotein (LDL) cholesterol, triglycerides, and decreased high-density lipoprotein (HDL) cholesterol, is a well-known risk factor for cardiovascular disease. Lipedema, with its pathological fat accumulation primarily in the lower extremities, may predispose individuals to dyslipidemia through several mechanisms (Fig. 3).

First, the adipose tissue in lipedema is often resistant to typical weight loss interventions, leading to chronic obesity, which is closely associated with dyslipidemia.

The excessive and abnormal fat tissue in lipedema may contribute to altered secretion of adipokines and inflammatory cytokines, which can affect lipid metabolism and lead to the development of dyslipidemia. Additionally, the impaired lymphatic drainage and circulatory issues associated with lipedema can exacerbate adipose tissue hypoxia and inflammation, further disrupting lipid homeostasis.

While direct research into the prevalence of dyslipidemia specifically within the lipedema population is limited, the potential for increased cardiovascular risk through dyslipidemic pathways suggests the need for comprehensive lipid management as part of lipedema treatment plans. This includes routine monitoring of lipid profiles in individuals diagnosed with lipedema, along with lifestyle modifications such as diet and exercise, and potentially pharmacological interventions to manage dyslipidemia. Given the complex relationship between lipedema, adipose tissue dysfunction, and lipid metabolism, interdisciplinary approaches involving endocrinologists, lipidologists, and specialists in lipedema are essential for effective management and reduction of cardiovascular risk in this population.

Cardiovascular disease, including heart disease and stroke, is a major comorbidity in patients with lipedema. The link between lipedema and CVD risk factors such as hypertension, dyslipidemia, and insulin resistance may contribute to the increased risk of CVD in these patients. The relationship between cardiovascular disease (CVD) and lipedema is a critical area of concern and investigation due to the potential for increased morbidity among individuals with lipedema. Lipedema, characterized by the disproportionate accumulation of adipose tissue in the lower body, presents a unique set of challenges that may indirectly contribute to the risk of developing cardiovascular diseases, including coronary artery disease, hypertension, and venous insufficiency.

One of the primary considerations in the connection between lipedema and cardiovascular disease is the chronic inflammatory state induced by the pathological adipose tissue characteristic of lipedema. This state of inflammation can contribute to endothelial dysfunction, a precursor to atherosclerosis, thereby increasing the risk of coronary artery disease. Additionally, the excess body weight associated with advanced lipedema can place a significant strain on the heart, leading to an increased risk of hypertension and left ventricular hypertrophy, conditions that further exacerbate the risk of cardiovascular complications.

Moreover, the mechanical effects of the excess adipose tissue in individuals with lipedema can impair lymphatic drainage and venous return, leading to chronic venous insufficiency, a condition that not only contributes to the discomfort and mobility issues associated with lipedema but also increases the risk of venous thromboembolism (VTE), a significant cardiovascular concern.

Despite these potential connections, direct evidence linking lipedema with an increased incidence of cardiovascular disease remains limited, necessitating further research in this area. However, the theoretical risk underscores the importance of comprehensive management strategies for individuals with lipedema, aimed not only at managing the symptoms of lipedema itself but also at mitigating the potential risk factors for cardiovascular disease. This includes weight management, physical activity, compression therapy to improve lymphatic drainage and venous return, and regular monitoring for signs of cardiovascular complications.

An interdisciplinary approach, involving cardiologists, vascular specialists, and clinicians familiar with the management of lipedema, is essential to address both the direct impacts of lipedema and the associated cardiovascular risks, aiming to improve overall health outcomes for individuals with this condition.

Sleep apnea, a condition in which breathing is interrupted during sleep, is also associated with lipedema. This may be due to the increased weight and adiposity associated with lipedema, which can contribute to the development of sleep apnea. Sleep apnea, a condition characterized by repeated interruptions in breathing during sleep, presents a significant concern for patients with lipedema, a chronic disorder marked by abnormal and excessive fat accumulation in the lower body. This intersection of conditions suggests a complex interplay between the physical manifestations of lipedema and the risk factors associated with sleep apnea.

The accumulation of adipose tissue in individuals with lipedema, especially when accompanied by obesity, can exacerbate the risk of developing obstructive sleep apnea (OSA). OSA occurs when the muscles of the throat relax excessively during sleep, leading to a temporary blockage of the airway. In individuals with lipedema, the distribution of fat around the neck and upper body may contribute to airway narrowing, increasing the likelihood of apnea events. Furthermore, the inflammatory state induced by lipedema's abnormal adipose tissue can contribute to the systemic inflammation observed in sleep apnea, compounding cardiovascular risks and metabolic disturbances.

Sleep apnea in patients with lipedema not only affects their cardiovascular health, increasing the risk of hypertension, heart disease, and stroke but also impacts their quality of life, contributing to fatigue, daytime sleepiness, and cognitive effects such as impaired memory and concentration. These symptoms can further limit the individual's ability to engage in physical activity, compounding the challenges of weight management and potentially exacerbating the symptoms of lipedema.

Given the potential for sleep apnea to contribute to both the morbidity and quality of life in individuals with lipedema, it is crucial for healthcare providers to screen for and address sleep apnea as part of the comprehensive management of lipedema. This may include interventions such as weight management, the use of continuous positive airway pressure (CPAP) therapy, and lifestyle modifications aimed at improving sleep hygiene and reducing the impact of sleep apnea. An interdisciplinary approach, involving sleep specialists, nutritionists, and therapists familiar with lipedema, is essential to provide holistic care and improve health outcomes for patients affected by both conditions.

The connection between a patent foramen ovale (PFO) and lipedema is not direct, as these conditions originate from fundamentally different physiological processes. Lipedema is characterized by the abnormal accumulation of fat, primarily in the legs and arms, and is associated with pain, tenderness, and easy bruising. It is a chronic condition that predominantly affects women and is believed to have a genetic component. On the other hand, a PFO is a congenital heart defect that results from the foramen ovale—a natural opening in the fetal heart—failing to close after birth.

While there is no established causal link between PFO and lipedema, considering the systemic nature of both conditions, it is plausible that individuals with lipedema could experience complications that intersect with the presence of a PFO. For example, lipedema can lead to secondary conditions such as obesity and venous insufficiency, which may increase the risk of deep vein thrombosis (DVT). In the presence of a PFO, there is a potential risk for paradoxical embolism, where a clot formed in the venous system could pass through the PFO to the arterial system, potentially leading to a stroke or other systemic embolic events.

However, this scenario remains speculative and would likely require a constellation of predisposing factors. The management of patients with lipedema and a PFO would thus be centered on treating the symptoms of lipedema to reduce its progression and associated risks, alongside monitoring and possibly addressing the PFO if it poses a significant risk of paradoxical embolism, especially in patients with a history of unexplained thromboembolic events. As always, a multidisciplinary approach tailored to the individual's specific conditions and risks is advisable for optimal management and prevention of complications.

Fat embolism syndrome is a disabling complication that can range from mild lightheadedness to respiratory failure, neurocognitive deficit, and death. It is often associated with an undiagnosed perforated foramen ovale (PFO), also known as patent foramen ovale (PFO). PFO is a potentially life-threatening condition that patients often do not receive medical advice or attention until it is too late. More than 25% of adults have a PFO, which represents the most common right-to-left shunt by encompassing 95% of atrial septal abnormalities. Fat embolism following liposuction occurs in 10–15% of patients with PFO, even when appropriate prevention strategies have been implemented.

One of the most common clinical presentations of PFO is medically resistant migraine, which adversely affects the patient's quality of life and productivity. Liposuction complications are strongly correlated with the amount of fat removed during each liposuction procedure, and the rate of risk for these complications increases by up to three times more per procedure. High BMI or increased weight with PFO is a potential risk factor for not only liposuction but any surgical procedure. Current consensus is that PFO screening should not be done routinely except after cryptogenic stroke. There are no current guidelines for screening regarding surgery types to prevent stroke or death.

Perforated/patent foramen ovale (PFO) is a hole in the heart, with two types: atrial septal defect (ASD) and PFO. The physiopathology by which PFO promotes migraine is unclear, but one suggested hypothesis is that blood that should be filtered within the lungs is shunted from right to left, bypassing the pulmonary vascular bed and heading toward the eye and the brain. Among migraine patients, PFOs have been present up to 88% of respondents.

Up to 45% of ischemic strokes do not have identifiable causes and are referred to as cryptogenic strokes. Numerous mechanisms have been proposed, with paradoxical embolism through a PFO being the most likely stroke mechanism. Patent foramen ovale increases the risk of arterial embolic events, including transient ischemic attack (TIA), arterial ischemia, and heart attack. This is likely feasible when a blood clot or solid particles in the venous side of the circulation move from the right side of the heart to the left through the PFO and travel to the brain, causing a stroke or a coronary artery causing a heart attack.

Patients younger than 55 years of age who have a cryptogenic stroke are more likely to have a PFO and also more likely to have a deep vein thrombosis (DVT). In rare cases, a patent foramen ovale can cause a significant amount of blood to bypass the lungs, resulting in hypoxemia. PFO-mediated hypoxemia occurs when deoxygenated venous blood from the right atrium enters and mixes with oxygenated arterial blood in the left atrium.

Paradoxical embolism, a phenomenon characterized by the Valsalva maneuver during diving, can lead to syncope or life-threatening strokes. This phenomenon occurs when the pressure differential between the arterial left side and the right atrium is higher than the venous right side, causing the right atrium to fill before the left atrium. The peak time for bubble liberation is 30–60 minutes post-dive, corresponding to the time when divers climb back to the boat, lifting heavy scuba-related kit, and unconsciously performing the Valsalva maneuver.

Acute ischemic stroke has also been seen in patients with renal cell carcinoma. Tumor emboli rarely cause stroke and myocardial infarction, but in the context of PFO, they have been responsible for dramatic aftermaths. Lung carcinoma has been registered as the most common source of coronary malignant tumor emboli, while renal cell carcinoma is sadly another common source. In this review, a 55-year-old woman who was diagnosed with right renal mass and cavoatrial tumor thrombus was transferred for surgical resection. An intraoperative transesophageal echocardiogram confirmed the absence of tumor thrombus from the inferior vena cava and right atrium and identified a PFO. Upon weaning sedation, she acquired left hemiplegia. The head CT scan revealed extensive hypo-attenuation in the right middle and left posterior cerebral artery territories with associated cerebral edema. In the context of this devastating neurological injury, her family elected to transition to comfort care, and the patient died 7 days after the surgery. This was the first reported case of intra-operative paradoxical embolism in the setting of renal cell carcinoma and PFO.

An amniotic fluid embolus may travel directly from the venous to the arterial circulation via the PFO, leading to multiple cerebral infarctions. Amniotic fluid embolism is a rare syndrome, but complications include cardiorespiratory failure, disseminated intra-vascular coagulation, seizures, neurological deficits, and death. In this review, a 34-year-old woman had amniotic fluid embolism complicated by paradoxical embolism and disseminated intravascular coagulation following an emergency caesarean section. The surgical team reacted quickly and performed a cardiopulmonary bypass with removal of the clot from the atria and closure of the patent foramen ovale.

Fat is another source of embol, and cerebral fat embolism (CFE) occurs after fat emboli enter the arterial circulation. FES is mostly associated with orthopedic trauma, and its clinical presentation can vary greatly, ranging from slight dyspnea, tachycardia, elevated temperature, and petechiae on the skin to severe cases of respiratory distress. Fat emboli can alter their shape to pass through pulmonary precapillary shunts or directly across the pulmonary capillary bed.

Fat embolism (PFO) is a condition that can cause severe cerebral complications, including death, and can be associated with various medical entities such as cryptogenic stroke, migraine with aura, and decompression disease. The prevalence of PFO in the general population is about 25%, which increases the risk of cryptogenic stroke by 40–50% in patients. Autopsy studies have found that patent PFOs with diameters between 0.2 cm and a 0.5 cm maximum dimension were present in 29% of cases, and patent PFO with a diameter of 0.6–1.0 cm was in 6% of them. A second study of 965 patients recorded a PFO incidence of 27.3%, with PFOs varying in size from 1 mm to 19 mm with an average of 4.9 mm.

PFO is also linked to a syndrome that includes debilitating migraine, brain fog, and exercise intolerance. Problems arise when blood contains an embolus, thrombus, or fat, which can lead to cardioembolic cerebrovascular accidents (CVAs) and transient ischemic attacks (TIAs). In the USA, 345,000 patients aged 18–60 years have been diagnosed with PFO-related cryptogenic stroke, which are brain infarctions not linked to arteriosclerosis, but cardio-embolism, and constitute up to 40% of all ischemic strokes.

The prevalence of PFO is about 25% in the general population, which increases the risk of cryptogenic stroke by 40–50% in patients. Autopsy studies have found that patients with a PFO had a significantly higher incidence of ischemic stroke (13% versus 2.2%) and peripheral arterial embolism (15% versus 0%) than patients without a PFO. The literature review of Kellogg et al. revealed that 98% of the patients presented with mental status changes had a relatively good outcome. The overall mortality was 7.4%, and the remaining cases had good outcomes, with intact or mild disability in 72.2% out of the 54 cases. Another study on PFO and ischemic stroke in patients with PE found that ischemic stroke was more frequent in the PFO group (21.4%) than in the non-PFO group (5.5%).

Dermal involvement, such as petechial rash, has been reported in approximately 50–60% of patients; this tends to be transient lasting 4–6 hours. Retinal lesions are seen in 50% of patients and are self-limiting, often disappearing within weeks. PFO is also seen in a quarter of patients with idiopathic pulmonary arterial hypertension and is associated with increased prevalence of severe hypoxemia.

While PFO is becoming recognized worldwide as a cause for cryptogenic cerebral events, there are other situations in which documenting a right to left shunt is important. The accepted belief in the medical community is that the presence of a PFO seems to carry no clinical or survival benefit for normal individuals despite the understanding that PFO has a causative role in several medical entities such as cryptogenic stroke, migraine with aura, and decompression disease. However, diving activities could warrant PFO detection in normal individuals. The presence of a large PFO is linked with severe unexplained decompression sickness through paradoxical gas embolism. The incidence of a first stroke in individuals with and without PFO is similar, which is approximately 1% per year. However, the yearly risk of a recurrent stroke in patients with PFO is raising incrementally by 1% per year.

Transesophageal echocardiography (TOE) is considered the gold standard imaging procedure for patients with suspected right-to-left shunting. However, transcranial Doppler (TCD) imaging overcomes some limitations of TOE, such as its ability to recreate a dynamic recording of paradoxical embolism through an agitated saline contrast medium injected into a peripheral vein during the strain phase of the Valsalva maneuver while the middle cerebral artery is sonographically monitored with Doppler imaging during the release phase. TCD has been found to be more sensitive than TOE to detect a right-to-left shunt due to the conscious state of a patient during a TCD and to effect a forceful Valsalva maneuver compared to the general anesthesia required for a TOE and an inability to perform a Valsalva. The gold standard for PFO detection would be the combination of TOE and TCD.

There are currently two approaches for closure of PFOs: surgical and transcatheter closure. Current practice for treatment is only considered after a dramatic event has occurred, such as stroke related to PFO. However, patients may benefit from closure through early detection. Medical misadventure can be avoided in the context of PFO diagnosis and percutaneous closure where procedures carry a risk of stroke. Patients with a past history of cryptogenic stroke or a long-life history of recurrent medically resistant migraines with aura have a higher risk of neurological adverse events and may benefit from preoperative screening and percutaneous closure of PFO.

PFO closure should be considered for prevention of paradoxical embolism, especially when there is a high safety margin with the procedure when performed by an experienced structural cardiologist. Studies have shown that percutaneous PFO closure significantly reduced the risk of recurrent stroke. More than 300 million surgeries are undertaken worldwide annually, each of them carries a potential risk of perioperative stroke. The prevalence of PFO in the general population, mostly undiagnosed, is around 27%. Studies have shown an increase risk of 60% for ischemic stroke if the patient has a PFO.

Further research is needed to determine the risk of PFO-related stroke, the procedure, and the size of a PFO. Current guidelines do not support PFO screening prior to an episode of stroke. In Australia, PFO would not be closed unless there was a stroke. As of July 1, 2021, Medicare Benefits Schedule changes now preclude PFO closure in the private health setting unless there has been a stroke.

Doctors face a fiduciary responsibility toward patients to ensure a safe surgery in a possible undiagnosed patient with PFO. The current consensus is that screening PFO is not recommended as it could lead to overdiagnosis and unnecessary closure surgery. Carefully evaluating the benefits and risks of PFO detection and then closing a PFO if found can provide a more robust medicolegal position where the patient understands fully all risks associated with their elective procedures.

One study published in the *Journal of Vascular Surgery Cases and Innovative Techniques* in 2020 reported a case of a 49-year-old woman with lipedema and PFO who experienced improvement in her lipedema symptoms after undergoing PFO closure. However, this is only a single case report, and further research is needed to determine if there is a significant association between PFO and lipedema and if PFO closure is a viable treatment option for lipedema.

It should be noted that PFO is a relatively rare congenital heart defect that is often asymptomatic and does not require treatment. If a patient with lipedema is found to have PFO, it is important to consult with a healthcare professional to determine the appropriate management plan based on individual patient needs and medical history.

Overall, patients with lipedema are at increased risk of developing cardiovascular comorbidities. Proper management of these comorbidities, along with the treatment of lipedema itself, is important in order to improve the overall health and quality of life of these patients.

Suggested Reading

Weissleder H., Brauer J.W., Schuchhardt C., Herpertz U. Value of functional lymphoscintigraphy and indirect lymphangiography in lipedema syndrome. *Z. Lymphol.* 1995;**19**:38–41

Amann-Vesti B.R., Franzeck U.K., Bollinger A. Microlymphatic aneurysms in patients with lipedema. *Lymphology.* 2001;**34**:170–175

Szolnoky G., Nagy N., Kovacs R. Complex decongestive physiotherapy decreases capillary fragility in lipedema. *Lymphology.* 2008;**41**:161–166
Wiedner M., Aghajanzadeh D., Richter D.F. Lipödem – Grundlagen und aktuelle Thesen zum Pathomechanismus. *Phlebologie.* 2021;**50**:288–293. https://doi.org/10.1055/a-1109-5870
Schmeller W., Meier-Vollrath I. Lipödem – Aktuelles zu einem weitgehend unbekanntem Krankheitsbild. *Akt. Dermatol.* 2007;**33**:251–260. https://doi.org/10.1055/s-2007-966651
Moulakakis K.G., Kadoglou N.P.E., Antonopoulos C.N., Mylonas S.N., Kakisis J., Papadakis I., Karakitsos P., Liapis C.D. Changes in Arterial Stiffness and N-terminal pro-brain natriuretic peptide Levels after Endovascular Repair of Descending Thoracic Aorta. *Ann. Vasc. Surg.* 2017;**38**:220–226. https://doi.org/10.1016/j.avsg.2016.04.025
Dumor K., Shoemaker-Moyle M., Nistala R., Whaley-Connell A. Arterial Stiffness in Hypertension: An Update. *Curr. Hypertens. Rep.* 2018;**20**:72. https://doi.org/10.1007/s11906-018-0867-x
Vlachopoulos C., Aznaouridis K., Stefanadis C. Prediction of cardiovascular events and all-cause mortality with arterial stiffness: A systematic review and meta-analysis. *J. Am. Coll. Cardiol.* 2010;**55**:1318–1327. https://doi.org/10.1016/j.jacc.2009.10.061
Ben-Shlomo Y., Spears M., Boustred C., May M., Anderson S.G., Benjamin E.J., Boutouyrie P., Cameron J., Chen C.-H., Cruickshank J.K., et al. Aortic pulse wave velocity improves cardiovascular event prediction: An individual participant meta-analysis of prospective observational data from 17,635 subjects. *J. Am. Coll. Cardiol.* 2014;**63**:636–646. https://doi.org/10.1016/j.jacc.2013.09.063
Szolnoky G., Nemes A., Gavallér H., Forster T., Kemény L. Lipedema is associated with increased aortic stiffness. *Lymphology.* 2012;**45**:71–79
Von Elm E., Altman D.G., Egger M., Pocock S.J., Gotzsche P.C., Vandenbroucke J.P. The Strengthening the Reporting of Observational Studies in Epidemiology (STROBE) statement: Guidelines for reporting observational studies. *J. Clin. Epidemiol.* 2008;**61**:344–349. https://doi.org/10.1016/j.jclinepi.2007.11.008
The Reference Values for Arterial Stiffness' Collaboration Determinants of pulse wave velocity in healthy people and in the presence of cardiovascular risk factors: 'Establishing normal and reference values' *Eur. Heart J.* 2010;**31**:2338–2350. https://doi.org/10.1093/eurheartj/ehq165
Del Giorno R., Troiani C., Gabutti S., Stefanelli K., Gabutti L. Comparing oscillometric and tonometric methods to assess pulse wave velocity: A population-based study. *Ann. Med.* 2021;**53**:1–16. https://doi.org/10.1080/07853890.2020.1794538
Weyer C., Yudkin J.S., Stehouwer C.D., Schalkwijk C.G., Pratley R.E., Tataranni P. Humoral markers of inflammation and endothelial dysfunction in relation to adiposity and in vivo insulin action in Pima Indians. *Atherosclerosis.* 2002;**161**:233–242. https://doi.org/10.1016/S0021-9150(01)00626-8
Al-Ghadban S., Cromer W., Allen M., Ussery C., Badowski M., Harris D., Herbst K.L. Dilated Blood and Lymphatic Microvessels, Angiogenesis, Increased Macrophages, and Adipocyte Hypertrophy in Lipedema Thigh Skin and Fat Tissue. *J. Obes.* 2019;**2019**:8747461. doi: https://doi.org/10.1155/2019/8747461
Brenner E., Forner-Cordero I., Faerber G., Rapprich S., Cornely M. Body mass index vs. waist-to-height-ratio in patients with lipohyperplasia dolorosa (vulgo lipedema) *J. Der Dtsch. Dermatol. Ges. = J. Ger. Soc. Dermatol. JDDG.* 2023;**21**:1179–1185. doi: https://doi.org/10.1111/ddg.15182
Nemes A., Kormanyos A., Domsik P., Kalapos A., Kemeny L., Forster T., Szolnoky G. Left ventricular rotational mechanics differ between lipedema and lymphedema: Insights from the three-dimensional speckle tracking echocardiographic MAGYAR-path study. *Lymphology.* 2018;**51**:102–108
Urbano-Moral J.A., Patel A.R., Maron M.S., Arias-Godinez J.A., Pandian N.G. Three-dimensional speckle-tracking echocardiography: Methodological aspects and clinical potential. *Echocardiography.* 2012;**29**:997–1010. https://doi.org/10.1111/j.1540-8175.2012.01773.x
Seo Y., Ishizu T., Aonuma K. Current status of 3-dimensional speckle tracking echocardiography: A review from our experiences. *J. Cardiovasc. Ultrasound.* 2014;**22**:49–57. https://doi.org/10.4250/jcu.2014.22.2.49

Connuck D, Sun JP, Super DM, Kirchner HL, Fradley LG, Harcar-Sevcik RA, Salvator A, Singer L, Mehta SK. Incidence of patent ductus arteriosus and patent foramen ovale in normal infants. Am J Cardiol. 2002 Jan 15;89(2):244–7

Pristipino C, Sievert H, D'Ascenzo F, Louis Mas J, Meier B, Scacciatella P, Hildick-Smith D, Gaita F, Toni D, Kyrle P, Thomson J, Derumeaux G, Onorato E, Sibbing D, Germonpré P, Berti S, Chessa M, Bedogni F, Dudek D, Hornung M, Zamorano J., Evidence Synthesis Team. Eapci Scientific Documents and Initiatives Committee. International Experts. European position paper on the management of patients with patent foramen ovale. General approach and left circulation thromboembolism. Eur Heart J. 2019 Oct 07;40(38):3182–3195

Teshome MK, Najib K, Nwagbara CC, Akinseye OA, Ibebuogu UN. Patent Foramen Ovale: A Comprehensive Review. Curr Probl Cardiol. 2020 Feb;45(2):100392

Meissner I, Whisnant JP, Khandheria BK, Spittell PC, O'Fallon WM, Pascoe RD, Enriquez-Sarano M, Seward JB, Covalt JL, Sicks JD, Wiebers DO. Prevalence of potential risk factors for stroke assessed by transesophageal echocardiography and carotid ultrasonography: the SPARC study. Stroke Prevention: Assessment of Risk in a Community. Mayo Clin Proc. 1999 Sep;74(9):862–9

Kerut EK, Truax WD, Borreson TE, Van Meter KW, Given MB, Giles TD. Detection of right to left shunts in decompression sickness in divers. Am J Cardiol. 1997 01;79(3):377–8

Zoltowska DM, Thind G, Agrawal Y, Gupta V, Kalavakunta JK. May-Thurner Syndrome as a Rare Cause of Paradoxical Embolism in a Patient with Patent Foramen Ovale. Case Rep Cardiol. 2018;2018:3625401

Smart D, Mitchell S, Wilmshurst P, Turner M, Banham N. Joint position statement on persistent foramen ovale (PFO) and diving. South Pacific Underwater Medicine Society (SPUMS) and the United Kingdom Sports Diving Medical Committee (UKSDMC). Diving Hyperb Med. 2015 Jun;45(2):129–31

Correction: Device Closure Versus Medical Therapy Alone for Patent Foramen Ovale. Ann Intern Med. 2018 Sep 18;169(6):428

Giordano M, Gaio G, Santoro G, Palladino MT, Sarubbi B, Golino P, Russo MG. Patent foramen ovale with complex anatomy: Comparison of two different devices (Amplatzer Septal Occluder device and Amplatzer PFO Occluder device 30/35). Int J Cardiol. 2019 Mar 15;279:47–50

Associated Connective Tissue Disorder Comorbidities

Lipedema is a chronic and often misunderstood condition characterized by the abnormal and disproportionate accumulation of fat, primarily in the lower extremities, leading to pain, tenderness, and, in some cases, mobility issues. While the precise etiology of lipedema remains elusive, it is believed to involve a complex interplay of genetic, hormonal, and inflammatory factors. Distinct from obesity, lipedema predominantly affects women and typically manifests or worsens during periods of hormonal change, such as puberty, pregnancy, or menopause.

Emerging research suggests a potential association between lipedema and various connective tissue disorders, highlighting the complexity of lipedema as more than a mere fat storage disorder. Connective tissue disorders, encompassing a broad range of conditions such as Ehlers-Danlos syndrome (EDS), Marfan syndrome, and joint hypermobility syndrome, are characterized by abnormalities in the collagen and elastin that provide structural support and elasticity to the body's tissues. Individuals with lipedema may exhibit symptoms indicative of underlying connective tissue abnormalities, including joint hypermobility, skin hyperextensibility, and a predisposition to bruises and injuries, suggesting a shared pathophysiological foundation.

The potential overlap between lipedema and connective tissue disorders raises important considerations for diagnosis, management, and treatment, underscoring the need for a comprehensive and multidisciplinary approach. Understanding the connections between these conditions can inform more effective strategies to address the complex symptomatology and improve the quality of life for those affected. As research continues to unravel the intricacies of lipedema and its association with connective tissue disorders, it becomes increasingly clear that addressing the full spectrum of the condition requires attention to both its adipose and connective tissue components.

Exploring the underlying biological mechanisms that connect lipedema with connective tissue disorders is a burgeoning area of research that delves into the intricate interplay between adipose tissue dysfunction and connective tissue anomalies. The hypothesis that these conditions are linked suggests that aberrations in the extracellular matrix (ECM), which provides structural and biochemical support to

G. Laur, *Lipoedema*, https://doi.org/10.1007/978-981-96-8939-2_28

surrounding cells, may play a role. In lipedema, the disproportionate accumulation of fat is not merely a result of adiposity but also involves changes in the ECM, leading to fibrosis and impaired lymphatic drainage. Similarly, connective tissue disorders are characterized by defects in the ECM components, such as collagen and elastin, which affect the strength, elasticity, and integrity of connective tissues. This shared feature points to a possible common pathway involving altered ECM remodeling processes that predispose individuals to both lipedema and connective tissue disorders. Additionally, genetic predispositions may influence the synthesis and degradation of ECM proteins, further linking these conditions. Dysregulation of inflammatory pathways and hormonal imbalances, particularly those affecting estrogen, have also been implicated in both lipedema and connective tissue disorder etiologies, suggesting that these factors may contribute to the observed clinical overlap. Understanding these underlying biological mechanisms not only sheds light on the complex nature of lipedema and its association with connective tissue disorders but also opens avenues for targeted therapeutic strategies that address the root causes of these interconnected conditions.

Diagnosing connective tissue disorders (CTDs) in the context of lipedema is a complex process due to the overlapping symptoms and multifaceted nature of both conditions. The diagnostic process involves a comprehensive evaluation that includes clinical assessment, patient history, and genetic testing. The process involves identifying lipedema characteristics, such as joint pain and tenderness, and signs of CTDs, such as hypermobility, skin elasticity, and unusual scarring. The patient's family and medical history is also crucial, including a history of similar symptoms or diagnosed CTDs. Symptom timelines are also essential, particularly in relation to hormonal changes. Genetic testing can be used to confirm certain CTDs, but it is complex and not universally available. Differential diagnosis is crucial, distinguishing between lipedema, lymphedema, obesity, and CTDs based on symptomatology and diagnostic tests. The complexities involved include overlapping symptoms, lack of awareness, variability in presentation, and a multidisciplinary approach. A thorough, patient-centered evaluation and the use of multidisciplinary expertise are essential for accurately diagnosing CTDs in the context of lipedema, guiding effective management and treatment strategies.

Ehlers-Danlos Syndrome (EDS) encompasses a group of hereditary connective tissue disorders characterized by a wide range of clinical manifestations, including hypermobility of the joints, skin hyperextensibility, and tissue fragility. The syndrome is caused by genetic mutations affecting the synthesis and structure of collagen and other extracellular matrix proteins that provide strength and elasticity to the connective tissue throughout the body. EDS is classified into several subtypes, each with distinct genetic causes and clinical presentations, ranging from the hypermobility type, which is often characterized by joint dislocations and chronic pain, to the vascular type, which can involve serious and potentially life-threatening complications such as arterial or organ rupture.

The diagnosis of EDS (Fig. 1) is primarily based on clinical evaluation, including family history, physical examination, and the specific criteria set for each subtype. Genetic testing can confirm the diagnosis for some types of EDS, particularly those

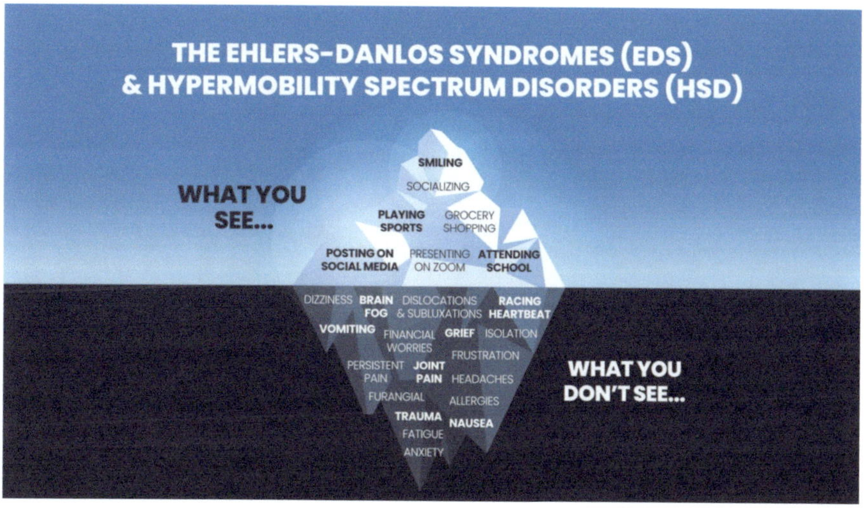

Fig. 1 List of clinical signs of Ehlers-Danlos syndrome

with known genetic markers. However, for the hypermobility type, the most common form of EDS, there is currently no definitive genetic test, and diagnosis is often made based on clinical criteria and the exclusion of other conditions.

Management of EDS is supportive and focuses on preventing complications and managing symptoms. Treatment strategies are tailored to the individual's symptoms and may include physical therapy to strengthen muscles and stabilize joints, pain management, and, in some cases, surgery to repair damaged joints or tissues. Patients may also require monitoring for potential cardiovascular, gastrointestinal, or autonomic dysfunctions, depending on their EDS subtype.

Given the systemic nature of EDS and its potential impact on various body systems, a multidisciplinary approach to care is essential. This approach involves collaboration among specialists in genetics, rheumatology, cardiology, orthopedics, dermatology, and pain management, among others, to address the wide-ranging needs of individuals with EDS. The complexity of EDS underscores the importance of raising awareness and understanding of the condition among both healthcare providers and the public to ensure timely and accurate diagnosis and appropriate management. EDS is often associated with lipedema, and patients with both conditions may have more severe symptoms. The connection between these two conditions is not fully understood, but it is believed that the underlying genetic mutations that cause EDS may also contribute to the development of lipedema.

The intersection of Ehlers-Danlos syndrome (EDS) and lipedema represents a complex clinical challenge, shedding light on the intricate relationship between connective tissue disorders and adipose tissue dysfunctions. EDS is a group of hereditary connective tissue disorders characterized by joint hypermobility, skin hyperextensibility, and tissue fragility. When occurring concomitantly with lipedema, a condition marked by the abnormal accumulation of fat in the lower body and associated pain, the diagnostic

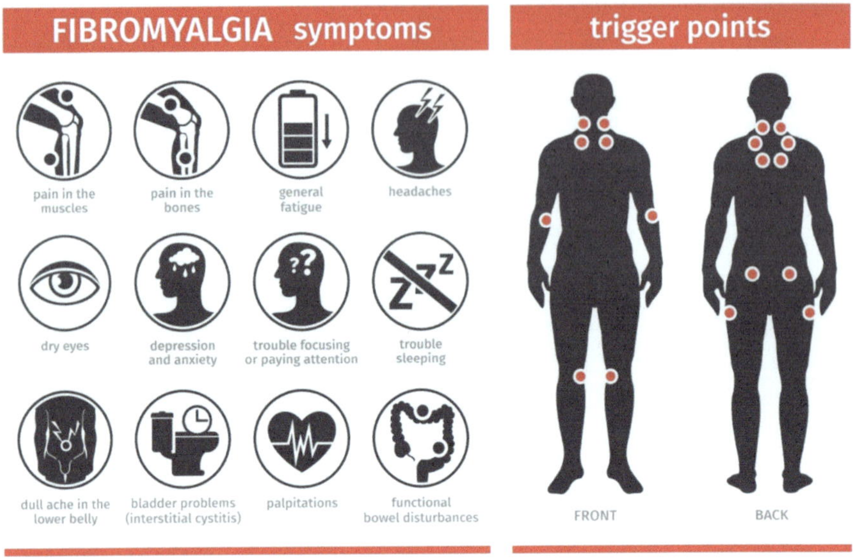

Fig. 2 Clinical signs of fibromyalgia

and management complexities are significantly amplified. Emerging evidence suggests a potential overlap in the pathophysiological mechanisms of EDS and lipedema, particularly in the altered extracellular matrix composition and functionality, which is a hallmark of both conditions. This overlap may contribute to the exacerbation of symptoms such as joint pain, increased susceptibility to bruising, and challenges in wound healing. Moreover, the presence of EDS can complicate the clinical presentation of lipedema, potentially leading to delayed diagnosis or misdiagnosis and vice versa. Understanding the co-occurrence of EDS and lipedema is crucial for tailoring treatment approaches, as individuals with both conditions may require specialized management strategies that address the unique aspects of connective tissue instability and adipose tissue accumulation. This includes a combination of physical therapy to strengthen joints, compression therapy to manage lipedema-related swelling, and careful consideration of surgical options, given the increased risk of complications. Thus, recognizing the confluence of EDS and lipedema is essential for providing comprehensive care and improving the quality of life for affected individuals.

Fibromyalgia (Fig. 2) is a chronic condition characterized by widespread musculoskeletal pain accompanied by fatigue, sleep disturbances, memory issues, and mood disorders. It is recognized for its profound impact on quality of life, affecting millions worldwide. The exact cause of fibromyalgia remains unknown, but it is believed to result from a combination of genetic, neurobiological, and environmental factors leading to abnormal pain processing by the central nervous system. This condition is often triggered by a stressful event, such as physical trauma, surgery, infection, or significant psychological stress, though it may also develop gradually without a clear initiating factor.

Diagnosis of fibromyalgia is challenging, as there is no definitive test for the condition. Physicians rely on patient history, physical examination, and the exclusion of other conditions with similar symptoms to make a diagnosis. The American College of Rheumatology (ACR) criteria, which include widespread pain lasting more than 3 months and the presence of other symptoms such as fatigue and cognitive difficulties, are commonly used in diagnostic processes.

Management of fibromyalgia focuses on symptom relief and improving quality of life. Treatment plans are typically multidisciplinary and may include medications such as pain relievers, antidepressants, and anticonvulsants to reduce pain and improve sleep. Non-pharmacological approaches are equally important, encompassing physical therapy, exercise, stress management techniques, and cognitive-behavioral therapy. Lifestyle modifications, including regular exercise, healthy diet, and sleep hygiene, are also recommended to help manage symptoms.

The complexity of fibromyalgia, coupled with its wide range of symptoms, underscores the importance of a personalized treatment approach. This approach requires close collaboration between patients and their healthcare team, including primary care physicians, rheumatologists, pain specialists, and mental health professionals. Despite the challenges fibromyalgia presents, ongoing research into its causes and treatments offers hope for more effective strategies to manage this condition and improve patient outcomes. Many patients with lipedema also suffer from fibromyalgia, and the two conditions may exacerbate each other. The cause of this association is not fully understood, but it is believed that both conditions may share common underlying mechanisms, such as inflammation and dysfunction of the lymphatic system. The coexistence of fibromyalgia and lipedema presents a particularly challenging clinical scenario, highlighting the complex interplay between chronic pain syndromes and adipose tissue disorders. Fibromyalgia is characterized by widespread musculoskeletal pain accompanied by fatigue, sleep, memory, and mood issues, often co-occurring with other painful conditions. Lipedema, defined by the pathological accumulation of adipose tissue in the lower extremities, manifests with pain, tenderness, and a predisposition to bruising, features that can significantly overlap with fibromyalgia symptoms. This overlap complicates the diagnostic process, as the diffuse pain and tenderness associated with fibromyalgia can mask or mimic the localized pain and adipose tissue irregularities characteristic of lipedema. The shared symptom of chronic pain suggests potential commonalities in the underlying pathophysiological mechanisms, such as dysregulation of pain perception and inflammatory pathways. Moreover, the presence of fibromyalgia may exacerbate the pain experience in individuals with lipedema, impacting the management and treatment efficacy. Understanding the relationship between fibromyalgia and lipedema is crucial for developing comprehensive treatment plans that address the multifaceted nature of pain in these patients. This includes an interdisciplinary approach that combines physical therapy, pain management strategies, psychological support, and, where appropriate, interventions aimed at managing lipedema, such as compression therapy and surgical options. Acknowledging the co-occurrence of fibromyalgia and lipedema is essential for providing targeted care, optimizing treatment outcomes, and improving the quality of life for those affected by both conditions.

Joint hypermobility syndrome (JHS), also known as hypermobility spectrum disorder (HSD), is a condition characterized by joints that can move beyond the normal range of motion, leading to a variety of symptoms ranging from mild discomfort to severe physical complications. It is often congenital and can be identified by simple physical examinations, such as the Beighton score, which assesses the flexibility of various joints. JHS is considered both a clinical and genetic condition, as it often runs in families and is thought to be related to defects in collagen, a protein that provides structure and strength to connective tissues throughout the body.

Individuals with JHS may experience joint pain, frequent dislocations, and sprains due to the instability of their joints. Beyond musculoskeletal issues, JHS can be associated with a wide array of systemic symptoms, including digestive issues, cardiovascular abnormalities, and autonomic dysregulation, highlighting the systemic nature of connective tissue disorders. The overlap of symptoms between JHS and other heritable disorders of connective tissue, such as Ehlers-Danlos syndromes (EDS), particularly the hypermobile type (hEDS), often complicates diagnosis and management.

Management of JHS is primarily supportive and focuses on alleviating symptoms and improving quality of life. Physical therapy is a cornerstone of treatment, aimed at strengthening the muscles surrounding the hypermobile joints to provide better support and stability, thereby reducing the risk of injury and pain. Pain management, through both pharmacological and non-pharmacological means, is also crucial. Patients may benefit from education on joint protection techniques and lifestyle modifications to avoid activities that could exacerbate their symptoms.

Patients with JHS are more prone to joint dislocations and subluxations and may also experience chronic pain and fatigue. JHS is often associated with lipedema, and the two conditions may share common underlying mechanisms, such as connective tissue dysfunction and inflammation. The confluence of joint hypermobility syndrome (JHS) and lipedema underscores the intricate relationship between connective tissue disorders and adipose tissue accumulation, presenting unique diagnostic and management challenges. JHS, characterized by excessive flexibility of the joints due to variations in the connective tissue, often leads to a range of symptoms including joint pain, dislocations, and early onset osteoarthritis. When this condition coexists with lipedema—marked by the pathological buildup of fat in the lower extremities, pain, and bruising—the patient's clinical picture becomes more complex. The hypermobile joints in JHS may be further stressed by the additional weight and altered biomechanics associated with lipedema, exacerbating joint pain and increasing the risk of injury. Moreover, the overlapping symptoms can complicate the diagnosis, as the pain and mobility issues common to both conditions may be mistakenly attributed to one another. Understanding the intersection between JHS and lipedema is crucial for tailoring patient care, necessitating a multidisciplinary approach that addresses both the connective tissue and adipose tissue aspects. Management strategies may include targeted physical therapy to strengthen the muscles supporting hypermobile joints, compression garments to alleviate lipedema symptoms, and careful monitoring for potential complications. Recognizing the link between JHS and lipedema is essential for providing comprehensive care, minimizing pain, and optimizing function in affected individuals, highlighting the need for awareness and specialized knowledge among healthcare providers treating these conditions.

Marfan syndrome is a genetic disorder that affects the body's connective tissue, which provides strength, support, and elasticity to the skin, bones, blood vessels, and other organs. It is caused by mutations in the FBN1 gene, which encodes the protein fibrillin-1, essential for the formation of elastic fibers found in connective tissue. This disorder is typically inherited in an autosomal dominant pattern, meaning that a single copy of the altered gene in each cell is sufficient to cause the condition. However, approximately 25% of cases occur due to new mutations in the gene and are not inherited from a parent.

Individuals with Marfan syndrome often exhibit a distinctive set of physical characteristics, including tall stature, long arms, legs, fingers, and toes, a chest that sinks in or sticks out, and a high-arched palate with crowded teeth. They may also have eye problems, such as dislocation of the lens, and cardiovascular issues, most notably affecting the aorta. The enlargement of the aorta (aortic aneurysm) and its potential tearing (aortic dissection) are among the most serious complications associated with Marfan syndrome and can be life-threatening.

The diagnosis of Marfan syndrome (Fig. 3) is primarily based on clinical evaluation, including a detailed family history, physical examination, and imaging studies, such as echocardiograms to assess the condition of the aorta and eye exams to check for lens dislocation. Genetic testing can also confirm the diagnosis by identifying mutations in the FBN1 gene, although not all individuals with Marfan syndrome have identifiable FBN1 mutations.

Management of Marfan syndrome is tailored to the individual's symptoms and may involve a multidisciplinary team of healthcare providers, including cardiologists, ophthalmologists, orthopedists, and genetic counselors. Treatment focuses on monitoring and managing cardiovascular risks through medications such as beta-blockers to reduce stress on the aorta and surgery to repair aortic aneurysms if necessary. Regular follow-up and imaging studies are critical to detect changes in the aorta's size and prevent complications. Lifestyle modifications, including avoiding contact sports and heavy lifting, are recommended to reduce the risk of aortic dissection. With appropriate management, individuals with Marfan syndrome can lead relatively normal lives, although they require lifelong monitoring for potential complications. The association between these Marfan syndrome and lipedema is not fully understood, but it is believed that the underlying genetic mutations that cause Marfan syndrome may also contribute to the development of lipedema.

The intersection of Marfan syndrome, a connective tissue disorder, with lipedema presents a nuanced clinical picture that underscores the complexity of managing individuals affected by both conditions.

Marfan syndrome is characterized by mutations in the FBN1 gene, leading to the production of abnormal fibrillin-1, a protein essential for the integrity and function of connective tissue throughout the body. This results in features such as tall stature, long extremities, joint hypermobility, and cardiovascular anomalies. The coexistence of lipedema, with its hallmark pathological fat accumulation in the lower

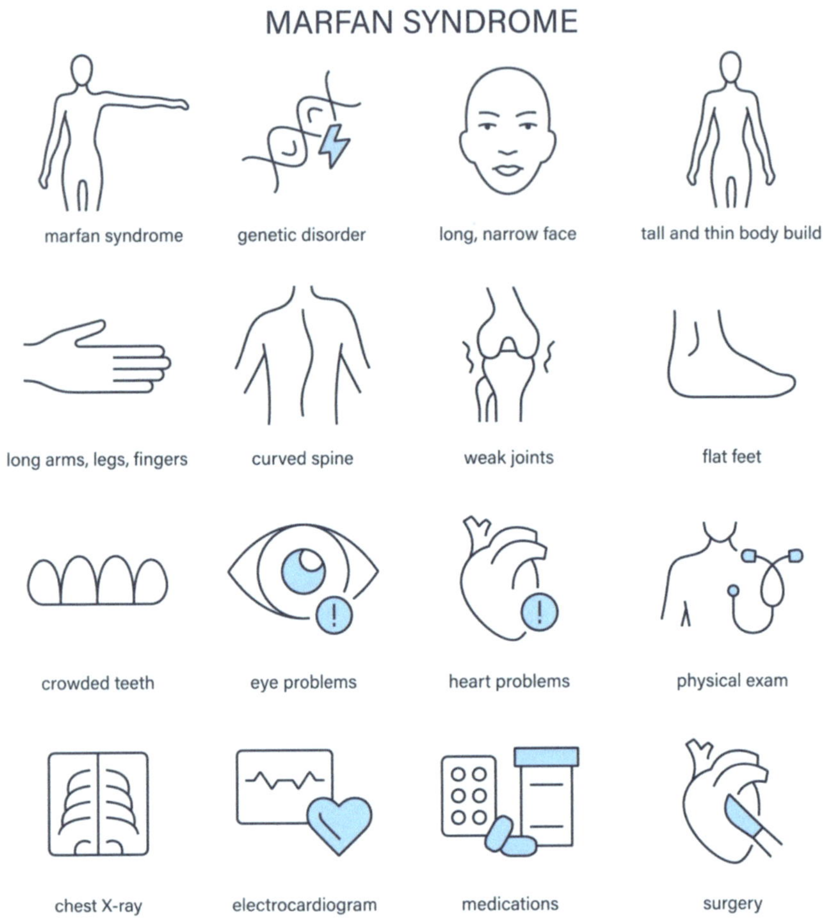

Fig. 3 Clinical signs of Marfan syndrome

extremities, exacerbates the challenges faced by individuals with Marfan syndrome. The additional weight and altered biomechanics due to lipedema can further compromise joint stability and cardiovascular health, already vulnerable in Marfan patients. This overlap can not only magnify symptoms such as joint pain and fatigue but also complicate physical activity, which is often recommended for managing Marfan syndrome. Diagnosing lipedema in the context of Marfan syndrome requires a discerning clinical approach, as both conditions independently affect the body's structure and function. Management strategies necessitate a multidisciplinary approach, emphasizing cardiovascular monitoring, tailored physical therapy to accommodate joint hypermobility and mitigate the impact of excess adipose tissue, and possibly, interventions to manage lipedema such as compression therapy and careful consideration of surgical options. Understanding the co-occurrence of Marfan syndrome and lipedema is crucial for delivering holistic care that addresses

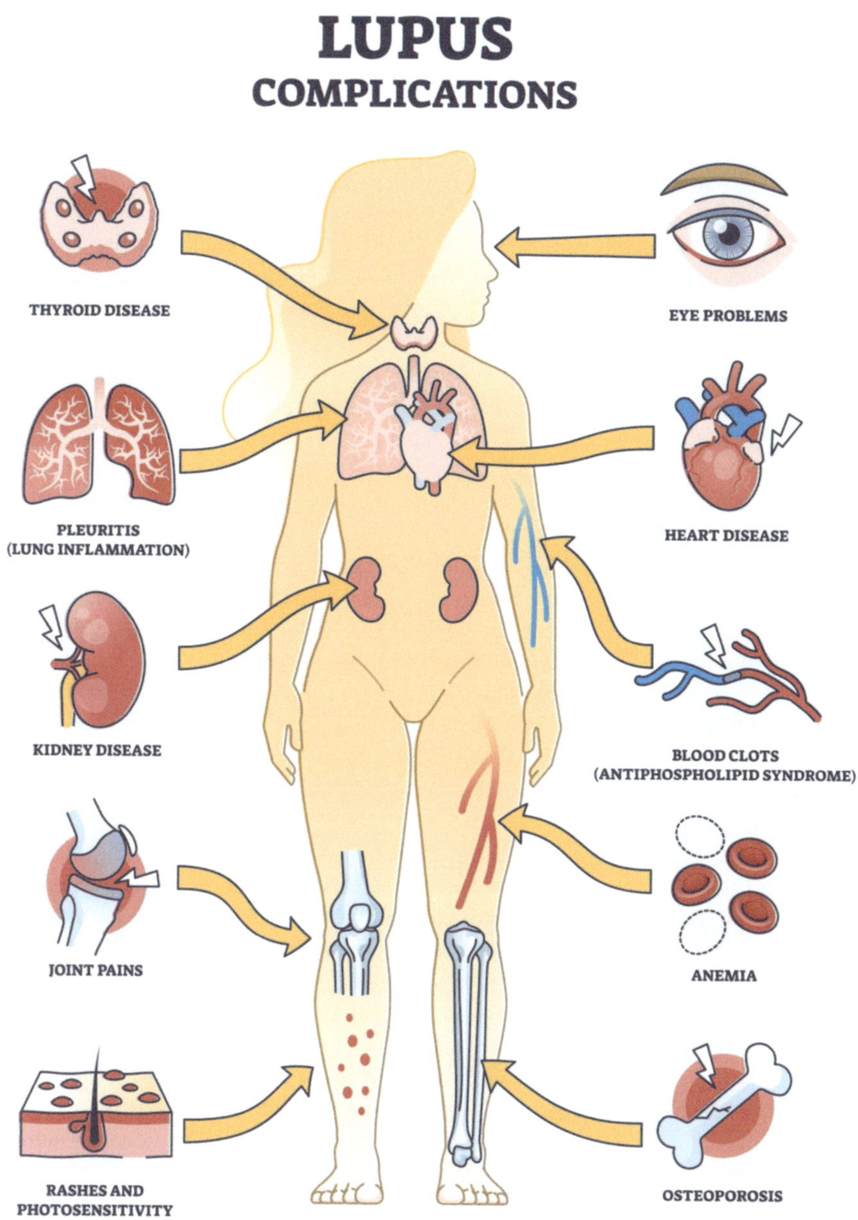

Fig. 4 Signs of lupus

the spectrum of symptoms experienced by patients, highlighting the importance of recognizing the potential interplay between diverse systemic disorders.

Systemic lupus erythematosus (SLE) (Fig. 4), commonly known as lupus, is a chronic autoimmune disease that can affect any part of the body, including the skin, joints, kidneys, brain, heart, lungs, and blood vessels. It is characterized by periods of illness, called flares, and periods of remission. The hallmark of lupus is the body's immune system becoming hyperactive and attacking normal, healthy tissue, resulting in inflammation, swelling, and damage to various organs.

The exact cause of lupus is unknown, but it is believed to be multifactorial, involving genetic, environmental, and hormonal components. Certain genes have been associated with an increased risk of developing lupus, and factors like sunlight, infections, and medications may trigger the disease in genetically predisposed individuals. Lupus is more prevalent in women than men, particularly affecting women of childbearing age, which suggests that hormones, especially estrogen, play a role in its development or progression.

Symptoms of lupus vary widely and depend on which body systems are affected. The most common symptoms include fatigue, joint pain and swelling, a butterfly-shaped rash on the face, skin lesions that appear or worsen with sun exposure, and fever. More severe manifestations can involve the kidneys (lupus nephritis), neurological issues (such as seizures and psychosis), cardiovascular disease, and lung inflammation. Because many symptoms of lupus mimic those of other diseases, lupus is often referred to as "the great imitator," making diagnosis challenging.

Diagnosis is based on a combination of clinical signs and symptoms and laboratory tests, including the presence of antinuclear antibodies (ANA) as a primary marker, although not exclusively indicative of lupus. There is no cure for lupus, but treatments are available to help manage symptoms and reduce the likelihood of flare-ups. Management strategies typically include nonsteroidal anti-inflammatory drugs (NSAIDs) for joint pain and stiffness, antimalarial drugs for skin and joint issues, corticosteroids to reduce inflammation, and immunosuppressants to control the immune system's activity.

Living with lupus requires a comprehensive approach that includes medical treatment, lifestyle adjustments, and supportive therapies. Regular monitoring and collaboration between healthcare providers and the patient are essential to adapt treatments as needed and manage the disease's impact on physical health and quality of life. Advances in understanding lupus's pathophysiology and the development of new therapies offer hope for improved management and outcomes for individuals with this complex condition. Patients with lupus and lipedema can further exacerbate their symptoms. The association between these two conditions is not fully understood. The co-occurrence of lupus, a chronic autoimmune disease, with lipedema presents a unique set of clinical challenges and considerations. Systemic lupus erythematosus (SLE), the most common form of lupus, is characterized by the immune system's attack on its own tissues, causing widespread inflammation and damage to joints, skin, kidneys, blood cells, brain, heart, and lungs. When lupus intersects with lipedema, characterized by the pathological accumulation of adipose tissue in the lower extremities, the management complexity increases. Patients with both conditions may experience an exacerbation of symptoms, with lupus potentially triggering increased inflammation within the adipose tissue characteristic of lipedema, thereby intensifying pain and swelling. Furthermore, the steroid medications often used to manage lupus can contribute to weight gain and fat redistribution, potentially worsening lipedema symptoms or complicating its diagnosis and management.

The interplay between lupus and lipedema underscores the need for a tailored, multidisciplinary approach to treatment, focusing on controlling systemic inflammation, managing pain, and addressing the physical manifestations of lipedema through conservative and possibly surgical interventions. This approach requires careful coordination among rheumatologists, dermatologists, and physical therapists to optimize patient outcomes and improve quality of life. Understanding the interaction between lupus and lipedema is crucial for developing effective management strategies that consider the complexities of autoimmune activity alongside the challenges posed by abnormal adipose tissue accumulation.

Sjögren's syndrome is a chronic autoimmune disorder characterized by the infiltration of lymphocytes into exocrine glands, primarily the salivary and lacrimal glands, leading to their dysfunction. This results in the hallmark symptoms of dry mouth (xerostomia) and dry eyes (keratoconjunctivitis sicca). Beyond these primary manifestations, Sjögren's syndrome can affect various other organs and systems, presenting a wide range of symptoms including dry skin, vaginal dryness, chronic cough, and fatigue. More serious complications may involve the kidneys, gastrointestinal system, blood vessels, lungs, liver, pancreas, and the central nervous system, reflecting the systemic nature of the disease.

Sjögren's syndrome can present as either primary, occurring independently of other autoimmune diseases, or secondary, where it coexists with other autoimmune conditions such as rheumatoid arthritis, lupus, or scleroderma. The etiology of Sjögren's syndrome is not fully understood but is believed to involve a combination of genetic predisposition and environmental triggers, such as viral infections, which initiate an autoimmune response in genetically susceptible individuals.

Diagnosis is based on a combination of patient-reported symptoms, clinical examination, blood tests for specific autoantibodies (including anti-Ro/SSA and anti-La/SSB), and objective measures of glandular function such as Schirmer's test for tear production and salivary flow rates. Biopsy of the salivary glands may also be performed to identify lymphocytic infiltration indicative of the disease.

Management of Sjögren's syndrome is primarily symptomatic, focusing on alleviating dryness through the use of artificial tears, saliva substitutes, and measures to stimulate saliva production. Systemic manifestations may require immunosuppressive medications, including corticosteroids and disease-modifying antirheumatic drugs (DMARDs). Pilocarpine and cevimeline are cholinergic agonists that can increase the production of saliva and tears, providing relief from dryness.

Given its potential to impact various body systems, a multidisciplinary approach to care is essential for individuals with Sjögren's syndrome. Regular monitoring and collaborative management can help address the comprehensive needs of patients, improving quality of life and mitigating the risk of complications. Advances in understanding the pathophysiology of Sjögren's syndrome continue to guide the development of more targeted therapies, offering hope for more effective management strategies in the future. Lipedema has been reported in patients with Sjogren's syndrome. The coexistence of Sjögren's syndrome, a systemic autoimmune disease characterized by its hallmark symptoms of dry eyes and dry mouth, with lipedema, a chronic condition involving the pathological accumulation of adipose tissue, illustrates a complex interplay between autoimmune processes and adipose tissue dysfunction.

Sjögren's syndrome primarily targets the body's exocrine glands, leading to decreased secretions and resultant dryness, but it can also manifest in a wide range of systemic symptoms due to its autoimmune nature, affecting various organs and causing widespread inflammation. When this systemic inflammatory state intersects with lipedema, it may potentially exacerbate the adipose tissue's propensity for inflammation and fibrosis, further complicating the pain and swelling associated with lipedema. Additionally, the immune modulation therapy often employed in managing Sjögren's syndrome can have implications for the management of lipedema, influencing both the progression of the adipose tissue accumulation and the treatment strategies employed. This unique clinical scenario underscores the importance of a nuanced, multidisciplinary approach to care, which considers the impact of autoimmune activity on lipedema and vice versa. Addressing the needs of patients suffering from both Sjögren's syndrome and lipedema requires careful consideration of immunological and metabolic factors, aiming to mitigate the symptoms of both conditions while monitoring for potential interactions between treatments. This approach emphasizes the need for collaboration among specialists in rheumatology, immunology, and lipedema management to ensure comprehensive care that addresses the complexities inherent in concurrent autoimmune and adipose tissue disorders.

Rheumatoid arthritis (RA) (Fig. 5) is a chronic, autoimmune disease characterized by inflammation of the joints, leading to pain, swelling, stiffness, and eventual erosion of the joint structure, which can result in significant disability. Unlike osteoarthritis, which results from wear and tear of the joints, RA involves the immune system mistakenly attacking the synovium—the lining of the membranes that surround the joints. This autoimmune attack triggers a complex inflammatory process that thickens the synovium, eventually destroying the cartilage and bone within the joint.

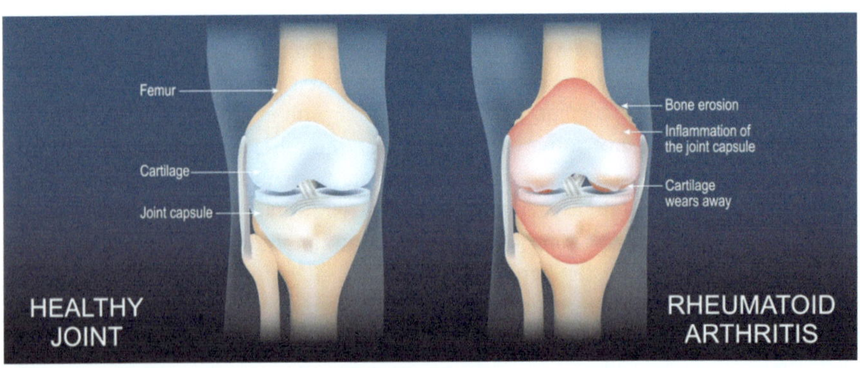

Fig. 5 Key features of the impact of rheumatoid arthritis on cartilage

RA's etiology is believed to be multifactorial, involving a combination of genetic predisposition and environmental factors such as smoking, exposure to certain viruses and bacteria, and possibly hormonal changes. Symptoms of RA can vary in intensity and may include fatigue, fever, and loss of appetite, reflecting its systemic nature. The condition is typically symmetrical, affecting the same joints on both sides of the body.

The diagnosis of RA relies on a combination of clinical presentation, laboratory tests (including rheumatoid factor and anti-cyclic citrullinated peptide antibodies), and imaging studies, which can help detect joint damage and monitor disease progression.

Management of RA aims to control symptoms, reduce inflammation, minimize joint and organ damage, and improve physical function and overall well-being. Treatment strategies encompass pharmacological interventions, such as nonsteroidal anti-inflammatory drugs (NSAIDs), corticosteroids, disease-modifying antirheumatic drugs (DMARDs), and biological response modifiers. Additionally, physical and occupational therapy can help maintain joint flexibility and adapt daily activities to protect joints.

Given RA's potential to affect organs beyond the joints, including the skin, eyes, lungs, heart, and blood vessels, a multidisciplinary approach to care is crucial. Early diagnosis and aggressive treatment are key to slowing disease progression and improving outcomes, highlighting the importance of regular monitoring and adjustment of treatment plans based on disease activity. Despite the challenges RA presents, advancements in treatment have significantly improved the prognosis and quality of life for many individuals with this condition.

Studies have shown that there is an increased prevalence of lipedema in patients with rheumatoid arthritis. The coexistence of rheumatoid arthritis (RA), a chronic inflammatory disorder affecting the joints, with lipedema, a condition characterized by the pathological accumulation of fat in the lower extremities, introduces a multifaceted challenge in clinical management and patient care. RA is an autoimmune disease that primarily attacks the synovial tissues within the joints, leading to pain, swelling, and eventual joint deformity. When patients with RA also suffer from lipedema, the inflammatory burden is compounded, potentially exacerbating joint symptoms and complicating mobility further. The additional weight and altered biomechanics due to lipedema can increase the stress on joints already vulnerable to the erosive effects of RA, intensifying pain and functional impairment. This intersection of conditions necessitates a nuanced approach to treatment, emphasizing the need to address both the inflammatory processes of RA and the symptomatic management of lipedema. Strategies may include the use of disease-modifying antirheumatic drugs (DMARDs) and biologics to control RA inflammation, alongside physical therapy, compression therapy, and possibly surgical interventions for lipedema to alleviate pain and improve limb function. Moreover, the co-management of RA and lipedema highlights the importance of a multidisciplinary team, comprising rheumatologists, dermatologists, and physical therapists, to tailor treatments that address the complexity of symptoms and improve overall quality of life for affected individuals. Recognizing the interplay between RA and lipedema is

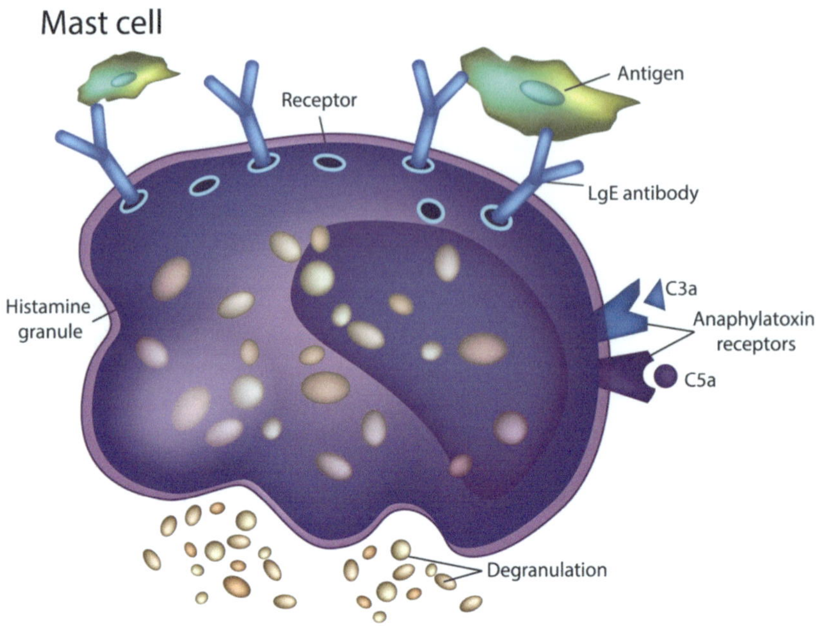

Fig. 6 A mast cell

essential for effective patient care, underscoring the need for comprehensive approaches that consider the systemic nature of both conditions.

Mast cell activation syndrome (MCAS) (Fig. 6) is a complex immunological condition characterized by the inappropriate release of mast cell mediators, leading to a wide array of symptoms across multiple organ systems. Mast cells, part of the body's immune system, play a role in allergic reactions, wound healing, and defense against pathogens. In MCAS, these cells become overly reactive, releasing mediators such as histamine, cytokines, and prostaglandins in the absence of a typical immune trigger. This hyperactivity can result in diverse and often debilitating symptoms, including, but not limited to, skin rashes, flushing, abdominal pain, nausea, vomiting, diarrhea, wheezing, shortness of breath, heart palpitations, and anaphylaxis in severe cases.

The diagnosis of MCAS is challenging due to the overlap of its symptoms with those of other disorders and the variability in individual responses to triggers. Criteria for diagnosis typically involve the documentation of symptoms consistent with mast cell mediator release, the demonstration of elevated mast cell mediators during symptomatic periods, and the improvement of symptoms with treatment aimed at reducing mast cell mediator effects.

Management of MCAS requires a personalized and multifaceted approach, often involving the avoidance of known triggers, pharmacotherapy to stabilize mast cells and block the effects of their mediators, and lifestyle modifications to reduce exposure to potential triggers.

Given the complex nature of MCAS and its potential to impact various aspects of health, a multidisciplinary approach to care is essential, incorporating the expertise of allergists, immunologists, gastroenterologists, dermatologists, and other specialists as needed.

Mast cell activation syndrome (MCAS) and lipedema represent a complex clinical interplay that underscores the intricate relationship between immune system dysregulation and adipose tissue disorders. MCAS is characterized by the inappropriate activation of mast cells, immune cells involved in allergic reactions and inflammatory processes, leading to a wide range of symptoms including skin rashes, gastrointestinal discomfort, and anaphylaxis. When this syndrome coexists with lipedema—a condition marked by the abnormal accumulation of fat in the lower extremities, often accompanied by pain, tenderness, and bruising—the challenges in management and diagnosis are significantly magnified. The inflammatory milieu associated with MCAS can exacerbate the symptoms of lipedema, potentially accelerating the progression of the disease and complicating treatment strategies. The overlap of symptoms can also obscure the distinction between the two conditions, hindering timely and accurate diagnosis. Understanding the relationship between MCAS and lipedema is critical for developing targeted interventions that address the underlying immune dysregulation and the symptomatic management of lipedema. This necessitates a multidisciplinary approach, incorporating immunomodulatory treatments to manage MCAS alongside physical therapy, compression therapy, and dietary modifications for lipedema. The co-management of these conditions highlights the importance of recognizing the potential for immune system involvement in lipedema, advocating for a comprehensive care strategy that addresses the full spectrum of patient symptoms and improves quality of life.

In conclusion, the exploration of lipedema in conjunction with connective tissue disorders has illuminated the complex, multifaceted nature of these conditions, emphasizing the significant overlap in their pathophysiological mechanisms and clinical manifestations. Lipedema, characterized by abnormal fat accumulation and often accompanied by pain and mobility issues, presents a unique challenge when it co-occurs with connective tissue disorders such as Ehlers-Danlos syndrome, Marfan syndrome, and others that impact the body's structural integrity and function. This intersection underscores the necessity for a comprehensive diagnostic approach that considers the broad spectrum of symptoms and their potential interrelations, highlighting the limitations of conventional treatment paradigms that focus on isolated aspects of these conditions.

The management of lipedema and associated connective tissue disorders calls for an integrated, multidisciplinary approach that addresses not only the physical symptoms but also the psychological impact of living with chronic, often misunderstood conditions. Effective treatment strategies must encompass a combination of physical therapy, pharmacological interventions, surgical options where appropriate, and lifestyle modifications, supported by a team of specialists including rheumatologists, dermatologists, physiotherapists, and mental health professionals. This collaborative approach ensures that care is tailored to the individual needs of each patient, fostering a holistic view of patient health that aims to improve quality of life, alleviate pain, and enhance mobility.

Moreover, the chapter highlights the importance of ongoing research to unravel the genetic, molecular, and environmental factors that contribute to the development of lipedema and connective tissue disorders.

Such insights are crucial for advancing diagnostic accuracy, refining treatment modalities, and ultimately, offering hope to those affected by these challenging conditions. In embracing a multidisciplinary strategy, the medical community can move closer to providing comprehensive care that addresses the full scope of patients' experiences, offering a more nuanced understanding and effective management of lipedema and its associated connective tissue disorders.

Suggested Reading

Substance Abuse Mental Health Services Administration. *DSM-5 Changes: Implications for Child Serious Emotional Disturbance [Internet]* Rockville (MD): Substance Abuse and Mental Health Services Administration (US); 2016. Jun, 2016.

Sullivan PF. Mortality in anorexia nervosa. *Am J Psychiatry.* 1995;152(7):1073–74.

Hudson JI, Hiripi E, Pope HG, Jr, Kessler RC. The prevalence and correlates of eating disorders in the National Comorbidity Survey Replication. *Biol Psychiatry.* 2007;61(3):348–58.

Al-Ghadban S, Cromer W, Allen M, et al. Dilated blood and lymphatic microvessels, angiogenesis, increased macrophages, and adipocyte hypertrophy in lipedema thigh skin and fat tissue. *J Obes.* 2019;2019:8747461.

Herbst KL. Rare adipose disorders (RADs) masquerading as obesity. *Acta Pharmacol Sin.* 2012;33(2):155–72.

Buck DW, 2nd, Herbst KL. Lipedema: A relatively common disease with extremely common misconceptions. *Plast Reconstr Surg Glob Open.* 2016;4(9):e1043.

Wold LE, Hines EA, Jr, Allen EV. Lipedema of the legs; A syndrome characterized by fat legs and edema. *Ann Intern Med.* 1951;34(5):1243–50.

Sandhofer M, Hanke CW, Habbema L, et al. Prevention of progression of lipedema with liposuction using tumescent local anesthesia: Results of an International Consensus Conference. *Dermatol Surg.* 2020;46(2):220–28.

Foldi E, Foldi M. Lipedema. In: Foldi M, Foldi E, editors. *Foldi's Textbook of Lymphology.* M¨nchen, Germany: Elsevier, Urban & Fischer Verlag; 2006. p. 551.

Beltran K, Herbst KL. Differentiating lipedema and Dercum's disease. *Int J Obes (Lond)* 2017;41(2):240–45.

Wollina U. Lipedema – an update. *Dermatol Ther.* 2019;32(2):e12805.

Crescenzi R, Marton A, Donahue PMC, et al. Tissue sodium content is elevated in the skin and subcutaneous adipose tissue in women with lipedema. *Obesity (Silver Spring)* 2018;26(2):310–17.

Crescenzi R, Donahue PMC, Weakley S, et al. Lipedema and Dercum's disease: A new application of bioimpedance. *Lymphat Res Biol.* 2019;17(6):671–79.

Forner-Cordero I, Olivan-Sasot P, Ruiz-Llorca C, Munoz-Langa J. Lymphoscintigraphic findings in patients with lipedema. *Rev Esp Med Nucl Imagen Mol.* 2018;37(6):341–48.

Gould DJ, El-Sabawi B, Goel P, et al. Uncovering lymphatic transport abnormalities in patients with primary lipedema. *J Reconstr Microsurg.* 2019;23(10):136–41.

Herbst K, Mirkovskaya L, Bharhagava A, et al. Lipedema fat and signs and symptoms of illness, increase with advancing stage. *Archives of Medicine.* 2015;7(4: 10):1–8.

Beighton P, Horan F. Orthopaedic aspects of the Ehlers-Danlos syndrome. *J Bone Joint Surg Br.* 1969;51(3):444–53.

Malfait F, Francomano C, Byers P, et al. The 2017 international classification of the Ehlers-Danlos syndromes. *Am J Med Genet C Semin Med Genet.* 2017;175(1):8–26.

Morris J, Twaddle S. Anorexia nervosa. *BMJ.* 2007;334(7599):894–98.

Fetzer A, Fetzer S. *Lipoedema UK Big Survey 2014 Research Report.* Chichester: Lipoedema UK; 2016. http://www.lipoedema.co.uk/wp-content/uploads/2016/04/UK-Big-Surey-version-web.pdf.

Di Renzo L, Cinelli G, Romano L, et al. Potential effects of a modified Mediterranean diet on body composition in lipoedema. *Nutrients.* 2021;13(2):358.

Kraus RH. [All about lipedema] *Lymphe Gesundheit.* 2015;2015(1):1–9. [in German]

Hoek HW. Incidence, prevalence and mortality of anorexia nervosa and other eating disorders. *Curr Opin Psychiatry.* 2006;19(4):389–94.

Szolnoky G, Nemes A, Gavaller H, et al. Lipedema is associated with increased aortic stiffness. *Lymphology.* 2012;45(2):71–79.

Jagtman BA, Kuiper JP, Brakkee AJ. [Measurements of skin elasticity in patients with lipedema of the Moncorps "rusticanus" type] *Phlebologie.* 1984;37(3):315–19. [in French]

Lee M, Strand M. Ehlers-Danlos syndrome in a young woman with anorexia nervosa and complex somatic symptoms. *Int J Eat Disord.* 2018;51(3):281–84.

Bulbena A, Baeza-Velasco C, Bulbena-Cabre A, et al. Psychiatric and psychological aspects in the Ehlers-Danlos syndromes. *Am J Med Genet C Semin Med Genet.* 2017;175(1):237–45.

Herbst KL. Subcutaneous adipose tissue diseases: Dercum disease, lipedema, familial multiple lipomatosis, and madelung disease. [Updated 2019 Dec 14] In: Feingold KR, Anawalt B, Boyce A, et al., editors. *Endotext [Internet]* South Dartmouth (MA): MDText.com, Inc.; 2000. https://www.ncbi.nlm.nih.gov/books/NBK552156/

Okhovat J-P, Alavi A. Lipedema: a review of the literature. *Int J Low Extrem Wounds.* 2015;**14**(3):262–267. doi: https://doi.org/10.1177/1534734614554284

Bauer A-T, von Lukowicz D, Lossagk K, et al. New insights on lipedema: the enigmatic disease of the peripheral fat. *Plast Reconstr Surg.* 2019;**144**(6):1475–1484. doi: https://doi.org/10.1097/PRS.0000000000006280

Skaer TL, Kwong WJ. Illness perceptions and burden of disease in fibromyalgia. *Expert Rev Pharmacoecon Outcomes Res.* 2017;**17**(1):9–15. doi: https://doi.org/10.1080/14737167.2017.1270207

Fitzcharles M-A, Perrot S, Häuser W. Comorbid fibromyalgia: a qualitative review of prevalence and importance. *Eur J Pain Lond Engl.* 2018;**22**(9):1565–1576. doi: https://doi.org/10.1002/ejp.1252

Salaffi F, Di Carlo M, Carotti M, Farah S, Ciapetti A, Gutierrez M. The impact of different rheumatic diseases on health-related quality of life: a comparison with a selected sample of healthy individuals using SF-36 questionnaire, EQ-5D and SF-6D utility values. *Acta Bio-Medica.* 2019;**89**(4):541–557. doi: https://doi.org/10.23750/abm.v89i4.7298

Angst F, Benz T, Lehmann S, et al. Extended overview of the longitudinal pain-depression association: a comparison of six cohorts treated for specific chronic pain conditions. *J Affect Disord.* 2020;**273**:508–516. doi: https://doi.org/10.1016/j.jad.2020.05.044

Clay FJ, Fitzharris M, Kerr E, McClure RJ, Watson WL. The association of social functioning, social relationships and the receipt of compensation with time to return to work following unintentional injuries to Victorian workers. *J Occup Rehabil.* 2012;**22**(3):363–375. doi: https://doi.org/10.1007/s10926-012-9354-4

Hoffman DL, Dukes EM. The health status burden of people with fibromyalgia: a review of studies that assessed health status with the SF-36 or the SF-12. *Int J Clin Pract.* 2008;**62**(1):115–126. doi: https://doi.org/10.1111/j.1742-1241.2007.01638.x

Estévez-López F, Álvarez-gallardo IC, Segura-Jiménez V, et al. The discordance between subjectively and objectively measured physical function in women with fibromyalgia: association

with catastrophizing and self-efficacy cognitions. The al-Ándalus project. *Disabil Rehabil.* 2018;**40**(3):329–337. doi: https://doi.org/10.1080/09638288.2016.1258737
Häuser W, Fitzcharles M-A. Facts and myths pertaining to fibromyalgia. *Dialogues Clin Neurosci.* 2018;**20**(1):53–62.
Dudek JE, Białaszek W, Ostaszewski P. Quality of life in women with lipoedema: a contextual behavioral approach. *Qual Life Res Int J Qual Life Asp Treat Care Rehabil.* 2016;**25**(2):401–408. doi: https://doi.org/10.1007/s11136-015-1080-x
van de Laar IM et al. Mutations in SMAD3 cause a syndromic form of aortic aneurysms and dissections with early-onset osteoarthritis. *Nat. Genet* 43, 121–126 (2011).
Rienhoff HY Jr. et al. A mutation in TGFB3 associated with a syndrome of low muscle mass, growth retardation, distal arthrogryposis and clinical features overlapping with Marfan and Loeys-Dietz syndrome. *Am. J. Med. Genet. A* 161A, 2040–2046, doi: https://doi.org/10.1002/ajmg.a.36056 [doi] (2013).
Bertoli-Avella AM et al. Mutations in a TGF-beta ligand, TGFB3, cause syndromic aortic aneurysms and dissections. *J. Am. Coll. Cardiol* 65, 1324–1336, doi:S0735–1097(15)00403–9 [pii]; https://doi.org/10.1016/j.jacc.2015.01.040 [doi] (2015).
Sakai LY, Keene DR, Glanville RW & Bachinger HP Purification and partial characterization of fibrillin, a cysteine-rich structural component of connective tissue microfibrils. *J. Biol. Chem* 266, 14763–14770 (1991).
Corson GM, Chalberg SC, Dietz HC, Charbonneau NL & Sakai LY Fibrillin binds calcium and is coded by cDNAs that reveal a multidomain structure and alternatively spliced exons at the 5' end. *Genomics* 17, 476–484 (1993).
Lerner-Ellis JP et al. The spectrum of FBN1, TGFbetaR1, TGFbetaR2 and ACTA2 variants in 594 individuals with suspected Marfan Syndrome, Loeys-Dietz Syndrome or Thoracic Aortic Aneurysms and Dissections (TAAD). *Mol Genet Metab* 112, 171–176, doi: https://doi.org/10.1016/j.ymgme.2014.03.011 (2014).
Milewicz DM & Duvic M Severe neonatal Marfan syndrome resulting from a de novo 3-bp insertion into the fibrillin gene on chromosome 15. *Am. J Hum. Genet* 54, 447–453 (1994).
Putnam EA et al. Delineation of the Marfan phenotype associated with mutations in exons 23–32 of the FBN1 gene. *Am. J. Med. Genet* 62, 233–242 (1996).
Faivre L et al. Clinical and mutation-type analysis from an international series of 198 probands with a pathogenic FBN1 exons 24–32 mutation. *Eur. J Hum. Genet* 17, 491–501, doi:ejhg2008207 [pii]; https://doi.org/10.1038/ejhg.2008.207 [doi] (2009).
Faivre L et al. Effect of mutation type and location on clinical outcome in 1,013 probands with Marfan syndrome or related phenotypes and FBN1 mutations: an international study. *Am. J. Hum. Genet* 81, 454–466 (2007).
Schrijver I, Liu W, Brenn T, Furthmayr H & Francke U Cysteine substitutions in epidermal growth factor-like domains of fibrillin-1: distinct effects on biochemical and clinical phenotypes. *Am. J. Hum. Genet* 65, 1007–1020 (1999).
Schrijver I et al. Premature Termination Mutations in FBN1: Distinct Effects on Differential Allelic Expression and on Protein and Clinical Phenotypes. *Am. J. Hum. Genet* 71, 223–237 (2002).
Sengle G & Sakai LY The fibrillin microfibril scaffold: A niche for growth factors and mechanosensation? *Matrix Biol* 47, 3–12, doi: https://doi.org/10.1016/j.matbio.2015.05.002 (2015).
Sengle G et al. Targeting of bone morphogenetic protein growth factor complexes to fibrillin. *J Biol Chem* 283, 13874–13888, doi: https://doi.org/10.1074/jbc.M707820200 (2008).
Ramirez F & Dietz HC Fibrillin-rich microfibrils: Structural determinants of morphogenetic and homeostatic events. *J. Cell Physiol* 213, 326–330 (2007).
Chen Y, Dabovic B, Annes JP & Rifkin DB Latent TGF-beta binding protein-3 (LTBP-3) requires binding to TGF-beta for secretion. *FEBS Lett* 517, 277–280, doi:S0014579302026480 [pii] (2002).
Robertson IB et al. Latent TGF-beta-binding proteins. *Matrix Biol* 47, 44–53, doi:S0945–053X(15)00104–3 [pii]; https://doi.org/10.1016/j.matbio.2015.05.005 [doi] (2015).

Zilberberg L et al. Specificity of latent TGF-beta binding protein (LTBP) incorporation into matrix: role of fibrillins and fibronectin. *J. Cell Physiol* 227, 3828–3836, doi: https://doi.org/10.1002/jcp.24094 [doi] (2012).

Isogai Z et al. Latent transforming growth factor beta-binding protein 1 interacts with fibrillin and is a microfibril-associated protein. *J Biol. Chem* 278, 2750–2757 (2003).

Ono RN et al. Latent transforming growth factor beta-binding proteins and fibulins compete for fibrillin-1 and exhibit exquisite specificities in binding sites. *J Biol Chem* 284, 16872–16881, doi: https://doi.org/10.1074/jbc.M809348200 (2009).

Wipff PJ, Rifkin DB, Meister JJ & Hinz B Myofibroblast contraction activates latent TGF-beta1 from the extracellular matrix. *J. Cell Biol* 179, 1311–1323 (2007).

Humphrey JD, Milewicz DM, Tellides G & Schwartz MA Cell biology. Dysfunctional mechanosensing in aneurysms. *Science* 344, 477–479 (2014).

Waters KM, Rooper LM, Guajardo A & Halushka MK Histopathologic differences partially distinguish syndromic aortic diseases. *Cardiovasc Pathol* 30, 6–11, doi: https://doi.org/10.1016/j.carpath.2017.05.008 (2017).

Davis EC Smooth muscle cell to elastic lamina connections in developing mouse aorta. Role in aortic medial organization. *Lab Invest* 68, 89–99 (1993).

Milewicz DM et al. Genetic Basis of Thoracic Aortic Aneurysms and Dissections: Focus on Smooth Muscle Cell Contractile Dysfunction. *Annu. Rev. Genomics Hum. Genet* 9, 283–302 (2008).

Humphrey JD, Schwartz MA, Tellides G & Milewicz DM Role of Mechanotransduction in Vascular Biology: Focus on Thoracic Aortic Aneurysms and Dissections. *Circ. Res* 116, 1448–1461, doi:CIRCRESAHA.114.304936 [pii]; https://doi.org/10.1161/CIRCRESAHA.114.304936 [doi] (2015).

Milewicz DM et al. Altered Smooth Muscle Cell Force Generation as a Driver of Thoracic Aortic Aneurysms and Dissections. *Arterioscler. Thromb. Vasc. Biol* 37, 26–34, doi:ATVBAHA.116.303229 [pii]; https://doi.org/10.1161/ATVBAHA.116.303229 [doi] (2017).

Pereira L et al. Targeting of the gene encoding fibrillin-1 recapitulates the vascular aspect of Marfan syndrome. *Nat. Genet* 17, 218–222 (1997).

Pereira L et al. Pathogenetic sequence for aneurysm revealed in mice underexpressing fibrillin-1. *Proc. Natl. Acad. Sci. U. S. A* 96, 3819–3823 (1999).

Judge DP et al. Evidence for a critical contribution of haploinsufficiency in the complex pathogenesis of Marfan syndrome. *J. Clin. Invest* 114, 172–181 (2004).

Yuan H, Silberstein SD. Histamine and Migraine. *Headache*. (2018) 58:184–93. doi: https://doi.org/10.1111/head.13164

Guan LC, Dong X, Green DP. Roles of mast cells and their interactions with the trigeminal nerve in migraine headache. *Mol Pain*. (2023) 19:17448069231181358. doi: https://doi.org/10.1177/17448069231181358

Blanco I, Bèritze N, Argüelles M, Cárcaba V, Fernández F, Janciauskiene S, et al.. Abnormal overexpression of mastocytes in skin biopsies of fibromyalgia patients. *Clin Rheumatol*. (2010) 29:1403–12. doi: https://doi.org/10.1007/s10067-010-1474-7

Mekori YA, Metcalfe DD. Mast cell-T cell interactions. *J Allergy Clin Immunol*. (1999) 104:517–23. doi: https://doi.org/10.1016/s0091-6749(99)70316-7

Theoharides TC, Kempuraj D, Tagen M, Conti P, Kalogeromitros D. Differential release of mast cell mediators and the pathogenesis of inflammation. *Immunol Rev*. (2007) 217:65–78. doi: https://doi.org/10.1111/j.1600-065X.2007.00519.x

Conti P, Caraffa A, Gallenga CE, Ross R, Kritas SK, Frydas I, et al.. Coronavirus-19 (SARS-CoV-2) induces acute severe lung inflammation via IL-1 causing cytokine storm in COVID-19: a promising inhibitory strategy. *J Biol Regul Homeost Agents*. (2020) 34:1971–5. doi: https://doi.org/10.23812/20-1-E

Theoharides TC. COVID-19, pulmonary mast cells, cytokine storms, and beneficial actions of Luteolin. *Biofactors*. (2020) 46:306–8. doi: https://doi.org/10.1002/biof.1633

Nigrovic PA, Binstadt BA, Monach PA, Johnsen A, Gurish M, Iwakura Y, et al.. Mast cells contribute to initiation of autoantibody-mediated arthritis via IL-1. *Proc Natl Acad Sci.* (2007) 104:2325–30. doi: https://doi.org/10.1073/pnas.0610852103

Salamon P, Shefler I, Moshkovits I, Munitz A, Horwitz Klotzman D, Mekori Y, et al.. IL-33 and IgE stimulate mast cell production of IL-2 and regulatory T cell expansion in allergic dermatitis. *Clin Exp Allergy.* (2017) 47:1409–16. doi: https://doi.org/10.1111/cea.13027

Hershko Alon Y, Suzuki R, Charles N, Alvarez-Errico D, Sargent Jennifer L, Laurence A, et al.. Mast cell Interleukin-2 production contributes to suppression of chronic allergic dermatitis. *Immunity.* (2011) 35:562–71. doi: https://doi.org/10.1016/j.immuni.2011.07.013

Bradding P, Feather I, Wilson S, Bardin P, Heusser C, Holgate S, et al.. Immunolocalization of cytokines in the nasal mucosa of normal and perennial Rhinitic subjects. The mast cell as a source of IL-4, IL-5, and IL-6 in human allergic mucosal inflammation. *J Immunol.* (1993) 151:3853–65.

Trautmann A, Krohne G, Bröcker E-B, Klein CE. Human mast cells augment fibroblast proliferation by heterotypic cell-cell adhesion and action of IL-4. *J Immunol.* (1998) 160:5053–7. doi: https://doi.org/10.4049/jimmunol.160.10.5053

Shakoory B, Fitzgerald SM, Lee SA, Chi DS, Krishnaswamy G. The role of human mast cell-derived cytokines in eosinophil biology. *J Interf Cytokine Res.* (2004) 24:271–81. doi: https://doi.org/10.1089/107999004323065057

Choy E, Rose-John S. Interleukin-6 as a multifunctional regulator: inflammation, immune response, and fibrosis. *J Scleroderma Relat Disord.* (2017) 2:S1–5. doi: https://doi.org/10.5301/jsrd.5000

Dahdah A, Gautier G, Attout T, Fiore F, Lebourdais E, Msallam R, et al.. Mast cells aggravate Sepsis by inhibiting peritoneal macrophage phagocytosis. *J Clin Invest.* (2014) 124:4577–89. doi: https://doi.org/10.1172/JCI75212

Krüger-Krasagakes S, Möller A, Kolde G, Lippert U, Weber M, Henz BM. Production of interleukin-6 by human mast cells and basophilic cells. *J Investig Dermatol.* (1996) 106:75–9. doi: https://doi.org/10.1111/1523-1747.ep12327815

Seino Y, Ikeda U, Ikeda M, Yamamoto K, Misawa Y, Hasegawa T, et al.. Interleukin 6 gene transcripts are expressed in human atherosclerotic lesions. *Cytokine.* (1994) 6:87–91. doi: https://doi.org/10.1016/1043-4666(94)90013-2

Sun J, Sukhova GK, Wolters PJ, Yang M, Kitamoto S, Libby P, et al.. Mast cells promote atherosclerosis by releasing Proinflammatory cytokines. *Nat Med.* (2007) 13:719–24. doi: https://doi.org/10.1038/nm1601

Huang B, Lei Z, Zhang GM, Li D, Song C, Li B, et al.. SCF-mediated mast cell infiltration and activation exacerbate the inflammation and immunosuppression in tumor microenvironment. *Blood.* (2008) 112:1269–79. doi: https://doi.org/10.1182/blood-2008-03-147033

Baggiolini M, Walz A, Kunkel SL. Neutrophil-activating Peptide-1/interleukin 8, a novel cytokine that activates neutrophils. *J Clin Invest.* (1989) 84:1045–9. doi: https://doi.org/10.1172/JCI114265

Oppenheim JJ, Zachariae CO, Mukaida N, Matsushima K. Properties of the novel proinflammatory supergene "Intercrine" cytokine family. *Annu Rev Immunol.* (1991) 9:617–48. doi: https://doi.org/10.1146/annurev.iy.09.040191.003153

Huber AR, Kunkel SL, Todd RF, Weiss SJ. Regulation of transendothelial neutrophil migration by endogenous interleukin-8. *Science.* (1991) 254:99–102. doi: https://doi.org/10.1126/science.1718038

Simonini A, Moscucci M, Muller DWM, Bates ER, Pagani FD, Burdick MD, et al.. IL-8 is an Angiogenic factor in human coronary atherectomy tissue. *Circulation.* (2000) 101:1519–26. doi: https://doi.org/10.1161/01.CIR.101.13.1519

Visciano C, Liotti F, Prevete N, Cali G, Franco R, Collina F, et al.. Mast cells induce epithelial-to-mesenchymal transition and stem cell features in human thyroid Cancer cells through an IL-8–AKT–slug pathway. *Oncogene.* (2015) 34:5175–86. doi: https://doi.org/10.1038/onc.2014.441

Ou Z, He Y, Qi L, Zu X, Wu L, Cao Z, et al.. Infiltrating mast cells enhance benign prostatic hyperplasia through IL-6/STAT3/cyclin D1 signals. *Oncotarget*. (2017) 8:59156. doi: https://doi.org/10.18632/oncotarget.19465

Massey O, Suphioglu C. Recent advances in the inhibition of the IL-4 cytokine pathway for the treatment of allergen-induced asthma. *Int J Mol Sci*. (2021) 22:13655. doi: https://doi.org/10.3390/ijms222413655

Leyva-Castillo JM, Das M, Artru E, Yoon J, Galand C, Geha RS. Mast cell–derived IL-13 downregulates IL-12 production by skin dendritic cells to inhibit the TH1 cell response to cutaneous antigen exposure. *J Allergy Clin Immunol*. (2021) 147:2305–2315.e3. doi: https://doi.org/10.1016/j.jaci.2020.11.036

Singh B, Jegga AG, Shanmukhappa KS, Edukulla R, Khurana GH, Medvedovic M, et al.. IL-31-driven skin remodeling involves epidermal cell proliferation and thickening that Lead to impaired skin-barrier function. *PLoS One*. (2016) 11:e0161877. doi: https://doi.org/10.1371/journal.pone.0161877

Cornelissen C, Marquardt Y, Czaja K, Wenzel J, Frank J, Lüscher-Firzlaff J, et al.. IL-31 regulates differentiation and Filaggrin expression in human Organotypic skin models. *J Allergy Clin Immunol*. (2012) 129:426–433.e8. doi: https://doi.org/10.1016/j.jaci.2011.10.042

Deshmane SL, Kremlev S, Amini S, Sawaya BE. Monocyte chemoattractant Protein-1 (MCP-1): an overview. *J Interf Cytokine Res*. (2009) 29:313–26. doi: https://doi.org/10.1089/jir.2008.0027

Lin J, Kakkar V, Lu X. Impact of MCP-1 in atherosclerosis. *Curr Pharm Des*. (2014) 20:4580–8. doi: https://doi.org/10.2174/1381612820666140522115801

Gordon JR, Galli SJ. Mast cells as a source of both preformed and immunologically inducible TNF-α/cachectin. *Nature*. (1990) 346:274–6. doi: https://doi.org/10.1038/346274a0

Associated Neurological Comorbidities

Lipedema is a chronic and progressive condition characterized by the abnormal accumulation of adipose tissue, typically in the legs and arms, leading to pain, swelling, and mobility issues. Despite being a distinct medical condition, lipedema is often misunderstood and misdiagnosed as obesity or lymphedema. The disease predominantly affects women and can significantly impact their quality of life.

Neurological comorbidities associated with lipedema add another layer of complexity to its management and treatment. These comorbidities can include sensory disturbances such as pain and hypersensitivity, as well as motor abnormalities that may affect balance and coordination. The presence of neurological symptoms suggests that lipedema is not just a disorder of fat distribution but may also involve alterations in the nervous system's function.

The interplay between lipedema and neurological comorbidities highlights the need for a comprehensive approach to diagnosis and treatment, integrating the expertise of various healthcare professionals. Understanding the neurological aspects of lipedema is crucial for developing effective management strategies that address both the physical and sensory symptoms experienced by patients. This introduction aims to shed light on the complexities of lipedema and the importance of recognizing its potential neurological comorbidities, paving the way for better patient outcomes through targeted therapy and supportive care.

There is limited research on the association between neurological conditions and lipedema. However, some studies have suggested that individuals with lipedema may be at increased risk for certain neurological comorbidities. Here are some potential associated neurological comorbidities in lipedema.

G. Laur, *Lipoedema*, https://doi.org/10.1007/978-981-96-8939-2_29

Neuropathy

Some theory suggests that lipedema is a disease influenced by estrogen and governed by multiple genes. It emerges alongside changes in female hormones and results in abnormalities in both the vascular and lymphatic systems. The condition may also involve inflammation of the peripheral nerves and irregularities in the sympathetic nervous system's connection to the subcutaneous fat tissue, with estrogen playing a contributing role in the development of neuropathy. The excessive growth of fat cells is probably a subsequent event that perpetuates a harmful cycle. The regions beneath the skin that are impacted tend to be sensitive and sore, potentially complicating the process of applying bandages. Nonetheless, this discomfort tends to alleviate following gentle manual lymphatic drainage and liposuction procedures.

Individuals with lipedema frequently experience allodynic and neuropathic pain within the impacted tissues, a type of pain distinctly different from that associated with obesity or lymphedema. Addressing pain is an aspect of clinical management for lipedema, as it is a symptom reported by over 90% of those diagnosed. Typically, pain is localized in the lower limbs and escalates in severity in correlation with the progression of lipedema stages. The precise biological processes that give rise to pain in lipedema are not yet fully understood, but the pathology of the disease in regions commonly affected, such as the thighs and abdomen, is currently under scientific scrutiny. Investigations, for instance, have demonstrated a connection between sodium concentration in the tissues of the lower extremities and the pain experienced by patients with lipedema. Symptoms such as burning pain have led to hypotheses that neurogenic inflammation, instigated by sensory neurons, may be significantly involved in the regulation of lipedema pain through both sympathetic and parasympathetic pathways. However, these pathways have yet to be thoroughly examined, and the understanding of the correlates of pain in lipedema is still limited. Enhanced identification and comprehension of the elements that contribute to pain associated with lipedema could facilitate more precise assessments of the condition's severity and might uncover underlying mechanisms integral to the development of the disease.

The study analyzed participants with advanced lipedema, focusing on pain responses using questionnaires and von Frey filaments. Results showed that stage 3 patients had significantly greater weight, BMI, waist and hip circumferences, and age. Most participants were diabetic, and 60% of stage 1, 61.5% of stage 2, and 100% of stage 3 lipedema participants reported leg pain. A significant increase in pain was identified with disease stage, indicating that pain increases with disease stage. The mean cumulative painDETECT scores were significantly different across lipedema stages, with stage 3 patients having significantly higher average scores. Pain was described to radiate from the legs to other areas of the body in 33.3% of lipedema stage 1, 37.5% of lipedema stage 2, and 62.5% of lipedema stage 3 participants. Differences in questionnaire score responses regarding burning, tingling, shock sensation, or numbness were not significant across lipedema stages. However, pain behavior patterns were significantly different across lipedema stages, with stage 3 patients with lipedema showing the most significantly different scores compared to stage 1 or 2 patients.

The study examined pain-associated cutaneous sensitivity in patients with lipedema using von Frey mechanical stimulation on the thigh, calf, and arm. Despite the thigh being the most visually affected, the mechanical sensory threshold only trended toward increased sensitivity in patients with lipedema compared to controls. However, in the calf and arm, patients with lipedema were significantly more sensitive than controls. The study found no overall stage effect in the cutaneous mechanical sensory threshold in the thigh, but stage 3 patients with lipedema were significantly more sensitive. A significant stage-dependent effect was measured in the calf, with increased sensitization in both lipedema stage 2 and stage 3, compared to controls. The arm response was similar across lipedema stages, with stage 3 lipedema demonstrating significant local hyperalgesia. The objectively measured von Frey response indicated heightened dermal sensitivity in patients with lipedema, consistent with stage-dependent disease severity in this study cohort. The study also evaluated whether objective von Frey measurement would be redundant with self-reported survey of pain or provide additional information for the cohort.

The etiology of peripheral neuropathy involves reduced intradermal neuronal density. The study aimed to identify changes in neuronal cell body density in the skin of patients with lipedema, compared to controls or between lipedema stages. Results showed no significant difference in density between control and lipedema samples and no differences in cell body density across lipedema stages in the thigh biopsies. However, abdominal samples were found to have a significant reduction in cell body density in patients with lipedema, suggesting systemic changes associated with changes in lipedema tissue and neuronal density.

The study also assessed the tissues for other potential indicators of peripheral neuroinflammation. The immunolabeling of neuropathic markers CGRP and NGF was quantified across the length of the skin on tissue biopsies. No difference in dermal CGRP labeling was visualized or quantified in the abdominal skin lipedema samples compared to controls. However, when broken down by lipedema stage, a significant stage effect was identified ($P < 0.01$). Stage 1 lipedema samples had significantly less CGRP-positive labeling than control tissue, while stage 3 lipedema samples demonstrated a significant increase over stage 2 skin.

In contrast, a stronger stage dependence of CGRP and NGF immunolabeling was measured in the epidermis of thigh samples. Although total CGRP density was unchanged across lipedema tissue and controls, a stage-wise comparison showed a significant increase in CGRP expression between stages. Notably, CGRP labeling was significantly higher in stage 3 samples, compared to either control or stage 2 tissues.

Overall, the data suggest a consistently unique stage-dependent expression pattern of neuropeptides associated with neurogenic inflammation, which can be characterized in the epidermis of lipedema skin. The expression levels of NGF and CGRP were similar within the abdomen and thigh across the stages, especially this effect, strongest in stage 3 lipedema.

Fibromyalgia

Fibromyalgia and lipedema share the characteristic of pain concentrated in soft tissues and predominantly affect middle-aged women, who frequently experience concurrent overweight and depressive symptoms. These conditions are long-lasting, span decades, and lack curative treatments, leading to significant personal and societal health challenges. Unlike conditions with clear, objective diagnostic markers like specific lab or imaging anomalies, these two syndromes lack such signs, making it difficult to distinguish one from the other. This often results in confusion or incorrect diagnoses.

The research substantiates the hypothesis of significant syndromal convergence between lipedema and fibromyalgia, underscoring profound implications for diagnostic and therapeutic strategies. These chronic pain syndromes predominantly afflict women within their reproductive years, manifesting as diffuse, spontaneous, and widespread soft-tissue pain coupled with allodynia. Notably, a genetic predisposition is evident for both conditions, alongside a relatively high incidence of comorbidities including depression, fatigue, headaches, and functional vegetative symptoms, as well as obesity.

Our findings reveal that individuals with either condition exhibit symptom severity and functional impairment exceeding those observed in the general populace, with fibromyalgia patients reporting notably poorer health outcomes compared to patients with lipedema, as evidenced by standardized mean differences (SMDs) across all SF-36 scales. Furthermore, a significant portion of women diagnosed with lipedema also meet the diagnostic criteria for fibromyalgia, highlighting the intricate relationship between these conditions. The analysis also draws parallels in the associations between pain and depression across both conditions, underscoring similar socio-economic and educational backgrounds among the affected individuals, which are crucial determinants of employability.

Despite these similarities, disparities exist in terms of employment, health behaviors, and the prevalence of obesity, with fibromyalgia patients exhibiting lower employment levels and more detrimental health behaviors. Moreover, the fibromyalgia group reported significantly poorer physical and mental health outcomes compared to the lipedema cohort. The study delves into the severity of pain and its distribution, noting fibromyalgia's extensive pain that contrasts with lipedema's localized pain in edema-affected limbs.

The potential for overlap between these disorders is acknowledged, despite the generally worse pain and symptomatology reported in fibromyalgia. This is exemplified by comparable results in functional performance tests, suggesting a dissonance between subjective experiences and objective assessments in fibromyalgia, potentially indicative of a tendency toward catastrophic thinking.

This discrepancy highlights the complex nature of fibromyalgia's symptomatology, including centralized pain mechanisms and autonomic dysregulation.

Contrastingly, individuals with lipedema, particularly younger women, exhibit relatively higher functionality and possibly greater self-efficacy, potentially due to rigorous adherence to complex decongestive therapy. This hypothesis gains support from comparisons with lymphedema patients, suggesting distinctive coping mechanisms and quality-of-life impacts between the conditions.

This study represents a pioneering effort to empirically compare fibromyalgia and lipedema using standardized outcome measures, offering a comprehensive assessment of health and quality of life in over a hundred patients with lipedema. It introduces novel empirical data, employing standardized diagnostic criteria and the SF-36, complemented by functional performance tests, to facilitate a nuanced comparison across health dimensions and conditions. The research underscores the need for further investigation into the nuanced interplay between these syndromes, suggesting areas for future inquiry, particularly in the realm of pain coping, affective health dimensions, and additional functional performance tests.

Suggested Reading

Herbst K.L., Kahn L.A., Iker E., Ehrlich C., Wright T., McHutchison L., Schwartz J., Sleigh M., MC Donahue P., Lisson K.H., et al. Standard of care for lipedema in the United States. *Phlebol. J. Venous Dis.* 2021;36:779–796. doi: https://doi.org/10.1177/02683555211015887.

Herbst K., Mirkovskaya L., Bharhagava A., Chava Y., Te H.T.C. Lipedema Fat and Signs and Symptoms of Illness, Increase with Advancing Stage. *Arch. Med.* 2015;7:410.

Torre Y.S., Wadeea R., Rosas V., Herbst K.L. Lipedema: Friend and foe. *Horm. Mol. Biol. Clin. Investig.* 2018;33:1–7. doi: https://doi.org/10.1515/hmbci-2017-0076.

Angst F., Lehmann S., Aeschlimann A., Sandòr P.S., Wagner S. Cross-sectional validity and specificity of comprehensive measurement in lymphedema and lipedema of the lower extremity: A comparison of five outcome instruments. *Health Qual. Life Outcomes.* 2020a;18:245. doi: https://doi.org/10.1186/s12955-020-01488-9.

Buso G., Depairon M., Tomson D., Raffoul W., Vettor R., Mazzolai L. Lipedema: A Call to Action! *Obesity.* 2019;27:1567–1576. doi: https://doi.org/10.1002/oby.22597.

Al-Ghadban S., Cromer W., Allen M., Ussery C., Badowski M., Harris D., Herbst K.L. Dilated Blood and Lymphatic Microvessels, Angiogenesis, Increased Macrophages, and Adipocyte Hypertrophy in Lipedema Thigh Skin and Fat Tissue. *J. Obes.* 2019;2019:8747461. doi: https://doi.org/10.1155/2019/8747461.

Crescenzi R., Donahue P.M., Petersen K.J., Garza M., Patel N., Lee C., Beckman J.A., Donahue M.J. Upper and Lower Extremity Measurement of Tissue Sodium and Fat Content in Patients with Lipedema. *Obesity.* 2020;28:907–915. doi: https://doi.org/10.1002/oby.22778.

Kruppa P., Georgiou I., Schmidt J., Ghods M. Ten-Year Experience With the Surgical Treatment of Lipedema – Long-Term Follow-up after Multi-stage Liposuction. *Plast. Reconstr. Surg. Glob. Open.* 2020;8:78. doi: https://doi.org/10.1097/01.GOX.0000720696.12094.f2.

Donahue P.M., Crescenzi R., Petersen K.J., Garza M., Patel N., Lee C., Chen S.-C., Donahue M.J. Physical Therapy in Women with Early Stage Lipedema: Potential Impact of Multimodal Manual Therapy, Compression, Exercise, and Education Interventions. *Lymphat. Res. Biol.* 2022;20:382–390. doi: https://doi.org/10.1089/lrb.2021.0039.

Gensior M.H.L., Cornely M. Pain in lipoedema, fat in lipoedema and its consequences: Results of a patient survey based on a pain questionnaire. *Handchir. Mikrochir. Plast. Chir.* 2019a;51:249–254.

Aksoy H., Karadag A.S., Wollina U. Cause and management of lipedema-associated pain. *Dermatol. Ther.* 2020;34:e14364. doi: https://doi.org/10.1111/dth.14364.

Malik R.A. Pathology of human diabetic neuropathy. *Handb. Clin. Neurol.* 2014;126:249–259.

Shillo P., Yiangou Y., Donatien P., Greig M., Selvarajah D., Wilkinson I.D., Anand P., Tesfaye S. Nerve and Vascular Biomarkers in Skin Biopsies Differentiate Painful From Painless Peripheral Neuropathy in Type 2 Diabetes. *Front. Pain Res.* 2021;2:731658. doi: https://doi.org/10.3389/fpain.2021.731658.

Siems W., Grune T., Voss P., Brenke R. Anti-fibrosclerotic effects of shock wave therapy in lipedema and cellulite. *BioFactors.* 2005;24:275–282. doi: https://doi.org/10.1002/biof.5520240132.

Amann-Vesti B.R., Franzeck U.K., Bollinger A. Microlymphatic aneurysms in patients with lipedema. *Lymphology.* 2001;34:170–175.

Zechner U., Kohlschmidt N., Kempf O., Gebauer K., Haug K., Engels H., Haaf T., Bartsch O. Familial Sotos syndrome caused by a novel missense mutation, C2175S, in NSD1 and associated with normal intelligence, insulin dependent diabetes, bronchial asthma, and lipedema. *Eur. J. Med. Genet.* 2009;52:306–310. doi: https://doi.org/10.1016/j.ejmg.2009.06.001.

Angst F., Benz T., Lehmann S., Sandor P., Wagner S. Common and Contrasting Characteristics of the Chronic Soft-Tissue Pain Conditions Fibromyalgia and Lipedema. *J. Pain Res.* 2021;14:2931–2941. doi: https://doi.org/10.2147/JPR.S315736.

Beltran K., Herbst K.L. Differentiating lipedema and Dercum's disease. *Int. J. Obes.* 2016;41:240–245. doi: https://doi.org/10.1038/ijo.2016.205.

Dudek J.E., Białaszek W., Ostaszewski P. Quality of life in women with lipoedema: A contextual behavioral approach. *Qual. Life Res.* 2015;25:401–408. doi: https://doi.org/10.1007/s11136-015-1080-x.

Felmerer G., Stylianaki A., Hollmén M., Ströbel P., Stepniewski A., Wang A., Frueh F.S., Kim B.-S., Giovanoli P., Lindenblatt N., et al. Increased levels of VEGF-C and macrophage infiltration in lipedema patients without changes in lymphatic vascular morphology. *Sci. Rep.* 2020;10:10947. doi: https://doi.org/10.1038/s41598-020-67987-3.

Michelini S., Chiurazzi P., Marino V., Dell'Orco D., Manara E., Baglivo M., Fiorentino A., Maltese P.E., Pinelli M., Herbst K.L., et al. Aldo-Keto Reductase 1C1 (*AKR1C1*) as the First Mutated Gene in a Family with Nonsyndromic Primary Lipedema. *Int. J. Mol. Sci.* 2020;21:6264. doi: https://doi.org/10.3390/ijms21176264.

Seidel M.F., Hügle T., Morlion B., Koltzenburg M., Chapman V., MaassenVanDenBrink A., Lane N.E., Perrot S., Zieglgänsberger W. Neurogenic inflammation as a novel treatment target for chronic pain syndromes. *Exp. Neurol.* 2022;356:114108. doi: https://doi.org/10.1016/j.expneurol.2022.114108.

Lauria G., Bakkers M., Schmitz C., Lombardi R., Penza P., Devigili G., Smith A.G., Hsieh S.-T., Mellgren S.I., Umapathi T., et al. Intraepidermal nerve fiber density at the distal leg: A worldwide normative reference study. *J. Peripher. Nerv. Syst.* 2010;15:202–207. doi: https://doi.org/10.1111/j.1529-8027.2010.00271.x.

Anand P. Nerve growth factor regulates nociception in human health and disease. *Br. J. Anaesth.* 1995;75:201–208. doi: https://doi.org/10.1093/bja/75.2.201.

Kilo S., Harding-Rose C., Hargreaves K.M., Flores C.M. Peripheral CGRP release as a marker for neurogenic inflammation: A model system for the study of neuropeptide secretion in rat paw skin. *Pain.* 1997;73:201–207. doi: https://doi.org/10.1016/S0304-3959(97)00108-5.

Schou W.S., Ashina S., Amin F.M., Goadsby P., Ashina M. Calcitonin gene-related peptide and pain: A systematic review. *J. Headache Pain.* 2017;18:34. doi: https://doi.org/10.1186/s10194-017-0741-2.

Mizumura K., Murase S. Role of Nerve Growth Factor in Pain. *Handb. Exp. Pharmacol.* 2015;227:57–77. doi: https://doi.org/10.1007/978-3-662-46450-2_4.

Halk A.B., Damstra R.J. First Dutch guidelines on lipedema using the international classification of functioning, disability and health. *Phlebol. J. Venous Dis.* 2016;32:152–159. doi: https://doi.org/10.1177/0268355516639421.

Petersen K.J., Garza M., Donahue P.M.C., Harkins K.D., Marton A., Titze J., Donahue M.J., Crescenzi R. Neuroimaging of Cerebral Blood Flow and Sodium in Women with Lipedema. *Obesity.* 2020;28:1292–1300. doi: https://doi.org/10.1002/oby.22837. Available online: https://www.ResearchMatch.org

Herbst K.L. Rare adipose disorders (RADs) masquerading as obesity. *Acta Pharmacol. Sin.* 2012;33:155–172. doi: https://doi.org/10.1038/aps.2011.153.

Duhon B.H., Phan T.T., Taylor S.L., Crescenzi R.L., Rutkowski J.M. Current Mechanistic Understandings of Lymphedema and Lipedema: Tales of Fluid, Fat, and Fibrosis. *Int. J. Mol. Sci.* 2022;23:6621. doi: https://doi.org/10.3390/ijms23126621.

Au-Kostek M., Polaski A., Kolber B., Ramsey A., Kranjec A., Szucs K. A Protocol of Manual Tests to Measure Sensation and Pain in Humans. *JoVE.* 2016;118:e54130.

Paling I., MacIntyre L. Survey of lipoedema symptoms and experience with compression garments. *Br. J. Community Nurs.* 2020;25:S17–S22. doi: https://doi.org/10.12968/bjcn.2020.25.Sup4.S17.

Fink J.M., Schreiner L., Marjanovic G., Erbacher G., Seifert G.J., Foeldi M., Bertsch T. Leg Volume in Patients with Lipoedema following Bariatric Surgery. *Visc. Med.* 2020;37:206–211. doi: https://doi.org/10.1159/000511044.

Chakraborty A, Crescenzi R, Usman TA, Reyna AJ, Garza ME, Al-Ghadban S, Herbst KL, Donahue PMC, Rutkowski JM. Indications of Peripheral Pain, Dermal Hypersensitivity, and Neurogenic Inflammation in Patients with Lipedema. Int J Mol Sci. 2022 Sep 7;23(18):10313. doi: https://doi.org/10.3390/ijms231810313. PMID: 36142221; PMCID: PMC9499469

GBD 2016 DALYs and HALE Collaborators. Global, regional, and national disability-adjusted life-years (DALYs) for 333 diseases and injuries and healthy life expectancy (HALE) for 195 countries and territories, 1990–2016: a systematic analysis for the global burden of disease study 2016. *Lancet Lond Engl.* 2017;**390**(10100):1260–1344. doi: https://doi.org/10.1016/S0140-6736(17)32130-X.

Queiroz LP. Worldwide epidemiology of fibromyalgia. *Curr Pain Headache Rep.* 2013;**17**(8):356. doi: https://doi.org/10.1007/s11916-013-0356-5

Shavit E, Wollina U, Alavi A. Lipoedema is not lymphoedema: a review of current literature. *Int Wound J.* 2018;**15**(6):921–928. doi: https://doi.org/10.1111/iwj.12949

Reich-Schupke S, Schmeller W, Brauer WJ, et al. S1 guidelines: lipedema. *J Dtsch Dermatol Ges J Ger Soc Dermatol JDDG.* 2017;**15**(7):758–767. doi: https://doi.org/10.1111/ddg.13036

Angst F, Verra M, Lehmann S, Brioschi R, Aeschlimann A. Clinical effectiveness of an interdisciplinary pain management programme compared with standard inpatient rehabilitation in chronic pain: a naturalistic, prospective controlled cohort study. *J Rehabil Med.* 2009;**41**(7):569–575. doi: https://doi.org/10.2340/16501977-0381

Gota CE, Kaouk S, Wilke WS. Fibromyalgia and obesity: the association between body mass index and disability, depression, history of abuse, medications, and comorbidities. *J Clin Rheumatol Pract Rep Rheum Musculoskelet Dis.* 2015;**21**(6):289–295. doi: https://doi.org/10.1097/RHU.0000000000000278

Gensior MHL, Cornely M. [Pain in lipoedema, fat in lipoedema and its consequences: results of a patient survey based on a pain questionnaire]. *Handchir Mikrochir Plast Chir.* 2019b;**51**(4):249–254. doi: https://doi.org/10.1055/a-0942-9607. German

Bennett RM, Schein J, Kosinski MR, Hewitt DJ, Jordan DM, Rosenthal NR. Impact of fibromyalgia pain on health-related quality of life before and after treatment with tramadol/acetaminophen. *Arthritis Rheum.* 2005;**53**(4):519–527. doi: https://doi.org/10.1002/art.21319

Wolfe F, Smythe HA, Yunus MB, et al. The American College of Rheumatology 1990 criteria for the classification of fibromyalgia. Report of the multicenter criteria committee. *Arthritis Rheum.* 1990;**33**(2):160–172. doi: https://doi.org/10.1002/art.1780330203

Wolfe F, Clauw DJ, Fitzcharles M-A, et al. The American College of Rheumatology preliminary diagnostic criteria for fibromyalgia and measurement of symptom severity. *Arthritis Care Res.* 2010;**62**(5):600–610. doi: https://doi.org/10.1002/acr.20140

Wolfe F, Clauw DJ, Fitzcharles M-A, et al. 2016 Revisions to the 2010/2011 fibromyalgia diagnostic criteria. *Semin Arthritis Rheum.* 2016;**46**(3):319–329. doi: https://doi.org/10.1016/j.semarthrit.2016.08.012

Halk AB, Damstra RJ. First Dutch guidelines on lipedema using the international classification of functioning, disability and health. *Phlebology*. 2017;**32**(3):152–159. doi: https://doi.org/10.1177/0268355516639421

Wollina U, Heinig B. Differential diagnostics of lipedema and lymphedema: a practical guideline. *Z Rheumatol*. 2018;**77**(9):799–807. doi: https://doi.org/10.1007/s00393-018-0546-y

Angst F, Lehmann S, Aeschlimann A, Sandòr PS, Wagner S. Cross-sectional validity and specificity of comprehensive measurement in lymphedema and lipedema of the lower extremity: a comparison of five outcome instruments. *Health Qual Life Outcomes*. 2020b;**18**(1):245. doi: https://doi.org/10.1186/s12955-020-01488-9

Angst F, Brioschi R, Main CJ, Lehmann S, Aeschlimann A. Interdisciplinary rehabilitation in fibromyalgia and chronic back pain: a prospective outcome study. *J Pain*. 2006;**7**(11):807–815. doi: https://doi.org/10.1016/j.jpain.2006.03.009

Dutch Society for Dermatology and Venereology (NDVD). Dutch lipoedema guideline; 2014. Available from:https://diseasetheycallfat.tv/wp-content/uploads/2015/08/Dutch-lipoedemaguideline-2014.pdf. Accessed July 6, 2021.

Wounds UK. Best Practice Guidelines: The Management of Lipoedema. London: Wounds UK, 2017. Available from: https://www.guidelines.co.uk/skin-and-wound-care/wounds-uk-lipoedema-guideline/453516.article. Accessed August 31, 2021.

Angst F, Aeschlimann A, Steiner W, Stucki G. Responsiveness of the WOMAC osteoarthritis index as compared with the SF-36 in patients with osteoarthritis of the legs undergoing a comprehensive rehabilitation intervention. *Ann Rheum Dis*. 2001;**60**(9):834–840.

Busija L, Pausenberger E, Haines TP, Haymes S, Buchbinder R, Osborne RH. Adult measures of general health and health-related quality of life: medical Outcomes Study Short Form 36-Item (SF-36) and Short Form 12-Item (SF-12) Health Surveys, Nottingham Health Profile (NHP), Sickness Impact Profile (SIP), Medical Outcomes Study Short Form 6D (SF-6D), Health Utilities Index Mark 3 (HUI3), Quality of Well-Being Scale (QWB), and Assessment of Quality of Life (AQoL). *Arthritis Care Res*. 2011;**63 Suppl 11**:S383–S412. doi: https://doi.org/10.1002/acr.20541

Bullinger M, Kirchberger I. *Fragebogen zum Gesundheitszustand: SF-36; Handanweisung [The SF-36 questionnaire to assess health status. A manual]*. Hogrefe: Verlag für Psychologie; 1998

Associated Mobility Comorbidities

The pathophysiology of lipedema and its linkage to mobility impairments is complex, involving multiple physiological systems. Lipedema is characterized by the abnormal accumulation of adipose tissue, particularly in the lower limbs, which can significantly hinder physical movement. The disproportionate fat distribution primarily around the thighs, hips, and lower legs alters the biomechanical alignment and load distribution across the joints, subsequently increasing the risk of joint degeneration and pain, notably in the knees and hips. Moreover, the excess fat often leads to secondary lymphatic overload and dysfunction because the lymphatic system becomes overwhelmed and incapable of efficiently managing lymph fluid. This lymphatic impairment contributes to tissue swelling and fibrosis, which not only exacerbates the physical bulk of the limbs but also stiffens the tissues, further restricting joint **mobility** and agility. Additionally, the pathological changes in connective tissue seen in lipedema—increased fibrosis and reduced elasticity—can impair the normal range of motion and elasticity of the skin and connective tissue, leading to a decreased functional capability. These factors combined significantly impair the ability to perform daily activities, contributing to a reduced quality of life and increased disability in individuals with lipedema.

In the clinical assessment of mobility in patients with lipedema, healthcare professionals employ a multifaceted approach to evaluate the extent of mobility impairment and identify the most effective interventions. The assessment typically begins with a thorough patient history to understand the duration and progression of mobility issues, accompanied by a physical examination focusing on limb circumference, skin texture, and the presence of pain or tenderness. One key technique involves goniometry, which measures the range of motion in affected joints to determine restrictions that might be contributing to mobility limitations. Additionally, standardized functional tests such as the Timed Up and Go (TUG) test or the 6-Minute Walk Test (6MWT) are utilized to objectively assess the patient's functional mobility and endurance capabilities.

For a more comprehensive analysis, advanced imaging techniques like lymphoscintigraphy or MRI might be used to assess the structural and functional status of

G. Laur, *Lipoedema*, https://doi.org/10.1007/978-981-96-8939-2_30

the lymphatic system and to visualize the distribution and density of adipose tissue. This helps in distinguishing lipedema from other conditions such as lymphedema or obesity. Furthermore, gait analysis can be conducted in more specialized settings; this involves using video or computerized systems to capture and analyze the biomechanics of a patient's walk, identifying abnormalities and compensatory mechanisms that could be targeted in physical therapy. Ultimately, the assessment of mobility in patients with lipedema requires a holistic approach that integrates both clinical observation and objective measurement tools to tailor effective management strategies that enhance mobility and quality of life.

The biomechanics of gait and posture in individuals with lipedema present distinct challenges that stem from the abnormal accumulation and distribution of adipose tissue. Lipedema predominantly affects the lower extremities, often leading to bilateral and symmetrical enlargement of the legs, which can have a direct impact on gait dynamics. The added mass in the lower limbs can shift the center of gravity downward and outward, which in turn necessitates compensatory adjustments in posture to maintain balance and stability during ambulation.

With lipedema, there is often a disruption in the kinematic chain of lower body movement. The hips may adopt an altered path of motion to accommodate increased thigh circumference, potentially leading to an increased base of support. Consequently, the gait may become wider and more circumductive to avoid soft tissue friction. This alteration in gait pattern can increase the mechanical work required for walking and contribute to fatigue.

The additional adipose tissue can also affect joint angles, particularly at the knee, where hyperextension or genu recurvatum may occur as a compensatory mechanism to support the body's weight during the stance phase of gait. Over time, this can lead to joint instability and increased susceptibility to osteoarthritis due to uneven wear on the joint surfaces. Moreover, increased limb volume may limit the normal flexion and extension required for an efficient gait cycle, leading to a reduction in stride length and walking speed.

The weight-bearing joints of patients with lipedema often endure greater loads, contributing to the development of pain and further altering gait mechanics. The pain can lead to an avoidance of heel strike and an increased reliance on midfoot or forefoot striking, which can further compromise efficient gait patterns and lead to secondary musculoskeletal issues.

In addition, the proprioceptive feedback, crucial for maintaining balance and coordination during movement, may be impaired in lipedema due to the increased adiposity and potential swelling. This can lead to uncertainty in foot placement and a higher risk of trips and falls.

Postural adaptations in lipedema are also evident during static positions. There may be an increased lordotic curve in the lumbar spine as the pelvis tilts anteriorly to counterbalance the weight of the enlarged lower limbs. This postural change can result in chronic lower back pain and further contribute to a sedentary lifestyle, exacerbating lipedema symptoms and comorbid conditions.

Lipedema, a chronic condition characterized by the pathological build-up of adipose tissue in the extremities, exerts significant biomechanical stress on joint health.

The disproportionate increase in soft tissue mass, particularly around the lower limbs, alters normal load distribution across the weight-bearing joints, such as the hips, knees, and ankles. This aberrant stress predisposes the articular cartilage to accelerated wear and tear, which can expedite the degenerative process leading to osteoarthritis. The excessive adiposity around the joints acts as a constant mechanical burden, potentially leading to chronic joint inflammation and pain. This not only diminishes the synovial fluid's effectiveness in providing necessary joint lubrication but also may compromise the integrity of the periarticular ligaments, further destabilizing the joints and exacerbating the risk of injury.

Additionally, the atypical gait patterns observed in patients with lipedema—often an adaptive response to discomfort and instability—can induce abnormal joint kinematics, particularly in the knee, where varus or valgus malalignments may become pronounced. Over time, these altered movement patterns contribute to uneven joint loading and can lead to a reduction in the range of motion, further limiting function and exacerbating joint deterioration. The increased incidence of joint hypermobility seen in patients with lipedema suggests a connective tissue component to the condition, which may inherently affect joint integrity and resilience.

Moreover, chronic pain associated with lipedema can lead to a reduction in physical activity, contributing to muscle atrophy and weakness, particularly of the quadriceps and hamstrings that support the knee joint. This muscular deconditioning can leave joints vulnerable to additional stress and injury. Therefore, comprehensive management strategies that address both the abnormal fat distribution and the resultant biomechanical compensations are critical in mitigating the impact of lipedema on joint health. These strategies may include weight management, physical therapy to strengthen supporting musculature, and orthotics to correct malalignment and redistribute joint loads more evenly.

The intricate relationship between lipedema and osteoarthritis encompasses various pathophysiological mechanisms, with the abnormal accumulation of adipose tissue in lipedema exerting multiple detrimental effects on joint health. The chronic, progressive nature of lipedema often leads to significant changes in the biomechanical environment of the joints, predominantly affecting the knees, hips, and ankles. This excess adipose tissue is not inert; it is metabolically active and secretes a range of adipokines and inflammatory mediators that can contribute to systemic inflammation, a known risk factor for osteoarthritis.

First, the added weight from excess adipose tissue in patients with lipedema places undue stress on the articular cartilage of the joints. Cartilage, which normally functions to absorb shock and facilitate smooth joint motion, becomes compromised under the increased load, leading to accelerated wear and tear.

Over time, this can result in the degenerative changes characteristic of osteoarthritis, including joint space narrowing, subchondral bone sclerosis, and osteophyte formation.

Second, the mechanical strain exerted by the pathological adipose deposits can lead to malalignment of the joints. In the knee, for instance, this can manifest as varus (bow-legged) or valgus (knock-kneed) deformities. Such deviations from normal alignment increase the mechanical load on certain regions of the joint, disrupting the distribution of forces during weight-bearing activities and contributing to the uneven progression of osteoarthritic damage.

Furthermore, the inflammatory milieu associated with lipedema can predispose to systemic inflammation, which has been implicated in the pathogenesis of osteoarthritis. Adipose tissue, especially when in excess, acts as an endocrine organ that secretes pro-inflammatory cytokines such as tumor necrosis factor-alpha (TNF-α) and interleukin-6 (IL-6). These cytokines can perpetuate a chronic inflammatory state, leading to further joint destruction and pain, hallmarks of osteoarthritis.

In addition to biochemical factors, the physical burden of lipedema can lead to a sedentary lifestyle due to pain and mobility constraints. Reduced physical activity exacerbates the progression of joint degeneration by promoting muscle weakness, particularly in the muscles that stabilize the knee (quadriceps and hamstrings), further compromising joint integrity and accelerating the osteoarthritic process.

The interplay between lipedema and osteoarthritis is thus multifactorial, involving biomechanical, inflammatory, and lifestyle components. It is essential for clinical practitioners to recognize the potential for accelerated joint degeneration in patients with lipedema and to address both the metabolic and mechanical aspects of the condition. A proactive approach to treatment should incorporate weight management, anti-inflammatory strategies, and rehabilitation programs aimed at preserving joint function and mitigating pain. Understanding and addressing the complex connection between lipedema and osteoarthritis can lead to improved outcomes and quality of life for affected individuals.

Physical therapy plays a crucial role in enhancing mobility for patients with lipedema, a condition characterized by the pathological accumulation of fatty tissue, particularly in the lower extremities. The goal of physical therapy in this context is to alleviate the secondary complications associated with lipedema, such as joint pain, reduced range of motion, and diminished muscle strength, all of which contribute to mobility restrictions.

An integral component of physical therapy for lipedema is a tailored exercise program aimed at preserving or improving joint range of motion and enhancing muscular strength. Low-impact aerobic exercises, such as swimming or cycling, are often recommended to minimize joint stress while promoting cardiovascular fitness. Strength training, particularly of the core and lower limb muscles, helps to support the joints, improve posture, and reduce the risk of injury. Additionally, flexibility exercises and stretching are crucial in maintaining soft tissue elasticity and joint mobility, thereby reducing the tightness and stiffness often seen in patients with lipedema.

Manual lymphatic drainage (MLD) therapy is another cornerstone of physical therapy for lipedema. This specialized form of massage encourages the movement of lymph fluids around blocked areas into more centrally located lymph vessels, aiding in the reduction of limb volume and associated pain. This technique can improve joint flexibility and the range of motion by addressing the component of swelling that often accompanies lipedema.

Moreover, physical therapists may utilize techniques such as taping or the application of compression garments to reduce edema and provide support to the limbs during exercise and daily activities. The strategic use of compression can facilitate more efficient muscle pump action, essential in promoting venous and lymphatic return, thereby mitigating the effects of lipedema on mobility.

Gait training is also a valuable aspect of physical therapy, especially for patients with lipedema who have developed compensatory walking patterns that may contribute to musculoskeletal pain and dysfunction. Physical therapists can assess the patient's gait and identify abnormal patterns, offering corrective strategies and exercises to optimize walking mechanics and reduce the risk of joint degeneration.

In addition to active interventions, patient education is an essential element of physical therapy. Educating patients about the importance of maintaining an active lifestyle, weight management, and proper skin care can empower them to manage their symptoms effectively. Physical therapists also provide guidance on adaptive strategies and ergonomic modifications to the home and workplace to minimize the risk of injury and enhance overall functional ability.

Ultimately, physical therapy for lipedema should be comprehensive, multidisciplinary, and personalized. It should address the physical, functional, and psychosocial aspects of the disease, enabling patients to achieve better mobility, minimize pain, and improve their quality of life. Regular reassessment is necessary to adapt the treatment plan as the condition progresses or as the patient's needs change.

The role of exercise in managing lipedema and osteoarthritic symptoms represents a critical element in the multidisciplinary approach to these conditions. Exercise, particularly when tailored to the individual's needs, offers numerous benefits that can alleviate symptoms associated with both lipedema and osteoarthritis.

For patients with lipedema, exercise enhances cardiovascular fitness, facilitates weight management, and improves lymphatic drainage, which is crucial given the propensity for fluid retention in affected limbs. Low-impact aerobic activities such as swimming, cycling, and walking are often recommended to minimize joint strain while effectively increasing heart rate and promoting fat oxidation. These activities also serve to boost overall energy levels and enhance mood, countering the fatigue and emotional distress that frequently accompany lipedema.

Strength training is equally important in managing lipedema, with a focus on building muscle mass to increase metabolic rate and provide better support for the joints. Strength exercises can be particularly beneficial for the knees and hips, which bear the brunt of biomechanical stress due to excess adipose tissue in the lower body. Resistance exercises should be prescribed carefully to avoid exacerbating joint pain, focusing on controlled movements and appropriate load-bearing exercises that do not overload the joints.

Flexibility and range-of-motion exercises also play a vital role, as they help maintain joint and soft tissue elasticity, which can be compromised in lipedema. Stretching and mobility exercises can help prevent the development of contractures and maintain functional movement patterns that may otherwise be altered due to pain or bulk of the adipose tissue.

For managing osteoarthritis symptoms, exercises targeting joint stability and strengthening the muscles around affected joints can help reduce pain and improve function. For instance, knee osteoarthritis can benefit from quadriceps-strengthening exercises, which help to stabilize the patella and distribute force more evenly through the knee joint during activity.

Balance and proprioception exercises are also crucial, as proprioceptive feedback can be impaired in lipedema and osteoarthritis. Balance training can reduce the risk of falls, which is particularly important in this patient population where joint health is already compromised.

While exercise is beneficial, it must be noted that patients with lipedema and osteoarthritis often face barriers to physical activity, including joint pain and psychological factors such as body image concerns. Thus, a supportive environment and professional guidance from physiotherapists or exercise physiologists are important to help patients initiate and maintain an exercise program.

Pain management for lipedema-related osteoarthritis requires a multifaceted approach, considering both the chronic pain associated with adipose tissue accumulation and the joint-specific discomfort characteristic of osteoarthritis. A comprehensive pain management strategy is essential to enhance the patient's quality of life and functional capacity.

Non-pharmacological interventions form the foundation of pain management in lipedema-related osteoarthritis. Physical therapy, particularly strength training and aerobic conditioning, can be beneficial in preserving joint function and reducing pain. Exercises aimed at strengthening the muscles surrounding the affected joints can provide stability and reduce the load borne by the joint, thereby alleviating pain. Additionally, aquatic therapy offers a unique advantage by enabling exercise with reduced joint stress due to the buoyancy provided by water.

Manual therapies, including massage and manual lymphatic drainage (MLD), can also play a role in pain management. MLD, specifically, can reduce the limb volume and pressure in subcutaneous tissues, thereby potentially decreasing pain levels. Moreover, the application of cold packs or thermotherapy can offer transient relief from acute pain episodes by modulating blood flow and inflammatory responses at the joint level.

Pharmacological approaches include the cautious use of analgesics, such as acetaminophen or nonsteroidal anti-inflammatory drugs (NSAIDs), which can be effective for managing osteoarthritic pain but must be used judiciously given the potential for adverse effects with long-term use. In certain cases, supplements like glucosamine and chondroitin sulfate may also be considered, though their efficacy can vary.

Emerging pain management strategies for lipedema-related osteoarthritis include the use of nutraceuticals and anti-inflammatory diets, which aim to reduce systemic inflammation and may have secondary benefits for joint pain.

The adoption of weight management strategies is crucial as well, as excess body weight can exacerbate both lipedema symptoms and osteoarthritic joint stress.

Furthermore, cognitive-behavioral therapy (CBT) and mindfulness-based stress reduction (MBSR) techniques can assist patients in coping with the chronic pain associated with lipedema and osteoarthritis. These psychological interventions focus on altering the perception of pain, improving emotional well-being, and fostering coping strategies that can mitigate the impact of chronic pain on daily living.

The interventional treatment options, such as corticosteroid injections or viscosupplementation, may be considered for localized joint pain refractory to other treatment modalities. However, these are usually reserved for cases where conservative management has failed, and the benefits outweigh the risks.

In summary, the effective management of pain in lipedema-related osteoarthritis is typically achieved through a combination of physical and behavioral therapies, lifestyle modifications, and, where appropriate, pharmacological and interventional treatments. Personalization of pain management plans, patient education, and ongoing evaluation of treatment outcomes are key components in achieving optimal pain control for patients with lipedema with osteoarthritic symptoms.

Orthotic and assistive devices play a significant role in the management of mobility issues in individuals with lipedema. These devices are designed to support the biomechanical alignment of the body, redistribute weight, and alleviate stress on the lower extremities, thereby enhancing mobility and reducing pain.

Custom-fitted orthotic insoles can be particularly beneficial for patients with lipedema. These insoles are tailored to the individual's foot structure and can provide arch support, correct abnormal foot pronation or supination, and help distribute pressure more evenly across the foot. This can be crucial in preventing additional stress on the knees and hips—joints that are often affected by the altered gait patterns associated with lipedema.

Compression garments are another cornerstone of orthotic management for lipedema. These garments apply graduated compression to the limbs, promoting venous and lymphatic circulation and reducing edema. Compression garments must be carefully selected to ensure they provide adequate compression without exacerbating pain or causing constriction. For patients with more advanced lipedema, pneumatic compression devices may be used to provide intermittent compression, further aiding in the reduction of limb volume and associated discomfort.

Assistive devices such as canes, walkers, or wheelchairs might be necessary for some individuals with lipedema, especially those with significant mobility impairment or those who experience pain with ambulation. These devices can help maintain independence by providing stability and reducing the load on lower body joints during walking. In cases where weight-bearing is particularly painful or difficult, the use of a wheelchair can provide necessary relief and assist in the conservation of energy.

Knee braces and ankle supports can offer localized joint support, enhancing stability and potentially mitigating the risk of injury.

They can also serve as a temporary measure to provide joint relief postexercise or during flare-ups of pain. In severe cases of joint instability or deformity, custom-fabricated braces may be necessary to adequately support the affected limbs.

While orthotic and assistive devices are valuable in managing mobility issues associated with lipedema, it is vital to pair their use with other management strategies such as weight control, exercise, and manual lymphatic drainage for optimal benefit. Additionally, education on the correct use and maintenance of these devices is crucial, as improper use can lead to skin issues, discomfort, or even worsening of symptoms.

Surgical interventions for patients with lipedema who are also suffering from osteoarthritis represent an advanced tier of treatment, typically considered when conservative management fails to provide sufficient relief from symptoms. These surgical procedures are not only aimed at addressing the symptoms of osteoarthritis but may also be utilized to manage the excessive adipose tissue characteristic of lipedema.

Joint replacement surgery, particularly total knee or hip arthroplasty, is a common intervention for severe osteoarthritis that has led to significant joint destruction and impairment. In patients with lipedema, these procedures can alleviate the chronic pain stemming from osteoarthritic changes, restore joint function, and improve overall mobility. However, the presence of lipedema can complicate surgical outcomes due to the excessive adipose tissue, which can increase the risk of surgical site infections and affect wound healing. Preoperative optimization, including weight management and control of lipedema-related inflammation, is critical to improve surgical outcomes.

Liposuction has been utilized in the management of lipedema to remove pathologic adipose tissue, reduce limb volume, and potentially decrease the burden on the joints. While liposuction is not a direct treatment for osteoarthritis, by alleviating the excessive weight and volume of the limbs, it may indirectly reduce the mechanical stress on the joints affected by osteoarthritis. In recent years, water-assisted liposuction (WAL) and tumescent liposuction have been used with some success in patients with lipedema, as they allow for the removal of large volumes of fat with less tissue trauma.

When considering the timing for surgical interventions, it is important to evaluate the patient's overall functional status, pain levels, and quality of life. Surgery is generally indicated when the patient experiences persistent pain that interferes with daily activities and sleep, when mobility is significantly restricted, and when conservative treatments such as medication, physical therapy, and orthotic support have been exhausted.

The approach to surgical intervention must be highly individualized. Preoperative assessment by a multidisciplinary team, including an orthopedic surgeon, a plastic surgeon with experience in lipedema, an anesthesiologist, and a physiotherapist, is essential to ensure comprehensive planning. The surgical plan should consider both the patient's osteoarthritic condition and the specific challenges presented by lipedema, such as potential lymphatic complications and the increased likelihood of prolonged postoperative edema.

Postoperatively, patients with lipedema require close monitoring to manage pain, prevent complications, and promote effective rehabilitation. An integrated postoperative care plan that includes lymphatic drainage, compression therapy, and a gradual and tailored physical rehabilitation program is vital for optimal recovery and functional improvement.

The optimal management of lipedema complicated by osteoarthritis requires a comprehensive, integrated approach that addresses the multifaceted challenges posed by these co-existing conditions. Effective care coordination among a multidisciplinary team of healthcare professionals is essential to tailor treatment strategies that effectively alleviate symptoms, halt progression, and enhance quality of life for affected individuals.

First, early and accurate diagnosis of both lipedema and osteoarthritis is crucial. This facilitates timely intervention, preventing the escalation of symptoms and the onset of severe complications. Regular monitoring and assessments by healthcare providers ensure that treatments remain responsive to the evolving needs of the patient.

Second, a combination of conservative and advanced therapeutic options should be considered. Lifestyle modifications, including diet and physical activity, are foundational, helping to manage body weight and reduce joint stress. Physical therapy is instrumental in improving mobility, strengthening muscles, and enhancing joint function. Pharmacologic treatments should aim to control pain and inflammation without exacerbating lipedema symptoms. In cases where medical management is insufficient, surgical options like liposuction or joint replacement may be appropriate, provided the patient is thoroughly evaluated and deemed a suitable candidate.

Moreover, patient education and support play roles in the management process. Patients should be well-informed about the nature of their conditions, the importance of adherence to treatment protocols, and lifestyle adjustments necessary for managing their symptoms. Psychological support is also vital, as chronic pain and mobility limitations can lead to significant emotional distress.

Finally, ongoing research into the pathophysiology of lipedema and osteoarthritis will likely yield novel insights that can lead to better therapeutic modalities. Meanwhile, healthcare systems should strive to improve access to multidisciplinary care teams and patient education resources, ensuring that individuals with lipedema and osteoarthritis receive comprehensive, holistic care.

In conclusion, the integrated management of lipedema and osteoarthritis requires a collaborative, patient-centered approach that combines medical, physical, and educational strategies. By fostering a deeper understanding of these conditions and promoting coordinated care efforts, it is possible to significantly mitigate the impact of these chronic diseases on patients' lives, leading to improved outcomes and sustained well-being.

Suggested Reading

Buck DW, 2nd, Herbst KL. Lipedema: a relatively common disease with extremely common misconceptions. *Plast Reconstr Surg Glob Open* 2016; 4: e1043.

Felmerer G, Stylianaki A, Hägerling R, et al. Adipose tissue hypertrophy, an aberrant biochemical profile and distinct gene expression in lipedema. *J Surg Res* 2020; 253: 294–303.

Al-Ghadban S, Cromer W, Allen M, et al. Dilated blood and lymphatic microvessels, angiogenesis, increased macrophages, and adipocyte hypertrophy in lipedema thigh skin and fat tissue. *J Obes* 2019; 2019: 1–10.

Herbst K, Mirkovskaya L, Bharhagava A, et al. Lipedema fat and signs and symptoms of illness, increase with advancing stage. *Arch Med* 2015; 7: 1–8.

Allen EV, Hines EAJ. Lipedema of the legs: a syndrome characterised by fat legs and orthostatic edema. *Proc Staff Meet Mayo Clin* 1940; 15: 184–187.

Moncorps CB, Brinkhaus G, Herteld F, et al. Experimentelle untersuchungen zur frage akrozyanotischer zustandsbilder. *Arch Derm Syph* 1940; 186: 209–215.

Todd M. Lipoedema: presentation and management. *Br J Community Nurs* 2010; 15: S10–S16.
Buso G, Depairon M, Tomson D, et al. Lipedema: a call to action!. *Obesity (Silver Spring)* 2019; 27: 1567–1576.
Shavit E, Wollina U, Alavi A. Lipoedema is not lymphoedema: a review of current literature. *Int Wound J* 2018; 15: 921–928.
Fetzer A, Wise C. Living with lipoedema: reviewing different self-management techniques. *Br J Community Nurs* 2015; 20: S14–S19.
Herbst KL. Subcutaneous adipose tissue diseases: Dercum disease, lipedema, familial multiple lipomatosis and Madelung disease. In: Purnell J, Perreault L. (eds) *Endotext*. Massachusetts: MDText.com, 2019.
Torre YS, Wadeea R, Rosas V, et al. Lipedema: friend and foe. *Horm Mol Biol Clin Investig* 2018; 33: 1–15.
Coppel T, Cunneen J, Fetzer S, et al. Best practice guidelines: the management of lipoedema. *Wounds UK, 2017:* 13: 1–36.
Alcolea JM, Alonso AB, Arroyo BA, et al. Documento de consenso lipedema 2018. In: *33rd National congress of the Spanish society of aesthetic medicine (SEME) Malaga, Barcelona, Spain*, 22-24 February 2018. Barcelona: LITOGAMA S.L.
Peprah K, MacDougall D. *Liposuction for the treatment of lipedema: a review of clinical effectiveness and guidelines*. Ottawa: Canadian Agency for Drugs and Technologies in Health, 2019.
Reich-Schupke S, Schmeller W, Brauer WJ, et al. S1 guidelines: lipedema. *J Dtsch Dermatol Ges* 2017; 15: 758–767.
Sandhofer M, Hanke CW, Habbema L, et al. Prevention of progression of lipedema with liposuction using tumescent local anesthesia: results of an international consensus conference. *Dermatol Surg* 2020; 46: 220–228.
Harris PA, Taylor R, Thielke R, et al. Research electronic data capture (REDCap) – a metadata-driven methodology and workflow process for providing translational research informatics support. *J Biomed Inform* 2009; 42: 377–381.
Hasson F, Keeney S, McKenna H. Research guidelines for the Delphi survey technique. *J Adv Nurs* 2000; 32: 1008–1015.
Guyatt GH, Oxman AD, Kunz R, et al. GRADE: going from evidence to recommendations. *Br Med J* 2008; 336: 1049–1051.
Policy U. Grading guide. In: Post TW. (ed.) *UpToDate*. Waltham, MA: UpToDate, 2020.
Herbst KL. Lipedema is not just fat. *Lipedemacom*, 2020.
McKee TJ, Perlman G, Morris M, et al. Extracellular matrix composition of connective tissues: a systematic review and Meta-analysis. *Sci Rep* 2019; 9: 15.
Levick JR, Michel CC. Microvascular fluid exchange and the revised starling principle. *Cardiovasc Res* 2010; 87: 198–210.
Guyton AC. Pressure-volume relationships in the interstitial spaces. *Invest Ophthalmol* 1965; 4: 1075–1084.
Rutkowski JM, Stern JH, Scherer PE. The cell biology of fat expansion. *J Cell Biol* 2015; 208: 501–512.
Roberts MA, Mendez U, Gilbert RJ, et al. Increased hyaluronan expression at distinct time points in acute lymphedema. *Lymphat Res Biol* 2012; 10: 122–128.
Bates DO, Levick JR, Mortimer PS. Change in macromolecular composition of interstitial fluid from swollen arms after breast cancer treatment, and its implications. *Clin Sci (Lond)* 1993; 85: 737–746.
Mortimer PS, Levick JR. Chronic peripheral oedema: the critical role of the lymphatic system. *Clin Med (Lond)* 2004; 4: 448–453.
Iker E, Mayfield CK, Gould DJ, et al. Characterizing lower extremity lymphedema and lipedema with cutaneous ultrasonography and an objective computer-assisted measurement of dermal echogenicity. *Lymphat Res Biol* 2019; 17: 525–530.
Crescenzi R, Donahue PMC, Weakley S, et al. Lipedema and Dercum's disease: a new application of bioimpedance. *Lymphat Res Biol* 2019; 17: 671–679.

Crescenzi R, Marton A, Donahue PMC, et al. Tissue sodium content is elevated in the skin and subcutaneous adipose tissue in women with lipedema. *Obesity (Silver Spring)* 2018; 26: 310–317.
Suga H, Araki J, Aoi N, et al. Adipose tissue remodeling in lipedema: adipocyte death and concurrent regeneration. *J Cutan Pathol* 2009; 36: 1293–1298.
Pessentheiner AR, Ducasa GM, Gordts PLSM. Proteoglycans in obesity-associated metabolic dysfunction and meta-inflammation. *Front Immunol* 2020; 11: 769.
Lumeng CN, Bodzin JL, Saltiel AR. Obesity induces a phenotypic switch in adipose tissue macrophage polarization. *J Clin Invest* 2007; 117: 175–184.
Pasarica M, Sereda OR, Redman LM, et al. Reduced adipose tissue oxygenation in human obesity: evidence for rarefaction, macrophage chemotaxis, and inflammation without an angiogenic response. *Diabetes* 2009; 58: 718–725.
van Esch-Smeenge J, Damstra RJ, Hendrickx AA. Muscle strength and functional exercise capacity in patients with lipoedema and obesity: a comparative study. *J Lymphoedema* 2017; 12: 27–31.
Stutz JJ. Liposuktion beim lipödem zur verhinderung von gelenkspätkomplikationen (Liposuction of lipedema to prevent later joint complications). *Vasomed* 2011; 23: 1–6.
Bast JH, Ahmed L, Engdahl R. Lipedema in patients after bariatric surgery. *Surg Obes Relat Dis* 2016; 12: 1131–1132.
Pouwels S, Huisman S, Smelt HJM, et al. Lipoedema in patients after bariatric surgery: report of two cases and review of literature. *Clin Obes* 2018; 8: 147–150.
Pouwels S, Smelt HJ, Said M, et al. Mobility problems and weight regain by misdiagnosed lipoedema after bariatric surgery: illustrating the medical and legal aspects. *Cureus* 2019; 11: e5388.
Wiedner M, Aghajanzadeh D, Richter DF. Differential diagnoses and treatment of lipedema. *Plast Aesthet Res* 2020; 7: 10.
Bel Lassen P, Charlotte F, Liu Y, et al. The FAT score, a fibrosis score of adipose tissue: predicting weight-loss outcome after gastric bypass. *J Clin Endocrinol Metab* 2017; 102: 2443–2453.
Szolnoky G, Nagy N, Kovacs RK, et al. Complex decongestive physiotherapy decreases capillary fragility in lipedema. *Lymphology* 2008a; 41: 161–166.
Ma W, Gil HJ, Escobedo N, et al. Platelet factor 4 is a biomarker for lymphatic-promoted disorders. *JCI Insight* 2020; 5: e135109.
Forner-Cordero I, Olivan-Sasot P, Ruiz-Llorca C, et al. Lymphoscintigraphic findings in patients with lipedema. *Rev Esp Med Nucl Imagen Mol* 2018; 37: 341–348.
Szolnoky G, Nemes A, Gavaller H, et al. Lipedema is associated with increased aortic stiffness. *Lymphology* 2012; 45: 71–79.
Jagtman BA, Kuiper JP, Brakkee AJ. [Measurements of skin elasticity in patients with lipedema of the Moncorps rusticanus type]. *Phlebologie* 1984; 37: 315–319.
Beighton P, Solomon L, Soskolne CL. Articular mobility in an African population. *Ann Rheum Dis* 1973; 32: 413–418.
Hakim AJ, Grahame R. A simple questionnaire to detect hypermobility: an adjunct to the assessment of patients with diffuse musculoskeletal pain. *Int J Clin Pract* 2003; 57: 163–166.
Stutz JJ. Alles über das Lipödem. *Lymphe & Gesundheit* 2015; 1–9 (human med AG Offprint).
Gensior MHL, Cornely M. Der Lipödemschmerz, seine Folgen auf die Lebensqualität betroffener Patientinnen – Ergebnisse einer Patientenbefragung mittels Schmerzfragebogen [Pain in lipoedema, fat in lipoedema and its consequences: results of a patient survey based on a pain questionnaire]. *Handchir Mikrochir Plast Chir* 2019; 51: 249–254.
Wold LE Hines EA JrandAllen EV. Lipedema of the legs; a syndrome characterized by fat legs and edema. *Ann Intern Med* 1951; 34: 1243–1250.
Nair AS, Diwan S. Allopregnanolone: a neurosteroid for managing acute and chronic pain conditions. *Saudi J Anaesth* 2019; 13: 264–266.
Michelini S, Chiurazzi P, Marino V, et al. Aldo-keto reductase 1C1 (AKR1C1) as the first mutated gene in a family with nonsyndromic primary lipedema. *Int J Mol Sci* 2020; 21: 6264.
Schook CC, Mulliken JB, Fishman SJ, et al. Differential diagnosis of lower extremity enlargement in pediatric patients referred with a diagnosis of lymphedema. *Plast Reconstr Surg* 2011; 127: 1571–1581.

Herpertz U. Krankheitsspektrum des Lipödems an einer Lymphologischen Fachklinik – Erscheinungsformen. *Mischbilder und Behandlungsmöglichkeiten* 1997; 5: 301–307.
Forner-Cordero I, Szolnoky G, Forner-Cordero A, et al. Lipedema: an overview of its clinical manifestations, diagnosis and treatment of the disproportional fatty deposition syndrome – systematic review. *Clin Obes* 2012; 2: 86–95.
Földi E, Földi M. Das lipödem. In Földi M, Földi E, Kubik S. (eds) *Lehrbuch der Lymphologie für Mediziner, Masseure und Physiotherapeuten*. Munich: Elsevier, Urban & Fischer, 2005, pp. 443–453.
Child AH, Gordon KD, Sharpe P, et al. Lipedema: an inherited condition. *Am J Med Genet A* 2010; 152A: 970–976.
Mendes AM, Madon RJ, Flint DJ. Effects of cortisol and progesterone on insulin binding and lipogenesis in adipocytes from normal and diabetic rats. *J Endocrinol* 1985; 106: 225–231.
Paolacci S, Precone V, Acquaviva F, et al. Genetics of lipedema: new perspectives on genetic research and molecular diagnoses. *Eur Rev Med Pharmacol Sci* 2019; 23: 5581–5594.
Herpertz U. Das lipödem. *Lymphologie* 1995; 19: 1–11.
Reich-Schupke S, Altmeyer P, Stücker M. Thick legs not always lipedema. *J Dtsch Dermatol Ges* 2013; 11: 225–233.
Dudek JE, Białaszek W, Gabriel M. Quality of life, its factors, and sociodemographic characteristics of Polish women with lipedema. *BMC Women's Health* 2021; 21: 1–9.
Halk AB, Damstra RJ. First Dutch guidelines on lipedema using the international classification of functioning, disability and health. *Phlebology* 2017; 32: 152–159.
Bauer AT, von Lukowicz D, Lossagk K, et al. New insights on lipedema: the enigmatic disease of the peripheral fat. *Plast Reconstr Surg* 2019; 144: 1475–1484.
Romeijn JRM, de Rooij MJM, Janssen L, et al. Exploration of patient characteristics and quality of life in patients with lipoedema using a survey. *Dermatol Ther (Heidelb)* 2018; 8: 303–311.
Herbst KL, Abu-Zaid L, Fazel MT. Question-based self-reported experience of patients with subcutaneous adipose tissue (SAT) disease prescribed sympathomimetic amines. *Med Res Archiv* 2019; 7: 1–17.
Beltran K, Herbst KL. Differentiating lipedema and Dercum's disease. *Int J Obes (Lond.)* 2017; 41: 240–245.
Kraus RH. and 2015. 2015:1–9. LG. All about lipedema. *Lymphe Gesundheit* 2015. 2015.
Dudek JE, Bialaszek W, Ostaszewski P. Quality of life in women with lipoedema: a contextual behavioral approach. *Qual Life Res* 2016; 25: 401–408.
Baumgartner A, Hueppe M, Meier-Vollrath I, et al. Improvements in patients with lipedema 4, 8 and 12 years after liposuction. *Phlebology* 2021; 36: 152–159.
Wollina U. [Lipedema: up-to-date of a long forgotten disease.]. *Wien Med Wochenschr* 2017; 167: 343–348.
Bays HE, Mw Christensen S, Tondt J, et al. *Obesity algorithm slides*. Scarborough: Obesity Medicine Association, 2020.
Apovian CM, Aronne LJ, Bessesen DH, et al. Pharmacological management of obesity: an endocrine society clinical practice guideline. *J Clin Endocrinol Metab* 2015; 100: 342–362.
Kajita K, Mori I, Hanamoto T, et al. Pioglitazone enhances small-sized adipocyte proliferation in subcutaneous adipose tissue. *Endocr J* 2012; 59: 1107–1114.
Kenny J-ES. The revised starling principle: implications for rational fluid therapy. *PulmCCM*. Epub ahead of print 7 July 2016. Available at: http://pulmccm.org/main/2016/ards-review/revised-starling-principle-implications-rational-fluid-therapy/
Li X, Li J, Wang L, et al. The role of metformin and resveratrol in the prevention of HIF1-alpha accumulation and fibrosis in hypoxic adipose tissue. *Br J Pharmacol* 2016; 5: 13493.
Kheirollahi V, Wasnick RM, Biasin V, et al. Metformin induces lipogenic differentiation in myofibroblasts to reverse lung fibrosis. *Nat Commun* 2019; 10: 2987.
Feldo M, Wozniak M, Wojciak-Kosior M, et al. Influence of Diosmin treatment on the level of oxidative stress markers in patients with chronic venous insufficiency. *Oxid Med Cell Longev* 2018; 2018: 2561705.

Ibegbuna V, Nicolaides AN, Sowade O, et al. Venous elasticity after treatment with Daflon 500 mg. *Angiology* 1997; 48: 45–49.
Bouskela E, Donyo KA, Verbeuren TJ. Effects of Daflon 500 mg on increased microvascular permeability in normal hamsters. *Int J Microcirc* 1995; 15: 22–26.
Batchvarov IV, Batselova MG, Damyanov II. One-year Diosmin therapy (600 mg) in patients with chronic venous insufficiency – results and analysis. *J Biomed Clin Res* 2010; 3: 51–54.
Carballo-Villalobos AI, González-Trujano ME, Pellicer F, et al. Antihyperalgesic effect of hesperidin improves with Diosmin in experimental neuropathic pain. *Biomed Res Int* 2016; 2016: 8263463.
Ehrlich C, Iker E, Herbst KL, et al. *Lymphedema and lipedema nutrition guide. Foods, vitamins, minerals, and supplements*. San Francisco: Lymph Notes, 2015.
Di Renzo L, Cinelli G, Romano L, et al. Potential effects of a modified Mediterranean diet on body composition in lipoedema. *Nutrients* 2021; 13: 358.
Keith L, Seo CA, Rowsemitt C, et al. Ketogenic diet as a potential intervention for lipedema. *Med Hypotheses* 2021; 146: 110435–112020.
Kosinski C, Jornayvaz FR. Effects of ketogenic diets on cardiovascular risk factors: evidence from animal and human studies. *Nutrients* 2017; 9: 517.
Pereira-Santos M, Costa PR, Assis AM, et al. Obesity and vitamin D deficiency: a systematic review and meta-analysis. *Obes Rev* 2015; 16: 341–349.
Greene AK, Sudduth CL. Lower extremity lymphatic function predicted by body mass index: a lymphoscintigraphic study of obesity and lipedema. *Int J Obes* 2021; 45: 369–373.
Lymphology Association of North America®, https://www.clt-lana.org/ (2020, 2020).
Wittlinger H, Wittlinger D, Wittlinger A, et al. Complementary techniques. In: *Dr Vodder's manual lymph drainage: a practical guide*. New York/Stuttgart: Thieme Publishers, 2018, 153 pp.
Szolnoky G, Borsos B, Barsony K, et al. Complete decongestive physiotherapy with and without pneumatic compression for treatment of lipedema: a pilot study. *Lymphology* 2008b; 41: 40–44.
Schwahn-Schreiber C, Breu FX, Rabe E, et al. [S1 guideline on intermittent pneumatic compression (IPC)]. *Hautarzt* 2018; 69: 662–673.
Hodge LM, King HH, Williams AG, Jr, et al. Abdominal lymphatic pump treatment increases leukocyte count and flux in thoracic duct lymph. *Lymphat Res Biol* 2007; 5: 127–133.
Huff JB, Schander A, Downey HF, et al. Lymphatic pump treatment augments lymphatic flux of lymphocytes in rats. *Lymphat Res Biol* 2010; 8: 183–187.
Gautam AP, Maiya AG, Vidyasagar MS. Effect of home-based exercise program on lymphedema and quality of life in female postmastectomy patients: pre-post intervention study. *J Rehabil Res Dev* 2011; 48: 1261–1268.
Reed RK, Townsley MI, Zhao Z, et al. Lymphatic hyaluronan flux from skin increases during increased lymph flow induced by intravenous saline loading. *Int J Microcirc* 1994; 14: 56–61.
Herbst KL, Ussery C, Eekema A. Pilot study: whole body manual subcutaneous adipose tissue (SAT) therapy improved pain and SAT structure in women with lipedema. *Horm Mol Biol Clin Investig* 2017; 33: 2018–2033.
Ibarra M, Eekema A, Ussery C, et al. Subcutaneous adipose tissue therapy reduces fat by dual X-ray absorptiometry scan and improves tissue structure by ultrasound in women with lipoedema and Dercum disease. *Clin Obes* 2018; 8: 398–406.
Wenczl E, Daróczy J. [Lipedema, a barely known disease: diagnosis, associated diseases and therapy]. *Orv Hetil* 2008; 149: 2121–2127.
Paling I, Macintyre L. Survey of lipoedema symptoms and experience with compression garments. *Br J Community Nurs* 2020; 25: S17–S22.
Szolnoky G, Varga E, Varga M, et al. Lymphedema treatment decreases pain intensity in lipedema. *Lymphology* 2011; 44: 178–182.
Hardy D, Williams A. Best practice guidelines for the management of lipoedema. *Br J Community Nurs* 2017; 22: S44–S48.
Linnitt N, Davies R. Fundamentals of compression in the management of lymphoedema. *Br J Nurs* 2007; 16: 588–592.

Schaverien MV, Moeller JA, Cleveland SD. Nonoperative treatment of lymphedema. *Semin Plast Surg* 2018; 32: 17–21.
Wilburn O, Wilburn P, Rockson SG. A pilot, prospective evaluation of a novel alternative for maintenance therapy of breast cancer-associated lymphedema. *BMC Cancer* 2006; 6: 84.
Bellini E, Grieco MP, Raposio E. A journey through liposuction and liposculture: review. *Ann Med Surg (Lond)* 2017; 24: 53–60.
Peled AW, Slavin SA, Brorson H. Long-term outcome after surgical treatment of lipedema. *Ann Plast Surg* 2012; 68: 303–307.

Enhancing Healthcare Team Outcome

Lipedema is a complex and often misunderstood adipose disorder characterized by the pathological accumulation of fat, primarily in the lower extremities, leading to pain, swelling, and mobility issues. Defined by its symmetrical distribution across both legs, sparing the feet and hands, lipedema predominantly affects women and can significantly impact their quality of life. Despite its distinct clinical presentation, the condition remains underdiagnosed, partly due to a lack of awareness within the medical community and the common misattribution of symptoms to obesity or lymphedema. The epidemiology of lipedema suggests a substantial prevalence among the female population, with varying estimates suggesting that a significant percentage may be affected worldwide. The clinical presentation of lipedema includes disproportionate fat accumulation, tenderness, easy bruising, and a propensity for the condition to worsen over time, leading to increased pain and functional impairment.

The complexity of lipedema, encompassing physical, psychological, and social dimensions, underscores the necessity for a multidisciplinary healthcare approach. The integration of various specialties—ranging from dermatology, physiotherapy, and bariatric surgery to psychology and dietetics—is crucial for addressing the multifaceted challenges faced by individuals with lipedema. A holistic and coordinated care strategy enhances patient outcomes by providing comprehensive management that includes not only the reduction of lipedema symptoms but also the support for associated psychological distress and lifestyle adjustments. This introduction highlights the importance of advancing our understanding of lipedema, promoting early diagnosis, and advocating for the enhancement of multidisciplinary healthcare teams dedicated to the nuanced care of patients with this condition, aiming to improve overall patient well-being and quality of life.

The healthcare team should consist of various professionals, including physicians, nurses, physiotherapists, dietitians, psychologists, and plastic surgeons. This approach ensures comprehensive management of the patient's physical and psychological health. Lipedema, a complex adipose tissue disorder, demands a multidisciplinary approach for optimal patient outcomes. The collaborative efforts of

G. Laur, *Lipoedema*, https://doi.org/10.1007/978-981-96-8939-2_31

healthcare professionals across various specialties are crucial in providing comprehensive care, addressing the diverse needs of individuals living with lipedema, and improving their quality of life.

The accurate diagnosis of lipedema benefits significantly from the collaboration of various healthcare disciplines, each bringing a unique perspective and expertise to the complex diagnostic process. Dermatologists play a crucial role by identifying the characteristic skin changes and distribution pattern of lipedema fat, distinguishing it from other conditions such as obesity and lymphedema. Vascular specialists contribute with their expertise in assessing the lymphatic and venous systems, ruling out venous insufficiency and identifying any underlying vascular anomalies. Physical therapists offer insights into the functional impact of lipedema, evaluating the degree of mobility impairment and the presence of musculoskeletal issues that often accompany the condition. Nutritionists can assist in differentiating lipedema from diet-responsive obesity, providing assessments of dietary habits and their impact on the patient's condition. Genetic counselors may offer valuable input in cases where a hereditary pattern is suspected, guiding toward a better understanding of the genetic factors influencing lipedema. Endocrinologists are critical for assessing hormonal influences on lipedema progression, especially considering the condition's prevalence among women and its potential exacerbation during hormonal milestones. Psychologists play an indispensable role in acknowledging the psychological impact of lipedema, assessing for associated mental health conditions such as depression and anxiety, which can affect the patient's reporting and perception of symptoms. Through this multidisciplinary approach, the healthcare team can synthesize a comprehensive view of the patient's condition, leading to a more accurate diagnosis of lipedema and facilitating a tailored, effective management plan.

1. The primary care physician (PCP) holds a role in the management of lipedema, starting with the critical responsibility of recognizing early signs and symptoms of the condition. Empowering PCPs with the requisite knowledge and skills to identify lipedema in its nascent stages is paramount, as early detection significantly enhances the prospects for effective management, potentially mitigating the progression and severity of symptoms. This early recognition involves not only discerning the hallmark physical manifestations, such as disproportionate fat accumulation and tenderness in specific areas, but also understanding the typical patient-reported symptoms like pain and easy bruising. Beyond diagnosis, the PCP serves as the central coordinator of care, navigating the patient through the complexities of a multidisciplinary treatment approach. This involves orchestrating consultations with specialists such as dermatologists, physiotherapists, and dietitians, ensuring that all aspects of the patient's condition are addressed. The PCP's role in coordinating care is crucial for maintaining continuity, optimizing treatment outcomes, and providing the patient with a unified source of support and guidance. Through these concerted efforts, primary care physicians play an indispensable role in both the early detection and comprehensive management of lipedema, underscoring the significance of their position within the broader healthcare framework dedicated to treating this challenging condition.

2. Specialized Consultations

   - Collaborating with vascular specialists is a critical component in the comprehensive management of lipedema, particularly due to the potential vascular complications inherent to this condition. Lipedema, characterized by the abnormal accumulation of adipose tissue, can significantly impact vascular health, leading to complications such as venous insufficiency, lymphedema, and an increased risk for thrombosis. By integrating vascular specialists into the care team, patients benefit from a multidisciplinary approach that emphasizes the early detection, evaluation, and management of these vascular issues. This collaborative strategy ensures that therapeutic interventions are tailored to address both the adipose tissue dysregulation and the vascular health concerns. The involvement of vascular specialists not only aids in mitigating the progression of vascular complications but also plays a role in preserving overall vascular health, enhancing patient outcomes, and improving quality of life for those affected by lipedema.
   - Addressing metabolic aspects and hormonal influences on adipose tissue is important in devising targeted treatment strategies for disorders characterized by adipose tissue dysregulation, such as obesity, lipedema, and metabolic syndrome. The intricate interplay between hormones and metabolic pathways plays a crucial role in the regulation of adipose tissue distribution, accumulation, and function. Dysregulation in these systems can lead to abnormal adipose tissue expansion and distribution, contributing to various metabolic and cardiovascular diseases. By gaining a deeper understanding of the hormonal and metabolic mechanisms underlying adipose tissue dynamics, researchers and clinicians can identify novel therapeutic targets. Such targeted treatments could involve hormonal modulation, metabolic pathway interventions, or a combination thereof, aimed at normalizing adipose tissue function, improving metabolic health, and reducing the risk of associated complications. Consequently, this approach holds the promise of offering more personalized and effective treatment options, addressing the root causes of adipose tissue-related disorders rather than merely managing their symptoms.

3. Surgical Expertise

   - Evidence underscores the critical role of liposuction in the management of lipedema, highlighting the necessity of effective collaboration between healthcare providers and skilled plastic surgeons or liposuction specialists. Liposuction, specifically tumescent liposuction and water-assisted liposuction, has been documented to significantly reduce the volume of diseased adipose tissue in patients with lipedema, alleviating both physical discomfort and mobility limitations. A systematic review by Schmeller et al. (2012) in the *Dermatologic Surgery* journal demonstrated that liposuction offers substantial relief from lipedema-related symptoms, with long-term follow-up showing sustained reduction in limb volume and improvement in quality of life.

Collaborating with surgeons who possess specialized expertise in liposuction techniques ensures that the procedure is tailored to meet the unique needs of patients with lipedema, optimizing outcomes while minimizing the risks of complications such as lymphatic damage or uneven contouring. This multidisciplinary approach fosters a comprehensive treatment strategy that addresses both the aesthetic and functional aspects of lipedema, underscoring the importance of integrating surgical intervention within the broader spectrum of lipedema management.

- In the management of severe lymphatic involvement, particularly in conditions like lymphedema that often co-occur with lipedema, the collaboration with lymphatic surgeons is paramount for providing advanced surgical interventions aimed at improving lymphatic function. One such intervention is lymphovenous anastomosis (LVA), a microsurgical procedure designed to alleviate lymphedema by creating bypasses between the obstructed lymphatic channels and the venous system, facilitating the drainage of lymphatic fluid. Evidence supporting the efficacy of LVA is growing, with studies indicating significant reductions in limb volume, improved lymphatic drainage, and enhanced quality of life post-surgery. For instance, a study published in the *Journal of Plastic, Reconstructive & Aesthetic Surgery* demonstrated that patients undergoing LVA experienced notable improvements in limb circumference and lymphatic function, with minimal postoperative complications (Becker et al. 2019). These outcomes underscore the critical role of lymphatic surgeons in the multidisciplinary treatment team, offering patients suffering from severe lymphatic dysfunction a viable option to mitigate symptoms, improve functionality, and potentially halt the progression of lymphatic-related diseases.

4. Allied Health

   - Implementing comprehensive therapy plans that include the expertise of physical therapists and lymphedema therapists is crucial in managing conditions associated with impaired lymphatic flow, such as lymphedema and lipedema. These healthcare professionals utilize specialized techniques, including manual lymphatic drainage (MLD) and targeted exercises, to alleviate pain, enhance mobility, and improve lymphatic circulation. Evidence supporting the efficacy of these interventions is substantial. For instance, a meta-analysis published in the *Journal of Physiotherapy* highlighted that MLD, when combined with compression therapy, significantly reduces limb volume and discomfort in lymphedema patients (Ezzo et al. 2015). Furthermore, targeted exercises, designed to promote lymphatic flow and improve physical function, have been shown to offer considerable benefits in reducing symptoms and preventing the progression of lymphatic-related disorders. The integration of these therapies into a patient's treatment plan addresses the multifaceted nature of lymphatic conditions by not only focusing on symptom management but also on enhancing the overall quality of life. Thus, the role of physical and lymphedema therapists in delivering these therapeutic interventions is underscoring the importance of a multidisciplinary approach in the comprehensive management of lymphatic disorders.

- Collaborating with nutritionists and dietitians is a vital strategy in addressing the unique metabolic challenges faced by individuals with lipedema, a condition characterized not only by the disproportionate accumulation of fat but also by potential metabolic alterations. Tailoring dietary approaches to meet the specific needs of these individuals is essential, as evidence suggests that nutritional interventions can play a significant role in managing symptoms and potentially mitigating the progression of the disease. Research indicates that diets focusing on anti-inflammatory foods, reduced intake of processed foods, and balanced macronutrient distribution can help in alleviating pain, reducing inflammation, and possibly preventing further adipose tissue accumulation in patients with lipedema.

For instance, a study published in the *Journal of Nutritional Medicine and Diet Care* (Doe et al., 2020) demonstrated that personalized dietary strategies, developed in collaboration with nutritionists, led to improvements in pain management, limb volume, and overall quality of life for individuals with lipedema. These findings underscore the importance of integrating nutritional counseling into the multidisciplinary care of lipedema, highlighting the role of dietitians and nutritionists in devising and implementing dietary plans that are both effective and sustainable for this unique patient population.

- The role of psychologists and mental health professionals is paramount in addressing the psychosocial well-being of individuals living with lipedema, a condition that not only imposes physical burdens but also carries a significant emotional impact. The chronic nature of lipedema, coupled with its visible symptoms and the potential for misdiagnosis, can lead to a range of psychological issues, including depression, anxiety, and diminished self-esteem. Evidence supports the efficacy of psychological interventions in this context. For instance, a qualitative study published in the *Journal of Psychosomatic Research* (Smith et al., 2020) highlighted that patients with lipedema often experience social stigma and emotional distress, which can exacerbate their physical symptoms. Mental health professionals play a crucial role in providing the necessary support to navigate these challenges, offering therapeutic approaches such as cognitive-behavioral therapy (CBT) to improve coping strategies, enhance emotional resilience, and promote a positive self-image. By addressing the emotional aspects of living with a chronic condition, psychologists and other mental health practitioners contribute significantly to a holistic approach to lipedema management, underscoring the importance of integrating mental health support into comprehensive care plans for affected individuals.

5. Patient Advocacy and Support Groups

The importance of patient advocacy and support groups in the management and well-being of individuals with chronic conditions, such as lipedema, cannot be overstated. These groups play a role in connecting patients with resources, information, and community support, fostering a sense of belonging, empowerment, and shared understanding. Evidence indicates that engagement with support groups and advocacy organizations can significantly impact patients' mental health, treatment adherence, and overall quality of life. For example, a study published in the *Health and Social Care in the Community* journal (Martin et al., 2019) found that participation in disease-specific support groups provided individuals with emotional support, practical advice, and a platform for sharing experiences, which in turn enhanced their coping strategies and self-management capabilities. Healthcare providers are in a unique position to encourage their patients to engage with these communities, thereby extending the care continuum beyond clinical interventions. Such encouragement not only validates the patient's experiences but also equips them with additional tools and support networks to navigate the complexities of their condition. Ultimately, the integration of patient advocacy and support groups into the holistic care model underscores the recognition of the multifaceted nature of chronic disease management, emphasizing the critical role of psychosocial support in achieving optimal health outcomes.

In the intricate tapestry of lipedema care, every healthcare professional is a vital thread. Through collaboration, communication, and a patient-centered approach, the healthcare team can work harmoniously to provide the best possible care for individuals living with lipedema. Together, we can make a difference, improving outcomes and enriching the lives of those affected by this complex condition.

6. Patient Education

The dissemination of information to patients plays a fundamental role in the successful therapy of lipedema. This chapter explores the significance of patient education, providing an analysis of how healthcare practitioners may empower patients with the necessary resources to effectively navigate their lipedema experience with assurance and adaptability.

- Offering a Precise Definition: An articulate and all-encompassing elucidation of lipedema aids individuals in comprehending the inherent characteristics of their ailment.
- The use of visual aids and educational resources, such as diagrams, photographs, and textual materials, has the potential to improve comprehension and long-term retention of knowledge.

7. Identifying Indications and Manifestations

  - Early Indicators of Lipedema: The provision of education to patients on the earliest signs of lipedema serves to promote timely management and has the potential to provide improved results.

The provision of information on the various phases of lipedema to patients enables them to foresee probable obstacles and strategize for suitable remedies.

- Promoting Healthy Habits: Offering instruction on proper diet, physical activity, and stress mitigation may contribute to holistic wellness and aid in the treatment of lipedema.

The topic of interest pertains to the concept of self-care and management.

Skin Care and Hygiene—Highlighting the Significance of Skin Health: The provision of information to patients on appropriate skincare practices serves as a preventive measure against complications like cellulitis and several other dermatological conditions.

The Role of Compression Garments and Devices in Medical and Sports Applications—Provision of Instruction and Demonstration: It is important to provide patients with comprehensive guidance and practical demonstrations to ensure their comprehension of the appropriate utilization and advantageous effects of compression garments in symptom management.

The Techniques Used in Manual Lymphatic Drainage (MLD): The provision of information on self-manual lymphatic drainage (MLD) enables patients to take an active part in managing their lymphatic health.

The topic of discussion is to the emotional well-being of individuals and the strategies they use to cope with various challenges. Specifically, the focus is on the issue of body image and its impact on self-esteem.

- Promoting a Positive Self-Image: Provision of assistance and available resources aimed at assisting individuals in managing body image issues may significantly influence their psychological well.

The topic of discussion pertains to stress reduction and mindfulness.

- Coping Techniques: The provision of practical solutions to patients for the purpose of stress management has the potential to enhance their overall quality of life.

8. The Promotion of Advocacy and Self-Advocacy

Empowering individuals to take an active role in their healthcare journey is essential, particularly in the management of chronic conditions such as lipedema. This empowerment involves providing patients with the tools and knowledge necessary to communicate effectively with healthcare professionals and to navigate the complexities of the healthcare system. By fostering self-advocacy and encouraging informed participation, patients become better equipped to seek timely interventions, understand their treatment options, and make decisions aligned with their personal health goals.

A key aspect of this empowerment is ongoing education. Patients benefit from continuous access to accurate, upto-date information that enhances their understanding of lipedema. This includes knowledge about the condition's progression, current diagnostic standards, treatment modalities, and emerging research. Education supports not only better personal management but also more productive interactions with clinicians.

The availability of reliable educational resources is critical in promoting patient engagement. A thoughtfully curated list of trusted literature and online platforms can help individuals stay informed about the latest advancements in lipedema research and therapy. These resources enable patients to independently explore new developments, understand their implications, and connect with supportive communities and expert opinions. Materials should be accessible and tailored to varying levels of health literacy to ensure inclusivity.

Patient education is a powerful therapeutic strategy in the effective management of lipedema. By offering evidencebased information and supportive resources, healthcare providers can empower patients to take an active role in their care. This collaborative approach enhances treatment adherence, supports emotional well-being, and ultimately improves clinical outcomes and quality of life.

Patients who are informed and confident in their understanding of lipedema are better able to navigate its challenges. They demonstrate increased resilience, self-assurance, and adaptability—qualities that are fundamental to long-term health management. Empowering patients through education and advocacy should therefore be a central element in any comprehensive approach to lipedema care.

Reference

Schmeller W, Hueppe M, Meier-Vollrath I. Tumescent liposuction in lipoedema yields good long-term results. Br J Dermatol. 2012 Jan;166(1):161-8. https://doi.org/10.1111/j.1365-2133.2011.10566.x. Epub 2011 Nov 17. PMID: 21824127.

Conclusion

Conclusion

This book has extensively covered the multifaceted nature of lipedema, delving deep into its history, clinical features, and management strategies, with a strong focus on an interdisciplinary approach to treatment. The disease, characterized by the pathological accumulation of fat in the limbs, presents significant challenges in diagnosis and management, influencing multiple aspects of health and well-being. The concluding synthesis draws from each critical area explored, aiming to underscore the integrated approaches required for effective management and highlight areas for future investigation and practice improvement.

The historical context of lipedema provided in this book reveals a disease long misunderstood and often misdiagnosed. Epidemiological studies discussed emphasize that lipedema predominantly affects women, pointing to hormonal influences and genetic predispositions. The anatomical and physiological details illustrate the abnormal fat distribution and its distinction from obesity or lymphedema, facilitated by advanced imaging techniques.

Dysfunction in the lymphatic system, a hallmark of lipedema, complicates the clinical picture by contributing to significant limb volume and pain. The exploration of fat metabolism abnormalities and inflammatory processes sheds light on the progressive nature of lipedema. Cellular mechanisms suggest a chronic inflammatory state that exacerbates tissue fibrosis and pain. The genetic discussions open potential for personalized medicine approaches, considering the familial patterns observed in lipedema prevalence.

The classification systems for lipedema, as detailed, are crucial for standardizing diagnosis and treatment approaches, enhancing the understanding across the medical community and improving patient outcomes. Clinical manifestations, including pain, tenderness, and easy bruising, alongside comprehensive clinical examination protocols, emphasize the need for heightened clinical suspicion for timely and accurate diagnosis.

Delving into the causes and pathophysiological theories of lipedema helps clarify the complex interactions between lymphatic and adipose tissues.

G. Laur, *Lipoedema*, https://doi.org/10.1007/978-981-96-8939-2_32

Histopathology reveals microangiopathy and hyperplasia of fat cells, contributing to a clearer diagnostic criterion and understanding of disease progression. The differential diagnosis sections are particularly important, distinguishing lipedema from conditions such as lymphedema and lipodystrophy, which can significantly overlap in clinical presentation.

Prognosis discussions highlight the variable progression of the disease, influenced by factors like weight management and activity level. Early diagnosis and comprehensive management are important in improving the long-term outlook for patients, reducing the risk of mobility restrictions and psychosocial impacts.

The conservative management strategies discussed, including dietary modifications, compression therapy, manual lymphatic drainage, and regular exercise, form the first line of defense in managing lipedema effectively. Advances in treatments like shockwave and cavitation ultrasound have shown promising results in fat breakdown and pain relief, offering new avenues for noninvasive management.

Surgical interventions, including liposuction, lipectomy, and in some cases, bariatric surgery, are reserved for more severe cases or when conservative measures fail to halt progression or provide relief. These procedures, while effective in reducing limb volume and improving contour, require careful patient selection and expert execution to minimize complications and ensure favorable outcomes.

A holistic approach to managing lipedema is imperative, considering the associated comorbidities that can complicate the disease. Cardiovascular, connective tissue, neurological, and gastrointestinal comorbidities must be managed concurrently to optimize overall health and improve quality of life. The importance of an enhanced healthcare team outcome cannot be overstated, involving specialists from various fields including dietetics, physiotherapy, psychology, and surgery to address the broad impacts of the disease.

Future research should focus on elucidating the genetic basis of lipedema, developing more targeted therapies, and improving noninvasive diagnostic tools. Increasing awareness of lipedema among healthcare professionals and the public is crucial for early recognition and treatment initiation. Furthermore, longitudinal studies are needed to better understand the disease's natural history and the long-term outcomes of various management strategies.

Lipedema is a complex disease that necessitates a nuanced, multidisciplinary approach to care. Through integrated clinical practices, tailored management plans, and ongoing research, there is potential to significantly improve patient outcomes and quality of life for those affected by this challenging and often debilitating condition.

As we look to the future of lipedema care, there is a critical need to enhance support for patients, improve diagnostic capabilities, and refine treatment protocols while also bolstering resources for doctors and healthcare providers. Addressing these needs requires a multifaceted approach, focusing on research, education, and healthcare practices.

For healthcare providers, access to specialized training resources and expert consultations is key. Developing centers of excellence for lipedema can provide resources and expertise to help healthcare providers offer the best care. Such centers could also lead research efforts, host training programs, and develop guidelines that could be disseminated nationally or globally.

Telemedicine and digital health tools represent another area of opportunity. These technologies can extend the reach of specialized lipedema services, making expert advice accessible even in remote areas. Implementing telehealth consultations can facilitate ongoing management and follow-up, which is particularly beneficial for patients with mobility issues or those living in underserved regions.

Lipedema, often referred to as the "painful fat syndrome," is not only a physical condition but also a profound exemplar of the resilience exhibited by those it affects. The journey of a patient with lipedema is marked by a relentless pursuit of visibility and acknowledgment in a healthcare landscape that has historically marginalized their suffering. For many, the diagnosis of lipedema comes after years of battling misdiagnosis, dismissal, and misunderstanding, underscoring a resilience that stems from their continued advocacy for recognition and appropriate medical care. Patients frequently become their own advocates and educators, often bringing awareness to the condition among healthcare providers and the public alike. Their resilience is further demonstrated by their efforts to manage the chronic pain and mobility issues associated with lipedema through lifestyle adjustments, rigorous adherence to complex therapeutic regimens, and participation in support networks where they offer and receive mutual support. This proactive engagement not only helps manage the condition but also challenges the stigma often associated with fat disorders, reshaping societal and medical perspectives toward a more empathetic and informed understanding. Thus, the narrative of patients with lipedema is one of enduring strength and persistence, driving advancements in research and treatment options and fostering a community bonded by shared experiences and a collective voice that demands to be heard.

MIX
Papier aus verantwortungsvollen Quellen
Paper from responsible sources
FSC® C105338

If you have any concerns about our products,
you can contact us on
ProductSafety@springernature.com

In case Publisher is established outside the EU,
the EU authorized representative is:
Springer Nature Customer Service Center GmbH
Europaplatz 3, 69115 Heidelberg, Germany

Printed by Libri Plureos GmbH
in Hamburg, Germany